Computer models of mind

Computational approaches in theoretical psychology

Margaret A. Boden, F.B.A.

Professor of Philosophy and Psychology, The University of Sussex

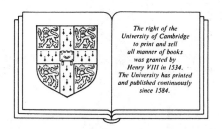

*The right of the
University of Cambridge
to print and sell
all manner of books
was granted by
Henry VIII in 1534.
The University has printed
and published continuously
since 1584.*

CAMBRIDGE UNIVERSITY PRESS

Cambridge

New York   New Rochelle   Melbourne   Sydney

Published by the Press Syndicate of the University of Cambridge
The Pitt Building, Trumpington Street, Cambridge CB2 1RP
32 East 57th Street, New York, NY 10022, USA
10 Stamford Road, Oakleigh, Melbourne 3166, Australia

© Cambridge University Press 1988

First published 1988

Printed in the United States of America

Library of Congress Cataloging-in-Publication Data

Boden, Margaret A.

Computer models of mind.

(Problems in the behavioural sciences)

Bibliography: p.
Includes index.

1. Psychology – Computer simulation.   2. Psychology –
Philosophy.   I. Title.   II. Series.
BF39.5.B63   1988   150'.724   87–25625

British Library Cataloguing in Publication Data

Boden, Margaret A.

Computer models of mind: computational approaches
in theoretical psychology – (Problems in the
behavioural sciences; 5).

1. Psychology – Experiments   2. Electronic
digital computers
I. Title   II. Series
150'.724   BF198.5

ISBN 0 521 24868 X hard covers
ISBN 0 521 27033 2 paperback

fon Earle

Problems in the Behavioural Sciences

Computer models of mind

Problems in the Behavioural Sciences

FOR IRA GALE

As regards the animals, Descartes was the first who, with a boldness worthy of reverence, ventured to think of the animal as a *machine*; our whole science of physiology is devoted to proving this proposition. Nor, logically, do we exclude man, as even Descartes did: our knowledge of man today is real knowledge precisely to the extent that it is knowledge of him as a machine.

Friedrich Nietzsche, The Anti-Christ, Section 14

Contents

vii

Preface

This book asks how computer models have been used, and might be used, to help us formulate psychological theories about the mind.

The models and concepts discussed here were selected for their psychological significance, not their technological promise. This is not a sharp divide, for even technologically motivated work may involve matters of psychological interest; "expert systems", for instance, raise questions about how people store and communicate knowledge, and how it is transformed as expertise grows. However, I have concentrated on computer models whose psychological relevance is comparatively direct. Usually, though not always, these models were intended by their creator as simulations of mental processes or tests of psychological theories.

The program-details of a few of the computer models mentioned in this book – specifically, scene-analysis programs and some very early simulations of language-understanding, problem-solving, and learning – were described in much greater detail in my *Artificial Intelligence and Natural Man* (first published in 1977; second edition, including a new "Postscript" chapter and additional bibliography, 1987). Most of the research discussed in this volume, however, was mentioned there only briefly – if at all. This is partly because some of it is very recent, but is owing also to the different aims of the two books. There, I concentrated on explaining just how AI-programs work, and referred in a very general way to the wider psychological, philosophical, and social implications of artificial intelligence. Here, I focus throughout on particular questions within theoretical psychology, ranging from domain-specific topics to more general methodological issues.

In short, I aim to clarify the ways in which practising psychologists can use computational ideas and computer-modelling to further their research.

M.A.B.

Brighton, England

ix

Acknowledgments

I am grateful to the following friends and colleagues for their helpful comments on various chapters (they should not be blamed for any mistakes which remain): Andy Clark, Gerald Gazdar, Geoffrey Hinton, David Hogg, Rudi Lutz, George Mather, Chris Mellish, Mike Scaife, Aaron Sloman, and Stephanie Thornton. Rickie Dammann drew my attention to the quotation I have used as the motto. Alison Mudd, with her usual good-humoured patience, undertook the chore of coaxing various computer printers to transfer my drafts from disc to paper. I am indebted to the Series Editor, Jeffrey Gray, for his constructive advice and encouragement. And I thank Jacqueline Korn, Jeremy Mynott, and Susan Milmoe, all of whose understanding and help have been invaluable.

I am obliged also to the Economic and Social Research Council for granting me a Personal Research Fellowship, and to the University of Sussex for allowing me a year's leave to take advantage of it.

1   Introduction

Computational psychology today is rather like the dragon in earlier times: of the people who are seeking it, not all agree on what they expect to find or how they hope to find it – while many others doubt that it exists to be found at all. My aim in this book is to explore the theoretical diversity of work in computational psychology, and the various controversial philosophical assumptions that underlie it. In doing so, I shall examine selected examples of psychological research using the methodology of computer-modelling.

Working models of living creatures are not new. They have existed as chic toys for many centuries: in the palaces of ancient Alexandria, the courts of medieval Islam, and the estates of the eighteenth-century European aristocracy. For over a hundred years they have cavorted in the pages of fiction, focussing cultural fears and fantasies of various kinds. But only very rarely in past centuries was the model-building motivated by the desire for theoretical understanding of men or animals. Even then (as in Vaucanson's nimble-fingered, fast-tongued flute-player), the focus was on bodily rather than mental processes. The attempt to build working models of intelligence that might help us to understand the nature and functioning of the mind is a very recent one.

By the mid twentieth century, speculative sketches of artificial animals could be found in the psychological literature. For example, in 1939 E. C. Tolman analysed trial-and-error learning in terms of an imaginary "schematic sowbug", and in 1943 C. L. Hull fantasized self-maintaining robots whose behaviour would be complex and adaptive like ours. The mathematician A. M. Turing was already discussing the logical properties of various possible types of computing machine in the 1930s [Turing, 1936]. With the rise of cybernetics in the early 1940s even purposive behaviour was characterized (by N. Wiener [1948] and others) as a basically mechanistic phenomenon.

At about the same time, K. J. W. Craik [1943] argued that psychological explanations should refer to cerebral models, conceived of as representational mechanisms (functioning "in the same way" as the phenomena being represented) capable of generating behaviour and thought of various kinds. But even Craik, influential though he was, could provide only the outlines of a new philosophical approach to psychology. He could not suggest any specific information-processing mechanisms which might be concerned, still less how such mechanisms might be built. Detailed theoretical hypotheses about mental representations had to await the development of the digital computer. Only then could mental modelling be seriously considered as a theoretical or practical enterprise.

The first such machines were being designed in the early 1940s, most importantly by J. von Neumann in the USA. (Turing and some others in England were tackling this problem too, and built the first electronic computer; but their work was top-secret for years because of its use in deciphering the ENIGMA code in the Second World War [Hodges, 1983].) In designing the digital computer, von Neumann was influenced not only by Turing's earlier work on the theory of computation, but also by some novel ideas about the logical functions of the brain. These were largely due to the physiologist and psychiatrist W. S. McCulloch and the mathematician W. H. Pitts [1943]. (Unlike McCulloch and Pitts, however, von Neumann did not believe that binary logic could model human thought: as he put it, "the language of the brain is not the language of mathematics"; his suggestion that thermodynamic probability is better suited has recently been revived, as we shall see in Chapter 7 [von Neumann, 1958, p. 80].)

In their paper "A Logical Calculus of the Ideas Immanent in Nervous Activity", McCulloch and Pitts [1943] compared the logical circuitry of digital computers with sets of interconnected neurones. Equating the on–off binary states of the computer to the all-or-none properties of nervous conduction, they claimed that the logical properties of the brain as a whole could be understood in terms of the logical properties of its constituent cells. Focussing on the computational or information-processing potential of neurones rather than their actual physiology, they argued that specific types of neuronal unit, functioning under particular constraints, would have specifiable logical properties.

For example, a certain simple arrangement of threshold-units would function as an "AND-gate", in which one cell in effect detects the simultaneous excitation of two others. Another primitive network embodies what logicians term exclusive OR, since one cell fires if and only if one (but not both) of two other cells is firing. Yet another computes AND-NOT, so that Cell 3 fires if and only if Cell 1 is firing and Cell 2 is not. More complex dispositions of units would compute not logical connectives such as AND, OR, and AND-NOT, but entire logical expressions – such as "A and (B or [C and D] but not both) and/or E and not-F". More generally, McCulloch and Pitts proved that every finite expression of the propositional calculus can in principle be computed by some neural network of the general type they described.

This paper, together with related work of McCulloch and Pitts [McCulloch, 1965], was very influential. The physiological psychologist D. O. Hebb [1949], introducing his seminal theory of *cell-assemblies,* saw "great potential value" in the McCulloch–Pitts project of describing the functional organization of the cerebral cortex in terms of mathematical analyses of the properties of groups of interacting neurones. Other psychologists were prompted to take an interest in computer models of various sorts. Very soon, attempts were made to build working models of mindlike functions, such as pattern-recognition, goal-directed behaviour, and logical thought. Early examples included Grey Walter's [1953] light-seeking tortoises and various computer simulations of neural nets, like F. Rosenblatt's [1958] *perceptrons,* reflecting physiological ideas (including Hebb's) about neural excitation and inhibition.

The late 1950s saw two distinct approaches to computer-modelling. Both owed much to the example set by McCulloch and Pitts. But whereas one stemmed from their (and Hebb's) ideas about the neurophysiological structure of the brain, the other owed more to their work on the embodiment of the propositional calculus in digital computers. On the one hand, there were early computer models of learning and pattern-recognition, inspired by Rosenblatt's work on perceptrons: O. G. Selfridge's [1959] Pandemonium was an influential example. On the other hand, there were early problem-solving computer programs such as the Logic Theorist [Newell, Shaw & Simon, 1957], and its successor the General Problem Solver (GPS) [Newell & Simon, 1961]. Crude though these early systems were, they raised some interesting theoretical problems. For example, it is still a controversial question (as we shall see) whether the essence of psychological processing was better represented by Pandemonium or by GPS.

Some of these pioneering models were described in *The Mechanization of Thought Processes* (1959), a report of a symposium (at the National Physical Laboratory) published by Her Majesty's Stationery Office and not easily accessible to the uninitiated, including most psychologists. But in the early 1960s, two books appeared that established the psychological visibility of this new way of thinking about thinking, and indicated some long-term goals.

One, significantly entitled *Computers and Thought,* was a collection of papers describing most of the then existing computer models of psychological interest [Feigenbaum & Feldman, 1963]. In addition to GPS, these included models of pattern-recognition, learning, concept-formation, geometrical reasoning, social interaction, and memory. It also contained more wide-ranging discussions, such as Turing's [1950] classic paper "Computing Machinery and Intelligence" and M. L. Minsky's [1961] speculations on the steps needed to achieve artificial intelligence in the future.

The other was *Plans and the Structure of Behavior* by G. A. Miller, E. Galanter, and K. H. Pribram [1960]. This book criticized S–R behaviourism, then the psychological orthodoxy, for ignoring what went on at the hyphen: namely, the unobservable mental processes intervening between stimulus and response. The authors looked to computer-modelling for concepts with which to describe these mental processes. They offered a sustained, if highly speculative, argument that the entire psychological spectrum – from instinct and motor control, through memory and language, to personality, psychopathology, and hypnosis – should be painted in computational colours. Strongly influenced by current advances in automatic problem-solving (notably GPS), they claimed that psychological explanations should specify hierarchical *plans* of various types. These plans are goal-directed procedures, and in conscious organisms many goal-states are represented and evaluated in the "image", a data-structure that reflects the individual's motivation and cultural interests. The proper aim of psychology, on this view, is the identification of procedures essentially comparable to computer programs.

Miller and his co-authors acknowledged an important intellectual debt to K. S. Lashley and N. Chomsky. Lashley had argued (in "The Problem of Serial Order in Behavior" [1951]) that all motor-skills – including speech – have a many-levelled hierarchical structure, which cannot be explained by Sherringtonian neurophysiology or behaviourism but requires us to postulate central controlling mechanisms in the brain. Chomsky [1957] too had stressed the hierarchical structure of language, and in a paper jointly written with Miller ("Finite State Languages" [1958]) had presented a mathematical proof of Lashley's insight that this cannot be explained behaviouristically. His *Syntactic Structures* [1957] had even offered a formal account of language in terms of a specific set of generative rules.

Nevertheless, the way in which Miller and his colleagues wished to explain language (and other psychological phenomena) differed significantly from Chomsky's approach. They thought of these phenomena as procedures, much like computer programs. But Chomsky's formal rules were not programs, nor were they primarily intended as specifications of actual psychological processes. Rather, they were abstract descriptions of structural relationships. They were "generative" in the timeless mathematical sense, whereby a formula is said to generate a series of numbers, not in the sense of being descriptions of a temporal process of generation. Similarly, his "transformations" were abstract mappings from one structure to another (as a square-root function transforms 9 into 3), not actual psychological changes or mental events. Likewise, his "finite-state and non-finite *machines*" were mathematical definitions (as are Turing machines), not descriptions of any actual manufactured systems that might conform to those definitions.

So in characterizing psychology as the study of plans, Miller and his co-authors were recommending a rather different sort of enterprise from Chomsky's. Many people would say that this was because they were psychologists whereas Chomsky was a linguist: they were interested in how language happens in the mind, whereas he was concerned only with language in itself. This is true, as far as it goes. But it obscures an important controversy. For some influential voices now argue that Chomsky's approach, rather than Miller's, is the more fundamental to a scientific psychology, that psychologists should focus primarily on *what* is computed, not on *how* it is computed. Like the controversy pitting Pandemonium against GPS, this dispute illustrates our main theme: the diverse theoretical and methodological assumptions informing computational psychology.

Computational psychology was compared, above, to dragons – about whose lineaments few agree and none is certain. Computational psychology is a broad church, whose members differ significantly about general methodology as well as specific detail. However, much as medieval bestiaries depicted their diverse dragons in broadly similar ways, so computational psychologists, despite their many differences, share certain very general philosophical assumptions about what it is they are looking for.

They all focus on the mind, considered as an informational not an energetic system, and take psychology to be the study of *mental* life. But so do many (non-behaviourist) psychologists who cannot be termed computationalists. And very many of them use computers – but again, so do many other psychologists (for calculating statistical significance, for example). The point is that computers – or rather, concepts drawn from computer science – play some central theoretical role in the computational psychologist's claims about what the mind is and how it functions. Accordingly, *computational* (as opposed to computer-using) psychologists share three characteristic ways of theorizing.

First, computational psychologists adopt a functionalist approach to the mind, in which mental states are abstractly defined in terms of their causal role (with respect to other mental states and observable behaviour). Functionalism is a philosophy of the late twentieth century in which the mind is conceived of in terms of the computational properties of universal Turing machines. Every psychological phenomenon (or at least every such phenomenon that is potentially capable of scientific explanation) is assumed to be generated by some *effective procedure,* some precisely specifiable set of instructions defining the succession of mental states within the mind. Since computer science is the study of effective procedures, this psychological approach takes computational concepts seriously.

Second, computational psychologists conceive of the mind as a representational system, and see psychology as the study of the various computational processes whereby mental representations are constructed, organized, interpreted, and transformed. A corollary is that they use *intentional* terminology (often including much of the vocabulary of everyday folk-psychology). That is, they think of (many) mental phenomena as having a meaning, or semantic content, as being directed upon some object or imaginary object outside the mind itself. (So, of course, do humanistic or hermeneutic psychologists, whose stress on intentionality and interpretation is closer in spirit to that of computational psychology than they believe.)

And third, they think about neuroscience (if they think about it at all) in a broadly computational way, asking what sorts of logical operations or functional relations might be embodied in neural networks. What the brain does that enables it to embody the mind is the main question, not what it is in itself as a physical system. As one such theorist has put it: "finding a cell that recognizes one's grandmother does not tell you very much more than you started with; after all, you know you can recognize your grandmother. What is needed is an answer to how you, or a cell, or anything at all, does it. The discovery of the cell tells one what does it, but not how it can be done" [Mayhew, 1983, p. 214].

These three process-oriented characteristics constitute a minimal definition of the family "computational psychology". In subsequent chapters we shall examine some fundamental ways in which the family members differ.

We shall see, for instance, that computational psychologists may mean rather different things by "computation" and by "representation". Whereas some theorists focus on symbol-manipulation defined in terms of formal rules, and take the (von Neumann) general-purpose digital computer as their inspiration, others emphasize parallel-processing computational networks whose behaviour is not defined by such rules. The former use a research methodology based on the ideas of orthodox artificial intelligence (AI), while the latter, no less sympathetic to computer-modelling in general, sometimes argue that these particular ideas have fundamentally misled us for the last quarter-century.

Artificial intelligence developed out of the mid-century experiments with complex programming mentioned above. Its goal is to understand, whether for theoretical or technological purposes, how representational structures can generate behaviour and how intelligent behaviour can emerge out of unintelligent behaviour. So AI-workers attempt to write computer programs (and/or to design machines) capable of performing complex information-processing tasks with a high degree of flexibility and context-sensitivity, like those faced by human and animal minds – such as perception, language, memory, motor-control, and thinking. This requires the rigorous expression of diverse symbolic processes, in terms of a rich variety of computational concepts specifically developed for managing informational complexity.

Computationally inclined psychologists in general see AI as potentially useful, largely because its conceptual focus is on representation and processes of symbolic transformation. (Perhaps one should rather say that these *appear to be* and *are generally taken to be* the conceptual focus of AI, so as not to beg the question, discussed in Chapter 8, whether a computer can properly be said to symbolize or represent anything in the full sense.) Moreover, they recognize that AI's emphasis on rigour encourages psychologists to be more precise, often pointing to unsuspected theoretical lacunae. And they appreciate that computer-modelling offers a manageable way of representing complexity, since the computational power of a computer can be used to infer the implications of a program where the unassisted human mind is unable to do so.

For these reasons, and for historical reasons too, many of the computer models discussed in the following chapters were developed in close relation to, or even within, artificial intelligence.

But this does not mean that all computational psychologists feel that AI has lived up to its early promise, or wish to be closely identified with it. As we shall see, some criticize AI as being "merely empirical", in the sense that it often achieves practical results by methods it does not understand and so cannot responsibly generalize. Such critics complain that there is, as yet, too little theoretical work in AI: too few proofs that a particular class of computation can or cannot work, given certain types of computational machine, and too few principled accounts of the advantages and disadvantages of distinct classes of program.

When these psychologists regard a program as interesting, they do so not because it achieves a particular result, but because the programmer attempts a general proof that results of this class can be computed by computational systems of this form, given certain specific constraints (which may apply to naturally evolved psychological systems). Indeed, there may not even be a program, but only an abstract analysis of the information-processing task in question. Such theorists agree with Chomsky in stressing the *what* of computation, rather than the *how*. Accordingly, they may use the term "computational" to refer not (as is more usual) to computational *processes*, but to the *abstract analysis of the task* facing the psychological system – irrespective of how it is actually performed. (This maverick non-procedural usage is introduced in Chapter 3, in relation to D. Marr's views on the "computational level" of explanation. When it is used in the succeeding chapters, the context or an explicit reference to Marr should prevent confusion with the more familiar sense of the term.)

Still less does the intellectual debt to AI mean that all computational psychologists favour the particular type of computer-modelling typical of orthodox AI-research (what J. Haugeland [1985] has termed GOFAI: Good Old-Fashioned AI). As mentioned above, some of them criticize mainstream AI for ignoring, at least until recently, the potential of types of computation that are not well-suited to the von Neumann machines traditionally used in AI. Instead, they recommend the study of parallel-processing, "connectionist", systems. These do not function by following explicitly represented rules, and concepts or representations are embodied in them as *patterns of activity* across entire networks of computational units. (At present, connectionist models have to be simulated on von Neumann machines; but connectionist hardware is being developed by various groups [e.g., Hillis, 1985].)

Another disagreement concerns the theoretical significance (for psychology) of neuroscience. Most computational psychologists (and AI-researchers) ignore physiology, arguing that computational questions are essentially distinct from questions of physical mechanism and so can be asked in their own terms. Indeed, the irrelevance of neurophysiology has acquired the status of a dogma in some circles. Heresy, however, abounds: there are opposing groups who champion the application of neurophysiological insights in formulating the basic outlines of their computer models.

The additional argument is often given (by the dogmatists) that we know so little about the neurophysiology of mental phenomena that it would be folly to try to constrain psychological theories and computer models by neurophysiological knowledge. The strongest counterexample concerns the physiology of some (low-level) aspects of vision. This is not only known to rest on massively parallel computation, but also involves cells (responsible for the early stages of visual processing) which are relatively accessible to neuroscientific investigations. Accordingly, it has prompted the formation of those connectionist psychological theories and computer models which attempt the most detailed neurophysiological interpretations. Parallelist theories of other mental processes (such as language or memory) are constrained by neurophysiology only in a much more general sense.

Again, some computationalists insist that the only intellectually responsible way to present a psychological theory is to embody it in a functioning computer model, whether von Neumann or not. Others see programming and model-building as largely irrelevant activities, although they plan their experiments and formulate their theories with computational questions in mind. People disagree, moreover, about how empirical data can be used to validate a theory presented in programmed form. And they differ over how we can decide which features of the program are really relevant to the theory concerned, and which are there only because the theorist had to write a program that would actually run.

Further controversy attends the question whether computational psychology can in principle explain the higher mental processes (such as problem-solving and memory). Many believe that it can. But others, who agree that problem-solving and memory are computational phenomena, hope for a scientific explanation only of peripheral processes. This controversy rests partly on varying ideas about what the aims of science are – specifically, whether they must include detailed prediction or detailed post-diction after the fact.

Finally, most computational psychologists trust that their approach will explain how representations function, and many believe it will even help to illuminate what representations are. But a few, together with many critics outside the computationalist camp, argue that computer models (and psychological theories grounded in them) in principle cannot exhibit or explain genuine *representation* (or *meaning*) at all.

Given these myriad disagreements, it is clear that computational psychology is a beast with many different incarnations. These species must be described in giving an account of the genus as a whole. So, if my theme is the nature – and the theoretical diversity – of computational psychology overall, my strategy is to proceed from the particular to the general.

In Chapters 2 to 7, various philosophical and methodological claims are introduced in relation to specific computer models of psychological processes, and to the psychological theories and experimental programmes associated with them. General concepts such as *representation, functional architecture, task-analysis, connectionism,* and *modularity* enter the text in the context of modelling imagery (Chapter 2) or low-level vision (Chapter 3), but appear also in the subsequent discussions of computer models of language (Chapters 4 and 5), problem-solving (Chapter 6), and learning (Chapter 7). Finally, Chapter 8 builds on this groundwork in drawing together some controversial issues in the foundations of computational psychology, and in asking whether it is possible at all.

For the sake of the sceptical reader who suspects at the outset that this dragon-hunt is doomed to failure – that computational psychology is not possible at all – it may be useful to make a Popperian point. Science advances not only by conjectures but also by refutations [Popper, 1963]. Even if we decided that a computational methodology is not appropriate to psychological modelling after all, we still should have learnt something. We should have some reasonably precise ideas about just what is faulty or inadequate in current models, and we might even have arrived at some notion of what sort of theoretical power is lacking.

However, this is an unnecessarily negative way of justifying the computational approach. We shall see that, despite all the difficulties and unsettled controversies, some distinct gains have been made for psychology by attempts to consider the mind as a computational machine.

2   Patterns, polyhedra, imagery

Work on vision includes some of the most fruitful psychological research inspired by computational ideas. It also exemplifies many of the general methodological controversies mentioned in Chapter 1. The discussion of computer vision (in this chapter and the next) will introduce topics such as the psychological relevance of neurophysiology, the need for new kinds of computation, the theoretical importance of programs as such, the role of orthodox AI, and the sense in which a psychological theory should be "computational". '

The philosophical background

The key problem for the psychology of vision is how our visual system enables us to gain reliable information about the environment. Implicit in this question are two others: How far does vision depend on high-level inferences as opposed to autonomous low-level processes? And do the low-level processes themselves actively construct a visual representation, or do they merely pick up information presented to the eyes? Insofar as one regards vision as the construction (at whatever level) of representations, one faces also a fourth question: What is the nature of visual representations? This, in turn, prompts enquiry into the nature of visual imagery.

Two theoretical poles from which to approach these questions were established by the seventeenth-century philosophers, and have informed experimental psychology since its inception a hundred years ago.

Empiricists (like Locke) stress low-level, automatic, processes rather than high-level judgments or control, and see these processes as passively reflecting the input information rather than transforming or interpreting it. Moreover, they assume a *tabula rasa* in the newborn organism, any interpretative activity being not only high-level but learnt. Images are merely less vivid copies of sense-impressions, which can be imaginatively combined, as when one pictures a unicorn.

Rationalist accounts, by contrast, stress the active construction of mental representations, and the contribution to vision of (unconscious) conceptual judgments. Descartes, for instance, said that though we think we see people walking down the street, all we really see is coats and hats moving. Although the connection between coats and people has to be learnt, rationalists assume that many structuring principles are innate. Imagination is

10

said to involve active thought, rather than being a repetition of a passive sensory experience.

In the experimental psychology of the early 1960s, a strong rationalist influence was exerted by (for example) R. L. Gregory and J. S. Bruner, according to whom the percept is actively constructed by high-level processes. Positing an analogy between perception and problem-solving, they claimed that the subject's mental schemata (F. C. Bartlett's term), or models (Craik's term), guide the search for cues in the input, and produce perceptual hypotheses which are then tested against the stimulus. Just how this guiding and testing are done, however, was left unclear.

The leading representative of the empiricist approach at that time was J. J. Gibson. He argued that many real-world features (texture, for example) can be recognized by low-level psychophysiological mechanisms, functioning without any control from high-level schemata or cerebral models. They respond to the rich information available in the ambient light, carrying out a direct, unanalysed, process of "information pickup". Further evidence for an empiricist position was furnished in 1960 by B. Julesz, whose random-dot stereograms showed that depth-perception does not absolutely require high-level control using knowledge about the stimulus-object. When the experimental conditions are such as to remove any scope for high-level control, stereopsis can occur without it (although it may be that such control is normally employed in depth-perception).

These two conceptual polarities dominated psychological debate well into the 1970s. The main issue of disagreement, as explained above, was the constructivist versus the non-constructivist nature of perception. It is because of their positions on this question that Gregory and Bruner count as rationalists and Gibson as an empiricist. On the issue of nativism (that is, whether perceptual capacities are innate), their positions did not fit these traditional philosophical labels. Indeed, the empiricist Gibson emphasized built-in psychophysiological mechanisms more than Gregory or Bruner did.

An interesting hybrid philosophical position had been suggested in the eighteenth century, by Kant. On this view, even the most basic sensory processes assign meaning to the input, in terms of real-world features such as object-identity, 3D-shape, and location. But (according to Kant) these interpretative processes are automatic, not derived from experience alone, and not open to conscious control. A few psychologists (such as J. Piaget) had attempted a compromise between rationalism and empiricism when discussing perception, but most mainstream experimentalists did not. The development of an influential hybrid psychology of vision had to await advances in computer-modelling.

These broad philosophical distinctions help us to identify four successive phases of computer-modelling, or AI-research, intended to throw light on the psychology of seeing. In this chapter we shall consider the first three, postponing discussion of the fourth (and most recent) to Chapter 3. These four phases are the *property-list* approach, the *picture-grammar* approach, the study of *scene-analysis,* and *connectionist* work on low-level computations in the visual system.

In terms of the distinctions outlined above, the first was empiricist in character, the second and third rationalist, and the fourth hybrid. The first two phases affected experimental psychology less significantly than the third and fourth did. Basically, this is because only the last two addressed the key theoretical issue: the interpretative relation between the visible world and the mind's representation of it.

Some people would feel uneasy about describing the fourth approach as a development of AI, albeit at the psychological end of the AI-spectrum. They would insist on calling it a development of computational psychology, *in contrast* with AI. This is not a mere terminological quibble, for it concerns controversial views about what sort of beast a scientific psychology should be. As we shall see in Chapter 3, one influential writer in the fourth group defined computational psychology in a way which differentiates it from most work in AI. His definition also excludes most psychology which, being influenced by computational ideas, qualifies as computational psychology in the very broad sense defined in Chapter 1. I shall continue (in the absence of explicit qualification) to use the term in this broad sense, since to do otherwise would be to beg some problematic methodological questions.

Computer vision: the first three phases

Property-list models (described in *The Mechanization of Thought Processes* and *Computers and Thought*) were developed in the 1950s and very early 1960s. Although this approach gave rise to many useful applications (such as automatic analysis of chromosome patterns), it had limited influence on psychological theories of vision. The prime reason for the lack of influence of property-models was that their task was not so much *vision* as *pattern-recognition* (a distinction explained below).

The type of pattern-recognition task performed by these models required the 2D-input or stimulus to be scanned for specific 2D-properties. For example, the scanner might look for spots or lines, or for line-junctions in certain places, or for dark regions of certain shapes. Different patterns were distinguished in terms of distinct lists of such properties. Usually, the property-lists were pre-defined by the programmer, but sometimes a specific pattern's property-list was learnt by the program itself.

For instance, L. Uhr and C. Vossler [1961] described "A Pattern Recognition Program That Generates, Evaluates, and Adjusts Its Own Operators", in which each operator was a 5×5 mini-matrix with a specific array of 0's and 1's in its cells. The stimulus was presented as a 20 × 20 matrix and scanned by the operators. These could be preprogrammed (to capture lines, curves, and the ends of vertical and horizontal bars) or randomly generated by the program itself. When an operator was used in a successful recognition-task, its probability of future use was increased. The program learnt to identify handprinted letters almost as well as people can, and arbitrary patterns better.

Property-list models were often regarded by their authors as interestingly analogous to biological visual systems. Like the perceptron systems mentioned in the previous chapter, they were early models of parallel processing in neural networks – albeit simulated on serial machines (only now are powerful parallel-processors becoming available).

Further, they seemed to fit well with the "feature-detectors" that had recently been discovered in the frog's retina and monkey's striate cortex. Uhr and Vossler [1963], for example, suggested that their "operators" were fundamentally analogous to neural nets of retinal cones converging on a single output, or to single cortical cells responding to lines of a specific orientation (the "bar-detectors" described by D. Hubel and T. Wiesel [1959; 1979]). Indeed, O. G. Selfridge's argument that pattern-recognition must involve analysis of the stimulus into distinct features (as in his computer model Pandemonium [Selfridge, 1959; Selfridge & Neisser, 1960]) had been partly responsible for these physiological studies being done in the first place. In their seminal paper "What the Frog's Eye Tells the Frog's Brain", J. Lettvin *et al.* [1959] explicitly acknowledged their debt to Selfridge's early computer-modelling. H. Maturana's discovery (in November 1958) of the first directional cells confirmed a hunch based on purely anatomical grounds (histological evidence of asymmetries in the connection-patterns of some ganglion-cells in the frog's retina). But Lettvin's knowledge of Selfridge's work helped him to see the importance of Maturana's finding, and prompted him immediately to change the main programme of research in his laboratory to a search for other functionally asymmetric retinal cells [Maturana, personal communication].

Some of the intuitions of the property-list phase were sound, such as the potential usefulness of analysing the stimulus into distinct significant features, and of simultaneously applying a number of different operators over the stimulus as a whole. Its influence on experimental psychology was evident, for instance, in N. S. Sutherland's [1957; 1968] work on the perception of horizontality and verticality in the octopus. Even U. Neisser [1967], who explicitly rejected this approach in favour of a constructivist "analysis-by-synthesis" account, allowed that feature-detectors broadly similar to those posited by Selfridge might be important at early stages of vision. And we shall see later that recent fourth-phase models have in some degree resurrected the first-phase aim of modelling parallel computations in neural networks.

CAT   HAT

Fig. 2.1. Example of visual ambiguity resolved by context.

But the property-list approach suffered from three essential limitations, because the distinction between pattern-recognition and perception was usually ignored. The first two of these limitations compromise its usefulness even for essentially 2D-phenomena, such as alphanumeric characters presented singly or in context. The third renders it useless for seeing objects in the real world.

First, the approach was strongly retinocentric, in that patterns had to be normalized for size, orientation, and position. Second, it was limited to patterns presented singly, since it offered no ideas about how to segment a picture into several distinct – perhaps even partially overlapping – forms. (Hence it could not deal with context-sensitivity, in which one and the same pattern is differently interpreted according to its surroundings, as in Figure 2.1.) And third, it was confined to the discrimination of patterns in two dimensions, making no provision for using a 2D-stimulus to provide information about a 3D-world. Insofar as this problem was borne in mind at all, it was simply assumed that a line in the stimulus-pattern must correspond to a physical edge in the world of material objects. But *why, how,* and *how far* this is true were not considered.

In the picture-grammar approach also, questions about how pictorial structures or visual input relate to 3D-scenes were ignored – or else were over-hastily assumed to have been answered, because the distinction between the picture itself and what it might be taken to depict was not clearly made. The focus was on how 2D-properties of images can be described in terms of various 2-D structures, concentrating not on independently defined properties, but on descriptions defined by reference to the structure of the stimulus as a whole.

For instance, in his paper "Pictorial Relationships – A Syntactic Approach", M. B. Clowes [1969] explicitly adopted the methodology of Chomsky's early work on syntax. Like Chomsky, Clowes relied on intuitions of paraphrase, ambiguity, and anomaly to suggest deep structural principles, or "grammars", generating surface (visible) forms. He discussed visually ambiguous stimuli in terms of distinct underlying spatial structures, and offered formal specifications of some of these. He argued, for instance, that the perceptual shift experienced in viewing the Gestaltists' sail/stingray figure (Figure 2.2) rests on the assignment of two different implicit axes around which to structure the picture as a whole.

Work on picture-grammars supported the Gestaltists' claim that one's phenomenal experience of a visual input can depend on the way in which

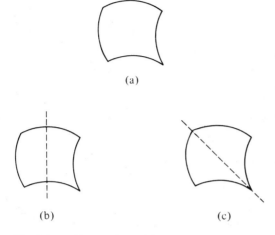

Fig. 2.2. Ambiguous figure (a), with imposed vertical and diagonal axes for inter-pretation as (b) sail and (c) stingray.

one implicitly structures it. Indeed, recent experiments drawing on compu-tational ideas, including these, have confirmed that one's ability to perceive significant properties of a visual input (such as symmetries and possible transformations) is determined by the axes and structural features one has assigned to it [Hinton, 1979]. However, in concentrating on the pictorial domain alone, picture-grammars suffered from an excessive concern with visual syntax at the expense of visual semantics.

By contrast, the scene-analysis work took semantics seriously, concen-trating on the mapping between 2D-picture and 3D-scene. Instead of tac-itly assuming that a picture-line can be interpreted as representing a scene-edge, scene-analysis provided explicit rules making clear whether or not a line of a certain sort is a *cue,* and if so how it can be used to assign a particular meaning to the stimulus. Not everything that is visible is a visual cue. A cue is an intentional, or subjective, concept, denoting part of a representational system. It is a stimulus-property that is assigned signifi-cance, that is interpreted as representing something else.

Scene-analysis showed that structural descriptions can be assigned to the input by a visual system, on the basis of specifiable cues. The more numer-ous the visual stimuli that can be treated as reliable cues, the more success-ful the visual system is likely to be (a point to be emphasized even more forcefully in the fourth-phase work). The choice of which stimulus-features or picture-properties to take as cues for which real-world phenomena is crucial. And the system of representation involved is theoretically under-stood (as opposed to being intuitively recognized) only if one appreciates *why* certain pictorial features can act as reliable cues while others cannot.

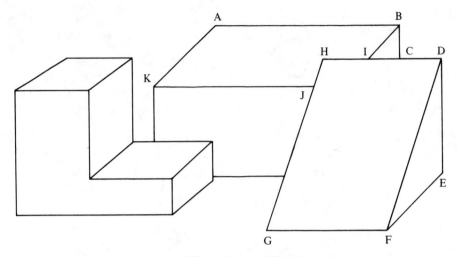

Fig. 2.3. HDFG, DEF, and BCI are approved polygons, but HDEFG and ABIHJK are not. Polygon BCI in a different context could depict the entire (triangular) face of an object, but in this context it does not, because of the occlusion of the rear cuboid by the wedge. (Notice that you, like the program, assumed the rear object to be a cuboid; but it *might* have a bite out of it at the five hidden corners.) By assuming that the lowest line in the picture (GF) is supported at ground level, Roberts' program can calculate all spatial dimensions in the scene. (Adapted from L. G. Roberts [1965], Machine Perception of Three-Dimensional Solids. In J. T. Tippett, D. A. Berkowitz, L. C. Clapp, C. J. Koester & A. Vanderburgh (eds.), *Optical and Electro-Optical Information Processing*. Cambridge, Mass.: MIT Press. P. 176.)

With successive developments in scene-analysis, these methodological morals were gradually clarified. The outline of scene-analysis given below focusses on these general matters, each of which is relevant to theories in other psychological domains, as we shall see. (I have described scene-analysis models in considerable detail in Boden, 1987 [chaps. 8 and 9].)

This third phase was initiated in the mid 1960s by L. G. Roberts' [1965] paper "Machine Perception of Three-Dimensional Solids". Roberts treated perception as a model-guided, constructive, activity. His program embodied models of various 3D-solids (cuboids, wedges, and hexagonal prisms) specifying mapping rules derived from projective geometry, which defined the complete range of images that could be associated with each solid given different viewing positions. The cues were regions of various types ("approved polygons"), and the program searched first for three cue-regions meeting at a point – though why was not made clear. The program used its models to arrive at a structural description of the picture whereby specific groups of regions were interpreted as depicting particular solid objects. Figure 2.3 shows a picture that could be interpreted sensibly by the program.

The "staircase" in Figure 2.3 had to be articulated by Roberts' program as a combination of two cuboids. This highlights an important limitation of all schema-driven models, including those written later by G. R. Grape [1969], G. Falk [1972], and P. H. Winston [1975] (some of which incorporated *line-labelling,* to be described presently). Such models can correctly assign shapes only to objects (or combinations thereof) of a type they already know about. The human visual system is not similarly constrained: we can perceive the shape of an object we have never seen before, without having to construct it out of constituent-objects. This fact was partly responsible for a reaction against scene-analysis models in the early fourth-phase work (though we shall see that prototypes crept back in at a later stage).

It may be objected here that this so-called limitation of schema-driven models is no limitation at all. For it is true of any perceptual system that it can perceive only objects constructed according to principles it already knows about, from primitives it already knows about. But the point is that the schemata and generative rules posited by scene-analysis were of a very high-level kind, representing a few specific classes of 3D-objects and excluding very many others. By contrast, the low-level principles and primitives to be discussed in Chapter 3 can in principle be used to construct representations of any 3D-object.

An attempt to generalize the power of machine-perception, by avoiding reliance on specific prototypes, formed the next step in scene-analysis: A. Guzman's SEE [Guzman, 1969]. This program could recognize any convex polyhedron as a solid object (but could not identify distinct classes of object). In Figure 2.4 for instance, it could correctly count 11 objects in the scene (but could not say what sorts of objects – cubes, wedges, or pyramids – they were).

Unlike Roberts' program, SEE worked bottom-up rather than top-down having no explicit stored models of prototype-objects. Its cues were vertices of various types, which were treated as evidence for linking the associated regions as pertaining to one and the same solid object (see Figures 2.5a and 2.5b). For example, a FORK-vertex in the picture suggested that the three regions sharing the FORK-lines as boundaries represented sides of the same 3D-object (compare Roberts' use of three regions meeting at a point). But Guzman's choice of cues and interpretative rules was intuitive and largely *ad hoc* rather than systematic, for he relied on representational relationships whose rationale he failed to appreciate. He implicitly assumed a model of a convex polyhedron but did not make this model, and its application, explicit. He did not ask why a FORK is such good evidence for an object-corner where three sides meet, or why his linking rules sometimes led to errors of interpretation. He tried to forestall such errors by specifying essentially syntactic rules about the form of legal and illegal pictures, without relating illegalities to physical impossibilities in the scenes putatively represented by anomalous pictures.

The need to ask these questions was recognized in the early 1970s, largely

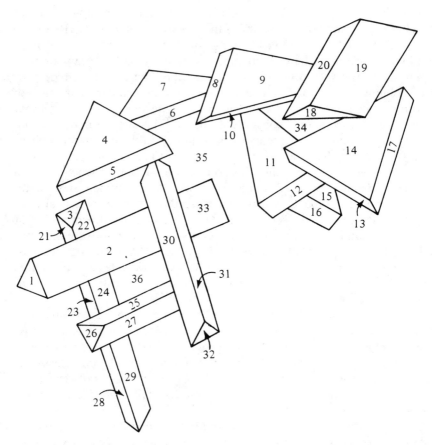

Fig. 2.4. Guzman's "HARD". All bodies are correctly identified by SEE, even though one (regions 6 : 7) has no "useful" visible vertices. The background (34 : 35 : 36) also is correctly found. (From A. Guzman [1969], Decomposition of a Visual Field into Three-Dimensional Bodies. In A. Grasselli (ed.), *Automatic Interpretation and Classification of Images*. New York: Academic Press. P. 273.)

because people wanted to understand the power of Guzman's system – and its (sometimes surprising) limitations, such as its inability to identify holes. The systematic representational relation between picture and scene was the theoretical focus of work done in the early 1970s by Clowes, D. A. Huffman, D. L. Waltz, A. K. Mackworth, and (more recently) S. W. Draper, whose analyses led to a series of increasingly powerful computer models. Their insights concerned the geometry of (polyhedral) physical objects in 3D-space and the associated projective geometry for mapping 3D-properties into 2D-images. The basic concept was *line-labelling,* which was later incorporated in *gradient-space* and *sidedness reasoning*.

The essence of line-labelling is that cue-lines are classified by the visual

L — Vertex where two lines meet.

FORK — Three lines forming angles smaller than 180 degrees.

ARROW — Three lines meeting at a
      point, with one of the angles
      bigger than 180 degrees.

T — Three concurrent lines, two of them
    collinear.

K — Two of the lines are collinear, and the
    other two fall on the same side of such
    lines.

X — Two of the lines are collinear, and the
    other two fall on opposite sides of such
    lines.

PEAK — Formed by four or more lines,
      when there is an angle bigger than
      180 degrees.

MULTI — Vertices formed by four or more
      lines, and not falling in any of the
      preceding types.

Fig. 2.5a. The vertex-definitions are Guzman's. FORK, ARROW, and PEAK can all be defined without reference to 180 degrees—for example, ARROW is a 3-line vertex, two of whose lines have the other two lying on the same side of it. (From A. Guzman [1969], Decomposition of a Visual Field into Three-Dimensional Bodies. In A. Grasselli (ed.), *Automatic Interpretation and Classification of Images*. New York: Academic Press. P. 251.)

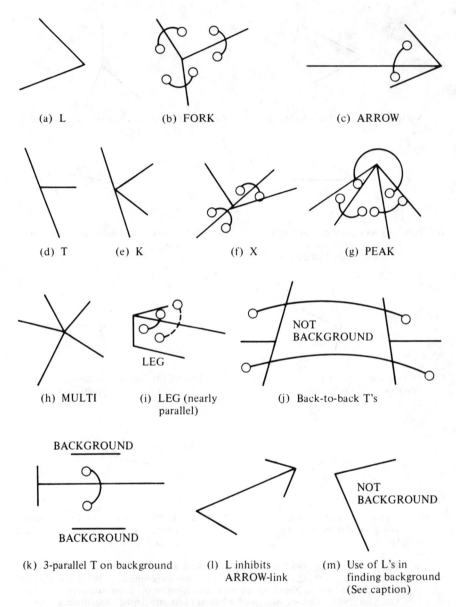

(a) L   (b) FORK   (c) ARROW

(d) T   (e) K   (f) X   (g) PEAK

(h) MULTI   (i) LEG (nearly   (j) Back-to-back T's
               parallel)

BACKGROUND

BACKGROUND

(k) 3-parallel T on background   (l) L inhibits   (m) Use of L's in
                                       ARROW-link   finding background
                                                               (See caption)

Fig. 2.5b. (a) to (h) show SEE's vertices, with strong region-links placed; (i) shows
weak link placed on ARROW by adjacent LEG; (j) and (k) show examples of
strong links placed on complex patterns; (l) shows example of link-inhibition by an
L-vertex (assumes convexity); (m) shows embodiment of convexity assumption in
use of L's when identifying background. Note that this interpretation of L's is an
ideal one: it can be overridden in contexts where L's are caused by the overlapping
of two bodies – see vertices of region 35 in Figure 2.4. (For a detailed discussion of
the difference between Guzman's "weak" and "strong" links, see Chapter 8 of

system in terms of the complete range of physical edges they could possibly depict, given a particular system of representation [Huffman, 1971; Clowes, 1971; 1973]. For example, given a polyhedral world and a representation based on the topological relations within projective geometry, this approach states explicitly that a FORK-vertex is reliable evidence for a convex or concave corner where three visible planar surfaces meet. This fact provides a theoretical explanation of the practical usefulness both of Roberts' primary cue (three cue-regions meeting at a point) and of Guzman's FORK-vertex (which led his program to interpret the three intermediate regions as surfaces of one and the same physical object). Roberts and Guzman had partially grasped the significance of FORK-vertices at an intuitive level but had not clearly recognized the theoretical basis of their intuitions.

Line-labelling allows for context-sensitivity in the interpretation of a picture, whereby potentially ambiguous picture-parts are disambiguated by reference to their surroundings. Each line in a picture is individually ambiguous, even if we know that it forms part of a vertex of a particular type. And some types involve more ambiguity than others: of the Clowes–Huffman set of vertices, the FORK is the most highly constrained (allowing only two physically realizable sets of line-labels), the ELL the most open (allowing six possible label-sets). But the physical feature which a given line represents must have determinate properties (some of which are relative to the viewpoint): if it is an edge, it must be concave *or* convex *or* occluding; and if it is a shadow (which could be represented in some later scene-analysis models, as we shall see), the illuminated surface must lie to one side *or* the other. In general, the theoretical basis of line-labelling makes it possible for local ambiguities in the picture to be resolved by coherence-rules that are grounded in specific physical constraints in the real world – not least, the constraint that a straight edge cannot be convex at one end and concave at the other.

For example, line-labelling tells us that if one end of a line contributes to a FORK-vertex, the line may represent either a concave or a convex (but not an occluding) edge. But the line-labelling theory explicitly guarantees that if one line in a FORK-vertex represents a convex (or concave) edge, then all three do. So if the labelling of one of the other lines contributing to this FORK-vertex has already been established as convex (say), then the line in question can immediately be taken as representing a convex edge too.

Anomalous pictures are not "illegal" (as Guzman would have it), nor "ungrammatical" (as Clowes put it in his picture-grammar phase). Rather,

Caption to Fig. 2.5b. (*cont.*)
M. A. Boden [1987], *Artificial Intelligence and Natural Man*. London and Cambridge, Mass.: MIT Press.) (In addition to my own data, adapted from A. Guzman [1969], Decomposition of a Visual Field into Three-dimensional Bodies. In A. Grasselli (ed.), *Automatic Interpretation and Classification of Images*. New York: Academic Press. P. 258. Also adapted from data in A. Guzman [1968], Computer Recognition of Three-Dimensional Objects in a Visual Scene. Ph.D. thesis, MIT.)

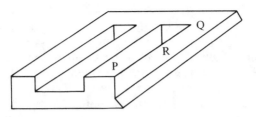

Fig. 2.6. Impossible object: "Devil's Pitchfork". (Adapted from M. B. Clowes [1971], On Seeing Things. *Artificial Intelligence*, 2, p. 105).

they are *uninterpretable* with respect to the real world. They depict impossible objects like the "Devil's Pitchfork" of Figure 2.6. Scene-analysis programs based on line-labelling could reject many anomalous pictures (including the "Devil's Pitchfork"), realizing that they do not depict any possible 3D-object, and could identify the specific pictorial contradictions involved. In Figure 2.6, for instance, the line PRQ has a FORK-vertex at P, which means it cannot represent an occluding edge; but it forms the cross-bar of a tee-junction at R, which means it must be labelled as an occluding edge.

The method of line-labelling was originally introduced in 1971 by Clowes and Huffman (independently) to distinguish between representations of convex edges, concave edges, and occluding edges with the visible surface to one side or the other. (Clowes also allowed for tee-junctions, which signalled one physical object passing behind another.) The semantics of line-labelling was later extended by Waltz [1975] to include the representation of cracks and shadow-boundaries (which made use of constraints about illumination).

Waltz also demonstrated a counterintuitive fact that has influenced work in computational linguistics and problem-solving, as well as the computer-modelling of vision; namely, although it appears *prima facie* that adding more information to a problem-representation must fuel the combinatorial explosion, it can in practice enable one to damp it down. The secret is to find some way of satisfying multiple constraints simultaneously. (Although Waltz was the first person to exploit constraint-satisfaction within scene-analysis, it had been used in *relaxation* models of vision essentially similar to those described in Chapter 3 [Rosenfeld, Hummel & Zucker, 1976], and also in problem-solving [Fikes, 1970]. Waltz employed sequential algorithms, but the next chapter will show how the same idea can be applied to parallel-processing too.)

Given the richer semantics of Waltz's representation (the larger number of line-labels available), a vertex considered in isolation is multiply ambiguous – even if only physically possible interpretations are allowed. A FORK-vertex, for instance, has five hundred sensible interpretations using Waltz's line-labels (not two, as in the Clowes–Huffman representation). To label each vertex independently (before comparing all pairs of neighbouring vertices) would have led to a combinatorial explosion in seeking a coherent interpretation of the whole picture.

So Waltz wrote a filtering algorithm that crawled around the picture deleting all labels except those which were physically consistent with the interpretations at the neighbouring, previously labelled, vertex. For instance, if the initial vertex-type determines that one of its component lines can have only five possible labellings, then only those five are allowed for the line at its other end (the next vertex), even though this second vertex considered in isolation might have allowed ten different labels for that line. This procedure was repeated (iterated), so that deletions made on the first round were fed back onto the initial starting-point, thus causing new deletions there.

Waltz expected this strategy to reduce the program's work, but was amazed to find that it cut down the combinatorics so drastically that in many cases it found a unique interpretation of the picture without further computation. When it did not, it reduced the possible alternatives to so small a number that they could be systematically examined.

This illustrates two important truths, relevant, as we shall see, not only to theories of vision but to computational psychology in general. First, iterative propagation of *local* constraints between neighbouring items in a representation sometimes suffices to find a unique *global* interpretation (in which each locally ambiguous element within the whole is disambiguated). Second, even our most strongly felt intuitions about the computational potential (or lack of it) of a particular procedure or method of representation may be mistaken. Certainly, people's intuitions differ: some might have been less surprised than Waltz was by the success of his filter. As this example suggests, good mathematical intuitions are especially useful in computational contexts, including those concerning psychological mechanisms. But it is true, and significant, that a functioning computer model may surprise us by showing that a given procedure can do something that even its programmer had assumed it could not do.ˌ

A still deeper understanding of the class of representations studied by scene-analysis was provided by Mackworth's [1973] definition of gradient-space. Gradient-space is a 2D-representation of 3D-objects that depicts surface-orientation. Points in gradient-space represent planes (surfaces) in 3D-space, lines represent intersections of planes (edges), and the position of a point represents the tilt of the equivalent surface relative to the picture-plane. Mackworth proved that if the tilt of some surfaces is known then the tilt of others can be inferred, and that information about the relative slopes of two surfaces meeting at an edge can be used in interpreting a line as depicting a convex or concave edge. He used this insight in writing a program that interpreted pictures of polyhedral worlds more reliably and economically than previous scene-analysis models had.

Even Mackworth's program was unable to interpret *all* polyhedral line-drawings sensibly. Some years later, S. W. Draper [1981] generalized gradient space in terms of another geometrical concept, dual space. Although dual space did improve the interpretation, it was not perfect either. Draper proved that the basic concepts of dual space could be expressed in an algebraic plane equation form, which would support a theoretically adequate scene-analysis program. However, such a program would be very difficult to work with, and psychologically implausible to boot. For plane equations are not readily intelligible in terms of familiar geometric ideas, nor of the line-labelling constraints from which they had ultimately been developed. Draper showed that the geometrical intuitions of line-labelling and dual space could be preserved, and the theoretical adequacy of plane equations equalled, by "sidedness reasoning". The greater power of this approach was due partly to the fact that it could translate individual line-labels into sidedness constraints, whereas Mackworth's program had needed pairs of connect-edges.

The detailed applications within computer-vision research of the mathematical work prompted by scene-analysis have recently been surveyed by Mackworth [1983]. Here, what is of especial – and general – psychological interest is the methodology used. Consider Mackworth's work on gradient-space, for example. In seeking to improve on previous models, Mackworth did not merely add a few new facts (about orientation) in an unprincipled fashion. This is what Guzman had done in outlawing "illegal pictures", and in classifying cue-vertices in the first place (and it is often done in AI to strengthen a program's performance). Rather, Mackworth developed a formal account of how orientation can be systematically represented, given certain optical constraints on the picture-taking process. And he proved that this representation can in principle be exploited in specific ways, to assign reliable interpretations in terms of particular real-world properties. Only after proving these matters abstractly did he turn to the problem of how to implement them in a particular computer program. The same is true of Draper's work; indeed, Huffman's first account of line-labelling was a purely abstract discussion, not yet implemented in any computer model. The general importance of this methodological approach will appear when I discuss the fourth phase of computer-modelling in Chapter 3.

Besides developing a deeper understanding of 2D-to-3D mapping, scene-analysis models became increasingly able to deal sensibly (though in a very limited way) with imperfect input, whose ubiquity was fully appreciated only when people tried to use programs to find the significant intensity-changes in real visual input. For instance, Roberts had suggested that a line-finder could be driven top-down by his system: if a predicted line was not found, the line-finder could be told where to lower its threshold for detecting intensity-changes. Some later scene-analysis programs exploited this idea so as to detect faint changes, to ignore strong ones, and even to hallucinate missing lines corresponding to badly illuminated edges. (Other examples are given in Boden, 1987 [chap. 9].) These schema-driven functions were sometimes compared with the *holistic* perceptions and *phenomenal closure* described by the Gestalt psychologists.

But whereas the Gestaltists had offered only the vaguest psychological (and false neurophysiological) "explanations" of such perceptual performances, scene-analysis provided specific computational mechanisms whereby its results could be generated. Whether closely comparable mechanisms are employed in human minds is of course another question. However, this third phase of computer-modelling was psychologically important less for its details than for its general approach. It suggested the *possibility* of clear explanations of puzzling facts about the phenomenology of vision, and influenced experimental psychology accordingly. Moreover, some of the concepts associated with scene-analysis were applicable to other mental capacities besides vision.

As regards the psychology of *vision,* scene-analysis research had two main effects. First, its constructivist and model-driven view of perception was consonant with the rationalist camp in perceptual psychology. For instance, the schema-based approach lent theoretical support to the experimental work already being done on so-called cognitive contours [Kanizsa, 1974], on selective feature-detection [Sutherland, 1968], and on the tracking of eye-movements insofar as they focus on salient points, or cues, in scenes or faces [Yarbus, 1967].

One of the first experimental psychologists to identify these models as support for the rationalist view of perception (which had embraced general information-processing ideas for some years) was Gregory. As early as the 1960s, he had argued that seeing-machines will necessarily suffer from illusions for the same sorts of reason that we do [Gregory, 1967]. And in the 1970s he cited scene-analysis programs as corroborative evidence for his long-standing view that many visual illusions occur because identifiable interpretative hypotheses mislead the system in specific ways [Gregory, 1977]. His first editorial in the new journal *Perception* (founded in 1972) described AI as an important source of ideas about vision, and later issues included many papers written from this point of view, including one by Mackworth [1976] called "Model-Driven Interpretation in Intelligent Vision Systems", which compared scene-analysis models with human perception.

Even while recommending scene-analysis models to psychologists, Gregory pointed out that they are less sophisticated, less knowledgeable, and less fast than human subjects.

Many people felt at the time that these drawbacks do not obviously call for a change of direction in research, but perhaps merely for more of the same. Like Gregory's patient S. B., whose sight was restored after fifty years of blindness [Gregory & Wallace, 1963], most scene-analysis programs confused shadow-boundaries with edges and were incapable of recognizing many 3D-shapes that present normal adults with no difficulty. According to the third-phase approach, these seeing-machines simply needed more knowledge about shadows and additional high-level schemata representing non-polyhedral objects.

Real-time functioning might be achieved, suggested M. L. Minsky [1975], by means of *frames* for seeing. (Minsky pointed out that the concept of frame is a general one: in Chapter 5 we shall consider its application in the computer-modelling of language-understanding.) Frames for seeing are hierarchically organized skeleton-schemas, such as might represent one's knowledge about the visual appearance of rooms (as opposed to one's knowledge of a particular room). They include computational pointers suggesting which unfilled *slot* should be examined next (which visual information should be sought), at various stages of perceptual processing. For example, a typical room has a roof (not the open sky), a floor (not a swimming pool), four walls (not six), one door in a wall (not a trap-door in the floor), and one or more windows in the walls (unlike some internal offices or bathrooms). If you want to find the door, the frame can suggest a strategy of locating a wall and looking for a door in it, passing to the neighbouring wall if no door appears. Frames also contain *default-values* for various slots, which function as assumptions that influence perception in the absence of evidence to the contrary. Thus you may seem to see a window in a wall even if there is no window there.

Frames were recommended by Minsky as being computational structures enabling perception, and action, to be fast (the idea was that you do not need to process all the details: if you see a tiger's head you assume it's got teeth – and you run). But recommendation is not implementation: Minsky and his colleagues did not provide frame-based computer models of vision that actually could function in real time.

However, perhaps a rather different approach was required for modelling real-time vision – one exploiting parallel-processing hardware, for instance? And perhaps types of computation radically different from those used in scene-analysis were needed also for the recognition of unfamiliar objects, and for the perception of real physical surfaces? Although high-level schemata may enable us to tune our sensitivity appropriately when familiar objects are being perceived (for instance by guiding us to look for distinctive features at specific points), they cannot explain our ability to perceive the shape of unfamiliar objects. Still less can they explain how we perceive the size, orientation, texture, and distance of such objects. As we shall see in the next chapter, it was these very general visual abilities which the very different fourth-phase models attempted to explain.

Images and analogues: conceptual preliminaries

The second major influence of scene-analysis on visual psychology, surprising though this may seem, was to encourage the nascent revival of psychological interest in images and imagery. These topics had been taboo in the behaviourist era. For an *image,* in the sense that is relevant here, is a *mental representation* – a concept for which behaviourism had no place. (A different sense of "image", which will figure in the discussion of fourth-phase work in the next chapter, connotes a set of *physical* events: the pattern of retinal excitation caused by the incoming light.) Scene-analysis did not merely support the anti-behaviourist belief that there are functionally significant mental representations associated with vision, and with the ability humans have to describe real or imaginary scenes as though they were actually looking at them when they were not. It also suggested the possibility of answering questions about their detailed nature: what they are like, how they function, and how they compare with other types of mental representations – including those associated with visual perception of existing things and those underlying the use of natural language.

But discovering what images actually are is made doubly difficult by conceptual confusion over what they conceivably might be. Psychological work on imagery has been bedevilled by conceptual unclarities, which have sometimes led to widespread misinterpretation of experimental results, as we shall see.

The prime reason for this state of affairs is that there is no adequate conceptual analysis of *image* or *imagery,* not even in the philosophical literature (which also was influenced by work in scene-analysis [Dennett, 1978, chap. 10; Block, 1981]. The difficulty of understanding *consciousness* or *experience* is not the only conceptual unclarity involved. If it were, theoretical psychologists could evade it (as they so often do) either by ignoring the specifically conscious aspect of images or by taking it for granted in a philosophically unanalysed way. Worse, theories about the abstract nature and the function of images (never mind consciousness) are problematic too, since their meaning – and so what sort of evidence could count for or against them – is unclear.

For example, the central question posed by the revival of concern with imagery in the early 1970s (soon to be encouraged by scene-analysis representations) was whether images are "iconic" – as opposed to being "symbolic", "verbal", or "propositional". As it was commonly put: Are images "like pictures", or "like descriptions"?

This dispute was not altogether well posed. Images are by definition in some sense like pictures (and imagery in some sense like vision). The question is, in what sense? Indeed, an additional question that needs asking is: What pictures? For pictures appear, *prima facie,* to represent in rather different ways: think of a Cézanne and a van Eyck, a stick-figure and a scale-diagram, a photograph and a caricature. One cannot assume without discussion that there is some core pictorial mode of representation common to all of these. A similar question arises with respect to descriptions: Do all descriptions represent in the same way? If not, do they nevertheless share some essential representational feature? (For example, are they all interpreted by way of *mental models*, like those to be discussed in Chapter 6?)

Moreover, even to ask whether *images* are like descriptions may be misleading, and might be better expressed as whether *imagery* involves representations that are (in some specific sense) like descriptions. For the former way of putting the question appears to take for granted that the concept of *having an image* is analysable as a person's *having x* – where *x* is an object with certain properties, to be determined. But perhaps *having x* is better analysed as a person's *being in a certain mental state* (*apt to produce behaviour of certain kinds*), the representational basis of which is to be determined. That is, *having an image* may be more fruitfully thought of as a predicate (applying to the person) than as a relation (between the person and a mental object). If so, then disputes over whether images are or are not like descriptions involve a category mistake. The question "Are images like descriptions?" should then be regarded as shorthand for "In what ways are the mental representations underlying imagery like, and unlike, descriptions?" This caveat should be borne in mind during the discussion below, which features the question "Are images like descriptions?" because this is the way in which the psychologists concerned usually posed the problem.

By the early 1970s (when scene-analysis was getting started), cognitive psychologists had already re-admitted imagery as a proper topic for debate. Computer-modelling in general had aided this resurrection, because it accepted internal mental processes and implied that specific types of representation or information-processing might have distinct psychological roles. For instance, Neisser had cited Newell, Shaw, and Simon when generalizing his account of perception to imagery.

But AI-work specifically on vision had not been important and was not widely known. It was not mentioned, for instance, in the two publications which (in 1971) were primarily responsible for reviving psychologists' interest in imagery. In his *Imagery and Verbal Processes* [1971], A. Paivio reviewed the experimental evidence suggesting that visual and verbal representations have different psychological functions, and different physiological substrates. He concluded that "iconic" and "linguistic" representations have different forms – *analogue* (*analogical*) and *symbolic* respectively – and rely on distinct (parallel as against serial) information-processing in the brain. His argument betrays some influence of computational work generally, but not of computer vision in particular. Similarly, R. N. Shepard and J. Metzler's influential paper "Mental Rotation of Three-Dimensional Objects" [1971] – which (as we shall see) appeared to provide some very specific, and surprising, information about the way imagery functions – sprang out of experimental psychology rather than computer vision.

However, the advent of third-phase work in the computer-modelling of vision did increase psychologists' newfound interest in imagery, not least because it suggested an approach different from that of Paivio and other iconicists. As we have seen, most of the structural descriptions generated by line-labelling models concerned non-metrical properties, such as convexity, occlusion, and shadowing. In the few cases where spatial distances were included (as in Roberts' program), they were represented by lists (or 2D-arrays) of numbers, not by things isomorphic with the objects represented. That is, scene-analysis appeared to imply that images are not analogue representations but symbolic descriptions (comparable to sentences in natural language or the strings of formal symbols manipulated by digital computers).

Before describing this controversy, something must be said about the terms of the debate. The notion of an *analogue* or *analogical* representation is not clearly understood, and is not used by all writers in the same way [Haugeland, 1981]. For example, it is sometimes, but not always, taken to mean that a representation is continuous, or non-discrete. And it is sometimes, but not always, taken to imply the existence of a special representational medium, whose intrinsic properties give the analogue form its significance. But common to all uses, as the etymology implies, is some (not necessarily well-defined) notion of *similarity* between the analogue-representation and the thing represented.

It is tacitly assumed – but, as we shall see, not always explicitly considered – that the similarity (whatever it is) is a *significant* one. That is, the similarity must somehow be specifically exploited in the interpretation of the representation. Otherwise, it would be a mere idle similarity: a matter of objective fact but of no psychological interest (like the similarity between the constellation Cassiopeia and the letter W).

Since significant similarity contributes to all senses of *analogical representation,* it may be regarded as the basic, minimalist, definition of the term. Indeed, some writers take it to be the only essential feature. For example, A. Sloman [1978, chap. 7] has defined an analogical representation as one in which there is an interpretative mapping, or significant isomorphism, between the structure of the representation itself and the structure of the thing represented. To understand an analogical representation is thus to know how to interpret it by matching these two structures, and their associated inference procedures, in a systematic way.

(Sloman contrasts analogical representations with *Fregean* ones, which are understood by some procedure essentially comparable to what the nineteenth-century logician G. Frege described as the application of logical *functions* to *arguments*. Accordingly, the structure of a Fregean description reflects not the structure of the thing represented, but the structure of the logical-computational procedure by which the representation is interpreted. Examples include English sentences, whose intrinsic structure enables them to be interpreted by logical-grammatical parsing-procedures (such as those to be described in Chapter 4). However, as Sloman points out, the analogical–Fregean distinction is neither exclusive nor exhaustive. For example, the sentences "Jehane drank her cocoa and went to bed" and "Jehane went to bed and drank her cocoa" mean distinctly different things, because of the analogical mapping between the temporal order of verb-phrases and the temporal order of the relevant events in the world.

Familiar analogical representations (in this minimalist sense) include maps, diagrams, and scale-models. Less familiar examples include computer models of vision in which inferences are made by successive interactions between neighbouring points in a visual array. B. V. Funt's [1980] program, for instance, can predict whether or not an irregularly shaped object, if tipped, would hit another object in the field of view. These predictions are made not by manipulating symbols (such as the differential equations of physics) but by taking successive "snapshots" of the local changes in the image-array that would ensue if the first object fell through the space separating it from the second. The significant similarity lies in the isomorphism between the hypothetical traversal of neighbouring points in real space by a physical object and the successive changes in the labels ("occupied" or "unoccupied") attached to neighbouring image-points.

The latter example shows that (as Sloman points out) a representation may involve both analogical and symbolic, descriptional, features. Given an image-array that is significantly similar to the points of physical space, the distinction between two significantly different states of an individual image-point may be coded (*sic*) by arbitrary labels. Likewise, the sentence "She drank her cocoa and went to bed" is a symbolic verbal representation with a strong analogue-element: the temporal order of the words maps onto the temporal sequence being represented (compare: "She went to bed and drank her cocoa"). So it may often be more convenient to distinguish analogue and symbolic *features* of a representation, rather than trying to classify what might reasonably be regarded as one representation as either analogue or symbolic. This is another reason for suspecting that the question "Are images like pictures or like descriptions?" is overly simplistic.

Some analogue-representations (using the term in the minimalist sense) depend on the availability of a special representational medium whose intrinsic properties are exploited in the functioning of the representation. Consider a plasticine-model of a planned building, for instance. An enlargement of the already planned rooms (without changing their topological relations) could be directly represented by stretching the plasticine. Extra rooms could be represented by being stuck onto the external surfaces, or inserted into the original plasticine-model. That is, the spatial properties, elasticity, and cohesiveness intrinsic to the plasticine are utilized by the manner of representation.

But analogue-representations (again, in the minimalist sense) do not necessarily require a distinctive medium. For instance, spatial arrays–like those in Funt's [1980; 1983] models–can be embodied in (simulated by) a general-purpose digital computer, just as verbal descriptions can.

So whether imagery involves representations that are (in the minimalist sense) analogue, and whether it exploits the intrinsic properties of a special medium of representation in the brain, are two different questions. It follows that arguments that images are analogue, rather than descriptional, are not necessarily arguments for their requiring a special representational medium. However, the distinction between these two questions may be obscured if "analogue representation"is understood in a stronger sense, as involving not only significant similarity, but also some special representational medium. In that case, to call imagery "analogue" or "analogical" commits one, on pain of contradiction, to answer "Yes" to both questions. We shall see that the main participants in the psychological debate about imagery often did use the term in this way. But they failed to realize that some of their arguments were relevant only to the *minimalist* sense. Consequently, some of their conclusions about the existence or nonexistence of a special medium were unfounded. (In what follows, I shall continue to use the term in its minimalist sense unless otherwise specified.)

Imagery in experiment and theory

The theoretical debate about imagery was initially focussed on Shepard and Metzler's research, since it seemed to many people to suggest that our visual representations, even of cubes and similar polyhedral objects, are analogical in nature. Shepard and Metzler's ingenious experiments were repeated and extensively varied throughout the 1970s, and–subject to the important qualification discussed below–all repetitions and variations gave similar results.

In a typical experiment, Shepard and Metzler showed their subjects line-drawings of pairs of complex 3D-objects, like those shown in Figure 2.7. The experimental task was to decide as quickly as possible whether the paired drawings were pictures of the same object, seen from different viewpoints.

In Figure 2.7, for instance, pair A depicts one and the same 3D-object rotated in the plane of the page, and pair B depicts one and the same 3D-object rotated "through" the page. Pair C, by contrast, cannot be interpreted as depicting one and the same object with any rotation whatever. Shepard and Metzler generated a wide variety of A-pairs and of B-pairs by varying the angle of rotation from zero to 180 degrees. (If only one direc-

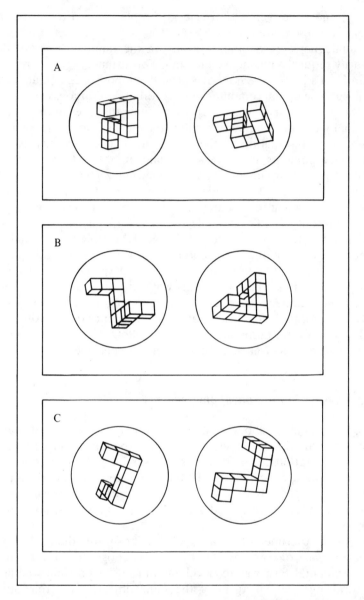

Fig. 2.7. Each of these six drawings represents a three-dimensional structure made up of 10 cubes stuck together. People were asked to look at pairs of drawings and to decide whether the drawings showed one and the same object (rotated) or two different objects. Three of the 1,600 pairs used are shown here. The A-pair and the B-pair show rotations (in the plane of the page and perpendicular to the page, respectively), but the C-pair does not. (Adapted from R. N. Shepard & J. Metzler [1971], Mental Rotation of Three-dimensional Objects. *Science,* 171, p. 702.)

tion of rotation is allowed, the range is zero to 360 degrees.) Their initial experiments used 1,600 drawing pairs, and practised subjects achieved 95 per cent accuracy.

The striking result was that subjects took more time to decide as the imagined rotation increased. Indeed, there was a precise linear relation between time and angle of rotation (see Figure 2.8). What is more, subjects often reported that they had been rotating images in their minds.

The experimenters drew what seemed – to them and many others – to be the obvious conclusions. Something internal, isomorphic with the object depicted, was really being rotated – or, at least, was undergoing real transformations analogous to actual rotation. That is to say, images are internal objects formed in a special medium of representation, in which quasi-spatial properties and transformations are inherent. ("Obvious" is not necessarily "correct": notice the logical jump here, from *isomorphism* to a *special medium*.)

Shepard and Metzler's experiments were seen as the leading challenge to the scene-analysis approach. Not surprisingly, then, their work was soon criticized. A radical attack on their basic theoretical assumptions (and Paivio's) was mounted by Z. W. Pylyshyn, in his paper "What the Mind's Eye Tells the Mind's Brain: A Critique of Mental Imagery" [1973].

Pylyshyn referred to AI-work on vision and other mental processes in criticizing the primitive ideas about possible forms of mental representation that were then current in experimental psychology. He argued that consciously accessible words and images cannot be the only mental representations (as was assumed by Paivio): there must be more abstract types of mental code underlying consciousness. And he pointed out that how empirical evidence should be used in evaluating competing hypotheses about different forms of mental representation was unclear: until this methodological problem was solved, no conclusions about such matters could be confidently accepted.

Images, said Pylyshyn, cannot helpfully be understood as mere internal pictures, isomorphic with external visual arrays, for this would require a further mind's eye to interpret them by another image, and so on *ad infinitum*. To pass from uninterpreted pictures (whether on the retina or in consciousness) to symbolic descriptions, suggestive of the things depicted by them, is to make a potentially explanatory move. To pass from one uninterpreted picture to another, virtually identical with it, is not.

Pylyshyn was correct to argue (what many philosophical discussions of imagery have also pointed out) that merely positing an image-simulacrum of the visual array can explain nothing. But the words "simulacrum" and (as in the preceding paragraph) "virtually identical" are crucial. We shall see in Chapter 3 that much useful image-processing at low levels of vision passes from one image to another image that is not identical with it.

However, this argument does not, as Pylyshyn seemed to imply, deny

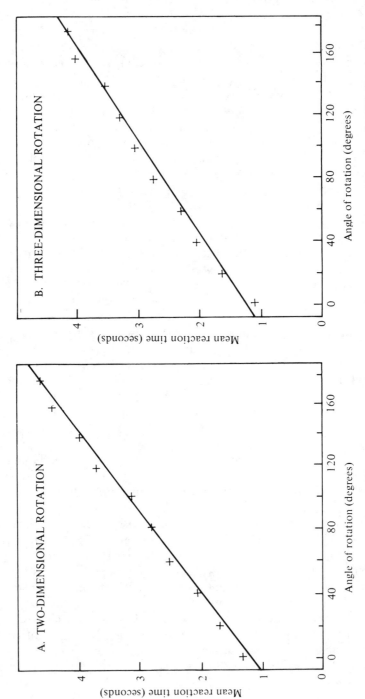

Fig. 2.8. Graphs showing the time needed to respond to stimulus-pairs like those in Fig. 2.7 (A and B) against the difference in degrees between the two pair-members. The maximum possible angular difference is 180 degrees, whether the stimuli are rotated on the plane of the page (as in the left-hand graph) or perpendicular to it (as in the right-hand graph). (Adapted from R. N. Shepard & J. Metzler [1971], Mental Rotation of Three-Dimensional Objects. *Science*, 171, p. 702.)

explanatory value to analogical representations in general. Merely to posit some unspecified analogue is indeed unhelpful. But if the significant (*sic*) structural analogies or isomorphisms are clearly identified, and their method of interpretation specified, talk of analogue-representations can be explanatory. They can even be programmed, as in Funt's model of analogue visual representation mentioned above. This is not to say that analogical representation is well understood, nor to deny that intellectually lazy appeals to "analogue representation" are too often made. But theoretical prejudice against analogue models *in general* is unjustified.

One reason for Pylyshyn's dissatisfaction with analogue accounts of imagery was that their proponents seemed to assume that isomorphism is enough. That is, they usually failed to realize that in identifying an isomorphism as a *significant* similarity, one must specify not only a representation's form, but also the way in which it can be used. One and the same form, interpreted (used) in different ways, can represent significantly different things. We have seen, for example that FORK-vertices were represented in the scene-analysis programs of Guzman, Clowes, and Waltz in much the same way (as a junction of three lines in which the angle subtended by the outer two lines, and enclosing the middle line within it, is more than 180 degrees), but that these three programs used, or interpreted, FORKS in significantly different ways. But psychologists often failed to recognize the theoretical necessity of explaining how a similarity is taken to be significant in a particular case. Even those iconicists who did not (trivially) posit icons exactly isomorphic with the visual array rarely faced the question of just how their hypothetical icons functioned.

By contrast, said Pylyshyn, we do have some specific ideas about what a description is – *and* about how it can be used. He saw the "greatest advantage" of the notion of a *description* as the fact that it had already been formalized in various computer simulation models.

In scene-analysis, for instance, the content and use of lists of descriptions had been defined rigorously enough to enable computers to interpret pictures of polyhedral objects. Vague remarks about quasi-spatial transformations of quasi-spatial internal pictures do not have comparably precise meaning. As yet, no computer model of analogue-representation existed. And no clear account had been given by Shepard and Metzler (or anyone else) of just how images are like – and unlike – their spatial analogues. *A fortiori*, Shepard and Metzler could not express their "theory" as a computer program, which would at least have shown the theory (whether true or false) to be both well defined and internally coherent.

But what of their experimental results? Even if Shepard and Metzler had not provided rigorous explanations, surely they had shown that imagery takes place within some special representational medium? – So it seemed to many people.

Pylyshyn countered that Shepard and Metzler's results, including their subjects' introspective reports, did not exclude the hypothesis that having an image is a matter of using mental representations that resemble descriptions (as opposed to having some internal object that is an analogue, in a spatial or quasi-spatial medium, of a real object). However, Pylyshyn's arguments in this early paper were relatively sketchy. (He was to develop them later, as we shall see.) And soon afterwards, his "descriptional" position appeared to suffer another blow. For in the early to mid 1970s, S. M. Kosslyn reported a number of experiments on naturalistic imagery which seemed – to many people – to support an analogue-account [Kosslyn, 1973; 1975; Kosslyn & Pomerantz, 1977].

Many of Kosslyn's experiments involved what is (tendentiously) called image-scanning. For instance, he got his subjects to memorize a map of a fictitious island (showing the church, the lighthouse, the river and its bridge, and so on). Next, he asked them to visualize the map in their minds and to focus on a certain place: the lighthouse, say. Then, they were told to imagine a spot moving from the lighthouse to the bridge (or the church), and to press a button as soon as the spot reached the destination. Amazingly (or so it seemed to Kosslyn), the time taken to press the button varied according to the distance on the map between the positions of lighthouse, bridge, and church.

Kosslyn concluded (invalidly, as we shall see) that there must be some image-property that is very like real distance, and some process of traversing an image that is very like the traversal of real space. It seemed to him, for example, that in image-traversal, as in actual traversal, all the intermediate points between two places have to be visited in getting from one to the other.

Indeed, studies done some years later led Kosslyn to describe images as three-dimensional. Subjects were asked to look at a 3D-scene and then to imagine it with their eyes shut. The time they took to scan from one imagined object to another increased in proportion to the actual 3D-distances between them, not the 2D-distances between objects that would have appeared in a photograph of the scene [Pinker, 1980]. Evidently, image-traversal can occur in three dimensions, as real movement in 3D-space can too.

Other experiments seemed – to many people – to show that there are mental objects, viz., images, with a spatial or quasi-spatial property analogous to real visual angle. Subjects were instructed by Kosslyn to visualize an elephant (or a dog) in the far distance and then to imagine walking towards it. They reported that the image of the animal grew larger (filled more of their imagined visual field) as they did this. In addition, all subjects eventually reported that the image of the animal had overflowed their visual field, so that they were no longer inspecting an image of the whole animal. As if all this were not enough, each subject's estimates of how far away the imagined creature was at the point of overflow made perfect sense in terms of the real size of elephants (or dogs) and the real visual angle each would subtend (at a given distance, small objects take up less of the visual field than large ones do).

Again, it seemed (to Kosslyn and to many others) that there must be some inner analogue of real vision, an image within a special representational medium that inherently possesses quasi-spatial properties. The image may not actually be spatial; as we shall see, Kosslyn claims it is not. But (seemingly) it has inherent properties allowing transformations that are isomorphic with spatial transformations. Likewise, even if symbolic representations are involved in the generation and semantic interpretation of imagery (Kosslyn claims they are), symbolic computation alone cannot explain it.

(Notice that the jump from "analogue" to "medium" in the first sentence of the preceding paragraph is inescapable only if "analogue" is understood, as it is by Kosslyn, in the strong sense defined above. If we adopt the minimalist sense, this jump expresses not a conceptual necessity but an empirical hypothesis – which requires justification for both clauses.)

Kosslyn's results were generally regarded as being even more sensational, even more surprising, than Shepard and Metzler's. To a large extent, however, they were only what was to be expected. Given the meaning of the concepts used in the experimental instructions, different results would have showed either that the subjects had not understood the instruction or that they had chosen not to obey it. For, whatever the psychological mechanism of imagery may be, the English verb "to imagine" means to represent something as though it were real. Thus imagining traversing a space entails imagining being successively at intermediate points – otherwise it would not be traversing that was being imagined (but rather hopping, or perhaps instantaneous transportation as in *Star Trek*). Likewise, imagining walking towards an elephant entails imagining seeing the elephant looming larger in one's field of view – for that is what happens when one walks towards something.

So Kosslyn's experiments, if not wholly unnecessary, discovered much less than he claimed. They showed that subjects can obey instructions of the type "Imagine doing *x*" – but we all knew that already. This is a special case of the fact that the results of some psychological experiments (especially in social psychology) are presented as surprising empirical discoveries, whereas in reality they are merely illustrations of well-known truths which conceptual analysis could have uncovered in the first place. (Pylyshyn's "countervailing" experiments on imagery, described below, were largely supererogatory for the same reason; but he did stress the importance of the meaning of the experimental instructions, as we shall see.) At best, Kosslyn's experiments discovered that people are rather better at obeying such instructions than one might have thought. The highly realistic changes in apparent visual angle, for example, were perhaps genuinely surprising.

However, we must distinguish between experimental results (the fact that subjects behaved in certain ways) and their theoretical interpretation. If Kosslyn's results were wrongly seen as remarkable, it does not follow that his interpretation of them was either uninteresting or invalid. Even the most familiar facts can have surprising implications. Do Kosslyn's conclusions – that images are not like descriptions (a "conclusion" prejudiced by the term *image-scanning*) and that imagery requires a special, quasi-spatial, representational medium – follow from his experimental results?

Recently, Pylyshyn [1984] has attempted to answer these points within a general theory of computational psychology. His view that all computational processes are, in essence, formal operations like those which occur in digital computers will be discussed (and rebutted) in Chapter 8. Here, our concern is with his views on imagery. In a nutshell, Pylyshyn's position is that experimental results that can be affected by the subject's knowledge and beliefs cannot force us to posit some special medium of representation. He expresses his argument in terms of two crucial concepts (defined below): *cognitive penetrability* and *functional architecture*. (He assumes – falsely, as later chapters will show – that these two terms are mutually exclusive and jointly exhaustive, that all representations are explicable by reference either to one or to the other. However, this assumption is irrelevant to the argument being considered here.)

By *cognitively penetrable* phenomena, Pylyshyn means those which are determined by the subject's tacit or explicit knowledge and so can be influenced, in rationally relevant ways, by changes in specific goals and beliefs. Our social perceptions, for example, are influenced by our knowledge (or beliefs) about other people; so our attitudes, roles, and attributions of intention are all cognitively penetrable. Social psychologists since the 1920s have explained social perceptions by referring to the subject's idiosyncratic or culturally shared "definition of the situation", a term which suggests verbal concepts or *descriptions*. Pylyshyn would regard this as no accident, because as he points out behaviour or experience generated by descriptive, or propositional, representations is in principle cognitively penetrable. The reason is that descriptions are symbolic representations (having semantic content) that can be transformed, by means of computational processes, in ways that are broadly rational with respect to the semantic content of other descriptions.

Functional architecture is a term drawn from computer science. In its original sense, it denotes those properties of the hardware of a computational system which make possible, and constrain, the information-processing going on. (A broader sense, which allows one to speak of a computer's *virtual* architecture, will be defined in later chapters.) Pylyshyn points out that psychological phenomena that are directly attributable to the functional architecture (rather than to computations carried out by means of it) will be cognitively *impenetrable*. The medium's inherent properties cannot be rationally influenced by computations, because they form the background information-processing architecture which makes computations possible. They can be altered only by biological, chemical, and maturational factors. (A computer might be able to change its own functional architecture, for example, by altering its voltages or switching some of its circuits on or off; but even if they were triggered by particular computations, these changes could not be rationally sensitive to a range of semantic contents, because voltage-levels and circuits do not have any semantic content.)

The concept of functional architecture provides Pylyshyn's criterion for *analogical representation*. Pylyshyn does not use this term in the miminalist sense favoured by Sloman, and explicitly excludes *continuity* from his definition. Rather, he says: "The essential idea behind the use of the term *analogue* by most psychologists is captured precisely by what I have been calling *functional architecture*" [1984, p. 209]. So to say that images are analogue representations, in this sense, is to say that they depend on some special representational medium in the brain. (Pylyshyn allows that this is a meaningful hypothesis, and that there may be more than one cerebral medium; his point is that the experiments done by Kosslyn and others do not prove that there is.)

The two concepts of cognitive penetrability and functional architecture, Pylyshyn believes, provide us with a methodology for finding out whether images are like descriptions. On the one hand, he says, (1) *if imagery involves descriptions, then it will be cognitively penetrable:* the experimental results will be rationally influenced by the subject's goals and beliefs. On the other hand, he claims, (2) *if images are quasi-spatial analogues, then the experimental results will not be cognitively penetrable.* We shall see that the first part of Pylyshyn's methodological claim here is correct (although its converse is not), but that the second part is less straightforward.

With reference to part (1) of the claim, Pylyshyn planned a series of experiments on imagery designed to test for cognitive penetrability. He wished to show that the experimental results so widely taken to prove the existence of images that really rotate actually prove nothing of the sort. So, for example, some of his experiments recalled Kosslyn's lighthouse-to-bridge and lighthouse-to-church problems. If Pylyshyn asked subjects to imagine a real spot moving, or to imagine that they were really walking, then the time taken to reach the destination varied with the distance, just as Kosslyn had claimed. But if he asked the subjects to imagine shifting their gaze as quickly as possible from the lighthouse to the bridge (or the church), and to press the button when they had done so, it did not. Moreover, if he asked subjects to imagine running (rather than walking) to the church, they pressed the button more quickly.

Pylyshyn argued that these experimental results are due to the subjects' knowledge, to their goals and beliefs. People know that running is faster than walking; and they know that shifting one's gaze from one place to another can always be done quickly, whereas the time needed to walk from one place to another depends on the distance between them. Likewise, most of Kosslyn's other *prima facie* persuasive results can be explained in terms of people's tacit knowledge of the properties and appearances of physical objects, and of the results of real actions. We all know that a large dog seen from afar appears the same as a small dog seen close-to, and that a dog and an elephant at a given distance take up differing proportions of one's visual field. Further, we know that examining the features of a small object often takes longer than inspecting a larger object (Kosslyn had reported that subjects took longer to "scan a small image" for its detailed features).

As for Shepard and Metzler's rotation-experiments, their results turn out not to be generalizable in the way one would expect if the effect were really due to some quasi-spatial simulacrum of a 3D-object. For example, as the shape of the imagined object is made more complex, the ability of experimental subjects to make correct judgments about its appearance under rotation decreases [Rock, 1973]. Likewise, people's capacity to imagine rotated objects, even simple cubes, depends crucially on what structural description of the object they are implicitly adopting [Hinton, 1979]. Subjects make systematic mistakes about how many corners of a cube would be visible after it had been rotated in certain ways: these mistakes should not happen if the subject were really rotating an internal quasi-cube, but they are intelligible if one takes into account the descriptions used in the experimental instructions. That is, the variation in experimental results shows that these phenomena are cognitively penetrable.

But what of the introspective reports given by Shepard and Metzler's subjects, to the effect that they were "rotating images in their minds"? Pylyshyn argued that these are unreliable. Experimental psychologists have long known that one cannot take at face value what people say about how they are using images, for subjects commonly report that they are doing something which the results show they cannot be doing. For instance, people report "scanning" or "reading off" a remembered array of letters, and can indeed recall the rows (left to right) and the columns (top to bottom); however, they are unable to "scan" the array diagonally, or to "read" the letters from bottom to top [Fernald, 1912]. Indeed, introspective reports in general must be treated with great caution. The reason is that introspections are self-perceptions, and so can be expected to be just as theory-laden, just as *descriptional,* as any other perception. Very general theories, or assumptions, about the nature of physical things or of mental processes are in principle capable of informing our perceptions – and our self-perceptions [P. M. Churchland, 1979; 1984]. It follows that introspections are themselves cognitively penetrable: if subjects believe (consciously or not) that imagery has certain properties, they will very likely experience their own imagery accordingly.

Pylyshyn was right when he said that imagery – and introspection – is cognitively penetrable. (But there are, as he admits, some difficult cases: for instance, people *ignorant of psychophysics* experience imaginary after-images in complementary colours [Finke & Schmidt, 1977; Pylyshyn, 1984, pp. 247–249]; similarly, people asked to imagine a grid moving away from them report "blurring" sooner if the grid-lines are oblique than if they are horizontal or vertical, which parallels an arcane finding of psychophysics.) But, for the reasons given above, his experimental findings should have been unsurprising. By definition, to *imagine* something happening is to represent it as though it really were happening. The only area for surprise is the detailed verisimilitude with which people are apparently able to do this.

It is strange that Pylyshyn did not realize this, for in criticizing Kosslyn, Shepard, and Metzler he stressed a closely related point: that the experimental instructions should make clear what task is to be performed. Pylyshyn distinguished two different tasks, with different criteria of success, that their subjects might undertake. They might try to solve a problem by using what they think of as a certain medium or mechanism. Alternatively, they might try to re-create as accurately as possible the sequence of perceptual events that (they believe) would occur if a real event were actually being observed. Instructions on image-scanning are often ambiguous as between these two tasks. But no experiment can be interpreted confidently if its task-demands are unclear. (A supposedly crucial experiment of Kosslyn's depends on asking subjects to *predict* how long a certain imagined object would take to rotate *if* they were to "simply rotate the image" [Kosslyn, 1983, p. 151]. Pylyshyn pointed out that the meaning of this instruction is highly problematic: just what should one do to imagine one's own imagining of a real object?)

Pylyshyn was right also to say, as in (1), above, that *if imagery involves descriptions, then it will be cognitively penetrable*. Descriptions are in principle cognitively penetrable, as we have seen. But the converse does not hold. If imagery is cognitively penetrable, we cannot infer (as does Pylyshyn) that it must be explained in terms of computations defined over descriptions – that is, in terms of *non-analogue* representation. To see why this is so, we must consider part (2) of Pylyshyn's methodological claim (namely, *if images are quasi-spatial analogues, then the experimental results will not be cognitively penetrable*).

Clause (2) is correct only under Pylyshyn's (non-minimalist) interpretation of *analogue*. On the minimalist interpretation, it is incorrect. Pylyshyn implicitly assumes that there are only two logical possibilities: that imagery involves either descriptions or analogues-in-a-special-medium. But there is a third possibility. Imagery could involve analogue-representations (whose function depends on *significant structural similarity*) that are not embodied in some special medium, or "cerebral plasticine". Moreover, his argument that an analogue-representation cannot be cognitively penetrable applies only to analogues-in-a-special-medium. If minimalist analogues exist in a medium of representation that can also support the computations involved in knowledge, then they might be cognitively penetrable. Structural isomorphisms stored in a digital computer, for example, could in principle be influenced by formal computations within the same machine. (This is so even if we accept Pylyshyn's questionable assumption that knowledge can depend only on computations defined over descriptions, not on analogue-representations.)

So Pylyshyn's methodology is flawed. To prove that imagery is cognitively penetrable (which in any event does not require experimental enquiry) shows only that it is not directly explicable in terms of functional architecture. It does not prove that imagery is not analogue in any psychologically interesting sense.

Pylyshyn's failure to appreciate this was partly due to his not distinguishing the minimalist sense of "analogue-representation" from his own, stronger, sense of the term. But it was due also to the fact that he focussed on the descriptional approach of the scene-analysis models discussed in the first half of this chapter. Some other (later) work in computer vision is analogical in that it exploits significant structural similarities, such as Funt's program already mentioned which in its most recent implementation [Funt, 1983, esp. p. 67] reproduces the time-relationships described by Shepard and Metzler (the more rotation, the more time taken by the subject to rotate). And the fourth phase of computer vision (described in Chapter 3) employs a form of computation that does not fit Pylyshyn's view of what *computation* is.

The history of the psychological debate on imagery raises another methodological issue, of relevance to computational psychology in general. Kosslyn was partly persuaded by Pylyshyn's critique, to the extent that he now allows that tacit knowledge of physics can influence imagery. Indeed, he uses this fact to explain his subjects' imagining inertial rotations, thus avoiding the implausible claim that there are inherently weighty images rotating through analogue space. Nevertheless, he still insists that quasi-spatial images are actually being rotated (the knowledge-based effects, he says, are superimposed on the basic image-form). A prime reason why Kosslyn feels he can insist on this point is that he has provided a computer model of his theory [Kosslyn, 1980; 1981; 1983]. This, he argues, gives a weight to his theoretical claims which previous psychological work on imagery lacked.

Kosslyn's computer model includes what he calls depictive representations. He grants that images cannot literally be inner pictures, and that they must be quasi-spatial, not really spatial. He compares them with the information about spatial matters that is stored permanently in a computer, information which can be manipulated and transformed in various ways, and which gives rise to fleeting displays on the VDU screen. That is, images exist both in active memory (when experienced) and in long-term memory.

The distinctive *medium* is modelled by a special matrix of cells, carrying the depictive information that can be displayed on a monitor-screen. This quasi-spatial matrix "functions like a space": it has a limited extent, a specified shape, and a "grain of resolution" (highest at the centre). The long-term storage includes both depictive and propositional components (the latter allows for a degree of cognitive penetrability). The long-term depictive representation consists of pairs of numbers: coordinates indicating where, in the matrix, the relevant image-point should be placed to depict the imaged object.

Kosslyn's computer model is highly complex, having been continually adjusted over several years to incorporate new empirical data. The ways in which the different long-term memory-structures are accessed, for instance, depend on a wide range of experiments done by Kosslyn and his associates. Decisions as to which type should be accessed reflect his results on "mental comparisons" (subjects asked to compare the size of two objects normally use imagery, but sometimes use propositional information about the objects concerned). Likewise, Kosslyn reports that the quasi-spatial properties of the matrix were dictated by his experimental findings.

Having produced a computer model, Kosslyn is immune to some of Pylyshyn's criticisms of Shepard and Metzler. One cannot complain that Kosslyn's ideas about "quasi-spatial" representations are hopelessly vague, nor that he offers no account of just how they are used. The program shows, too, that his theory is neither unclear nor inconsistent, and that it is compatible with the empirical evidence.

Why, then, is Pylyshyn so critical of Kosslyn's work? To be sure, Pylyshyn favours symbolic-descriptional accounts, and avoids analogue-theories in general. But he is after all a computational psychologist, and Kosslyn has provided a computer model. Why does Pylyshyn not allow Kosslyn's theory to be (at least) a candidate account of imagery?

The time is long past when one could expect psychologists to be deeply impressed by just any computer model whose input–output performance mimics aspects of human behaviour. Computer models are no longer like a dog walking on its hind legs, of which Dr Johnson said that the wonder is not that it does it well but that it does it at all. Computational psychologists, in the broad sense defined in Chapter 1, take it for granted that many, perhaps all, mental functions can be simulated by computational processes. A mere input–output simulation, then, is not necessarily of any great interest to them.

To be sure, when someone produces the first simulation of performance in a particular domain, people will be intrigued. Pylyshyn himself acknowledges that there are "numerous excellent ideas" in Kosslyn's pioneering model (about how structures are accessed, and how classes of transformation differ). And he praises Kosslyn's "clever experiments", many of which were planned to help decide on detailed features of the computer model. His quarrel is not with Kosslyn's data, nor – with one important qualification – with his computer model, but with the specific theoretical interpretation Kosslyn puts on them.

The qualification is that Pylyshyn is unimpressed by the model's ability to predict the experimental results. Indeed, "predict" is perhaps the wrong word. As mentioned above, the program was continually adapted (Kosslyn would say "improved" or "extended", Pylyshyn would say "patched") so as to take account of new experimental evidence. Up to a point, this is admissible, even laudatory – but only if the adaptations make coherent theoretical sense in terms of the guiding principles of the model. Pylyshyn complains that Kosslyn's model is "more like an encyclopedia than a theory" [Pylyshyn, 1984, p. 254]. Because it is essentially *ad hoc,* the fact that it "predicts" the empirical evidence is hardly surprising.

The Pylyshyn–Kosslyn debate has occasionally been criticized on the ground that it, like other disputes about representation, is irresolvable. J. R. Anderson [1976; 1979] argued that it is impossible, in principle, to discriminate empirically among various forms of representation. (More recently, Anderson has said that he was speaking of the *notations* used to express representations, not the *processes* defined in relation to them: the latter, he has said, are indeed empirically distinguishable [Anderson, 1983, p. 46].) More generally, it is often said by opponents – and, indeed, by sensible proponents – of the computational approach, that just because a computer program produces the same input–output performance as a human subject, it does not follow that the human being does it in the same way.

Pylyshyn replies with a familiar point from the philosophy of science: all scientific theories (not only psychological theories about representations) are radically underdetermined by the evidence. It is always possible, no matter how many data we have, that another theory might be found which predicts the data equally well. Likewise, it is always possible that a different computer program might fit the evidence better. Methodological caution is therefore required. But if physics can live with this situation, so can psychology.

Setting aside the inevitable underdetermination of theories, then, how can we actually evaluate computer models of mental processes? How can we decide which programs are acceptable as psychological theories, and which merely mimic behaviour in a psychologically uninteresting way?

Various answers will be considered in this book. One, explored in Chapter 6, depends on distinguishing the fixed constraints of a given information-processing system (its functional architecture) from the processes or algorithms running on it. Another is considered in the following chapter, which describes fourth-phase work on vision. We shall see that much of this work rests on a view of computational psychology that is very different from Pylyshyn's, but which would likewise regard Kosslyn's computer model, and many others, as psychologically irrelevant.

3   Connectionist models of vision

The fourth phase of computer-modelling of vision, like the third, focusses on the interpretative mapping betweeen 2D-input and 3D-world. But it can be contrasted with the scene-analysis tradition in a number of ways. Fourth-phase work stresses low-level computations (though high-level schemata are sometimes included too); it employs realistic input (as opposed to line-drawings) in many cases; it makes use of detailed knowledge of physical optics (to describe the process of image-formation); it involves massive parallel-processing; its representations are often distributed (in a way to be described) over whole networks of computational units; it takes some account of neurophysiology; and its preferred (though not, yet, its usual) implementation is in dedicated hardware rather than general-purpose machines.

The connectionist core

Fourth-phase models are parallel-processing systems which are broadly labelled *connectionist,* because they rely on co-operative computation based on simultaneous local interactions between interconnected units. Connectionism has many varieties, ranging from the pioneering work of D. O. Hebb [1949], O. G. Selfridge [1959], and F. Rosenblatt [1958] to the more complex systems now being developed [Hinton & Anderson, 1981; Rumelhart & McClelland, 1986a]. Indeed, there are potentially many more types yet to be conceived.

An increasingly influential class of systems falling within this general approach to computer-modelling is "PDP-theory": the abbreviation standing for "parallel distributed processing". In PDP-models, a representation is embodied as the pattern of activity over the network as a whole, and in this sense is *distributed* over the whole system. Indeed, in most PDP-models, it is not possible to attach any clear meaning to the activity of an individual unit, or "neurone", in the network. In these cases, each unit represents not any familiar concept (as do the units in some connectionist models) but some abstract aspect or relationship, which contributes to the more readily intelligible feature that is represented by the overall activity-pattern. For example, we shall see that each unit in a PDP-system modelling stereopsis codes *a comparison between the light falling on corresponding points on the two retinae;* it is the overall pattern of many such abstract point-comparisons which represents the *depth,* or *distance,* of the object being looked at. (Stereopsis is the ability to see how far away an object is by comparing the images it presents to the left and right eyes; objects at different distances from the observer provide image-pairs in which the two images are horizontally shifted to different degrees.)

The versions of connectionism described in most detail here, those due to D. Marr and G. E. Hinton, have been chosen because they raise significant questions about psychological method in general. Since connectionism is *a way (or set of ways) of doing computation,* connectionist systems can in principle compute many different things: semantic interpretations of sentences, planned bodily movement . . . whatever. In Chapter 7, for example, we shall consider a general specification of a possible class of connectionist learning-systems [Hinton & Sejnowski, 1986] and a specific PDP-system which learns the morphology of the past tense of English verbs [Rumelhart & McClelland, 1986b]. However, connectionism is introduced, in this chapter, by reference to the psychology of vision.

All connectionist visual systems posit a visual mechanism made up of locally communicating computational units functioning in parallel, where (because of excitatory and inhibitory connections) the state of any one unit depends largely on the states of its neighbours. The specific connections are carefully chosen so as to embody powerful physical constraints on 2D-to-3D mapping (which was not the case for property-list models or early simulations of "neural nets"). The excitatory and inhibitory connections fulfil a role somewhat analogous to the Waltz filter, for they constrain the interpretation of one part of the input according to the probable properties of the neighbouring parts.

In D. L. Waltz's scene-analysis program, only those potential interpretations of a vertex were allowed which were consistent with the previously accepted interpretations of the neighbouring vertex. And once a decision was made, it could not be unmade. In the simple world of perfect line-drawings of polyhedra, this hardly mattered (although it prevented any solution being found when, as in the Necker cube, several are possible). But in more realistic worlds, where many constraints are probabilistic rather than all-or-none, such a method is too inflexible. It leads to an inferential gangrene, for a whole set of potential choices (many of which may be correct) is blocked off if one choice has already been made which is inconsistent with any of them.

In complex and noisy (that is, real-life) domains, where the individual criteria incline but do not necessitate, one needs methods of consistency-testing wherein decisions can be tentatively explored and can be undone if they do not work out well. The first such method was called *relaxation* [Rosenfeld, Hummel & Zucker, 1976]. All connectionist models use some computational technique based on or similar to relaxation. (This is true given the broad sense of "connectionism" that is common today: the term used to be understood in a narrower sense, which excluded relaxation-models.)

Relaxation allows continual adjustments to be made in (varying-strength or binary) decisions, so that a mutually consistent set is eventually reached. If each tentative decision were taken in isolation, there would often be an explosive depth-first search. (That is, each possible alternative for each individual decision would be examined in turn, at successively deeper inferential levels; in practice, the system might never finish considering the implications of the very first alternative to be considered.) But relaxation allows each decision to be influenced by the effects of other decisions, changing in a way that is likely to turn out right. Although some sets of mutual constraints would lead to interminable oscillations, others allow the system to converge towards a set of mutually supportive decisions. In practice, then, one must identify convergent sets of constraints relevant to the problem concerned.

Relaxation in the original sense can be illustrated by the example of a class of schoolchildren who are required to reach a communal decision. (Later, in the final sections of this chapter and of Chapter 7, I shall describe three further classrooms, which represent differing forms of connectionism.)

In this classroom (let us call it Classroom A), no child can think about all aspects of the problem, but each can consider a small part of it. No two children concern themselves with the same problem-part. Each child talks continuously to her immediate neighbours, adjusting her opinion slightly with every interchange in the light of what she hears. This goes on for some time, so that the opinion of the child in the left-hand corner of the back row will indirectly influence the opinion of every other child (though the children in the front row will never know precisely what their friend's opinion was, as it comes to them mediated by the varying opinions of the children in the intermediate rows). Although individual opinions change, no new information is introduced. Eventually (if it is a convergent case), all the children will be stating opinions that are consistent with each other. At this stage the opinion-forming process has stabilized, and this is taken to be the class-decision.

To design a connectionist computer model, one must specify the basic computational units (the children), and the nature and strength, and modes of variation, of each of the connections between them.

In principle, all connectionist systems could be modelled by programming a general-purpose, serial, computer to act in the requisite way. However, since any realistic system involves vast numbers of units, a full-scale simulation on a von Neumann machine would often be unacceptably slow, or even in practice impossible. Moreover, it would fit ill with the neurophysiological emphasis of connectionism. Cells in the retina and visual cortex, and several other cortical areas, appear to function in parallel and to be dedicated to specific functions (although some cortical neurones may be general-purpose mechanisms).

Connectionists therefore think in terms of parallel, dedicated, hardware. In a dedicated machine, the basic units are engineered (not programmed) so as to compute certain things: light-intensity, for example. And the computational connections are implemented as hardwired links, whose state of excitation (whether continuously varying or binary) can be influenced by the activity of the linked units. Fourth-phase modellers have already designed dedicated parallel machines for implementing certain aspects of low-level vision, and others are currently being built [Hillis, 1985]. Meanwhile, however, many of their ideas have to be tested by simulating (toy) connectionist systems on traditional von Neumann computers.

The connectionist account of perception was described in Chapter 2 as a broadly Kantian hybrid of empiricism and rationalism, because it is both *data-driven* and *interpretative*.

Like Gibson, fourth-phase modellers emphasize the richness of the information that is normally available in the visual array. Although some connectionist systems (such as those discussed at the end of this chapter) work only on highly restricted artificial examples, others can use the ambient light in natural images to extract 3D-information about shape, orientation, and depth. In the third phase, such information could have been inferred only, if at all, *top-down* from high-level knowledge of the familiar objects in the scene. (Roberts' and Mackworth's programs were among the very few scene-analysis programs which could deal with orientation, for instance.) Like Gibson too, fourth-phase workers stress the extent to which visual information is picked up by data-driven *bottom-up* processes. Their computer models can derive a significant amount of 3D-information even about unfamiliar objects. But this is done by low-level interpretative procedures (edge-detectors, for example) which can be thought of as applying schemas hunting top-down, though at a very low level, for specific local structures. For unlike Gibson, who posited an unanalysed function of "information pick-up", these workers insist that even the lowest-level visual processes involve specifiable computations whereby the retinal image caused by the stimulus-light is interpreted in terms of its real-world significance.

This theoretical emphasis on real-world interpretation distinguishes the fourth phase of computer vision from the first. Like connectionism, the property-list approach aimed at computations that were low-level, done in parallel, and neurophysiologically plausible. It might even be regarded as an embryonic form of connectionism – but one in which issues of ecological validity were not taken seriously.

One of the best-known and most-elaborated examples in this fourth category – though by no means the earliest – is due to Marr. Besides being an example of connectionism in the general sense described above, Marr's work is of interest to psychologists (and physiologists) in two other ways. First, it has produced testable hypotheses about specific aspects of vision, some of which have already led to experimental research (on stereopsis and apparent motion, for instance). Second, it offers a novel, and controversial, account of the nature of a scientific psychology *in general.*

Computational psychology according to Marr

Marr argued that an adequate psychology will comprise explanations at three distinct but interrelated levels: computational, algorithmic, and hardware. He regarded the first level (also called the top level because it is the most abstract) as theoretically fundamental, in that its insights should determine the questions asked at the other two, increasingly concrete, levels. Despite his regarding a specific sort of computational explanation as theoretically basic, Marr's account challenges not only non-computational positions but much of what is normally termed computational psychology too.

This approach to theoretical psychology evolved through the late 1970s in Marr's research papers, and formed the central theme of his book *Vision,* published posthumously in 1982. (For Marr's earlier, non-technical, introduction see Marr & Nishihara, 1978; for an excellent recent overview see Mayhew & Frisby, 1984.)

Marr's approach, like most novel insights, was not absolutely new. The basic idea was independently arrived at by T. Poggio. A somewhat similar claim about psychological methodology had been made – in a different, and arguably less confusing, terminology – by A. Newell and H. A. Simon (whose work will be discussed in Chapter 6). And pioneering studies of image-optics had been done by B. Horn in the mid 1970s. But Marr made these and related ideas part of an integral view of psychology.

His three-level description was intended by him as a definition of psychology in general, and in later chapters we shall consider whether it is overly restrictive when applied to non-visual domains. Here, I shall outline his theoretical approach to vision, indicate how he related it to experimental evidence and to work in computer vision, and ask whether even vision can be adequately captured by his preferred methodology. (I shall concentrate on his views as finally expressed, ignoring the history of their changes. His final definitions of "primitives" and of the "2½D Sketch", for example, differ from his earlier position.)

The top level – which Marr calls the *computational* level – is not what one might expect, given the most familiar usage of the term "computational", for it is not concerned with process: it identifies what the system as a whole is doing, not how it is doing it. It is concerned with what N. Chomsky had earlier defined as *competence,* rather than *performance,* or with what Newell and Simon had termed *task-analysis.* The computational level, then, provides an abstract formulation of the information-processing task which defines a given psychological ability, together with a specification of the basic computational constraints involved. Where vision is concerned, these constraints are grounded in the structure of the physical world, as we shall see. They provide the necessary and sufficient computational basis for any creature (man, monkey, Martian – or machine) faced with the task in question.

The second, algorithmic, level takes account of these constraints in specifying the psychological processes, or computations, by means of which the task is actually performed, which may differ in men and Martians. These processes are defined in terms of a particular system of representation, which can be proved to be reliable (to yield the relevant information) by reference to the top-level constraints. (Marr's specifications of *three* levels is over-simplified in that it ignores the concept, explained in Chapter 6 below, of the *virtual* machine; and some critics have argued that the first two of his three explanatory levels are not so clearly separable as he implied [Morgan, 1984].)

The term "algorithm" need not imply the sort of sequential program familiar in traditional AI. Connectionist algorithms can define processes of self-organization occurring over a whole network of computational units. Again, an algorithm need not be defined in terms of (essentially syntactic) formal rules of symbol-manipulation, although algorithms for execution by general-purpose computers (the machines most commonly used in AI) are so defined. Connectionist systems can embody radically different types of computation. (Some people argue that they are not really examples of *computational psychology* at all; this claim will be discussed in Chapter 8.)

The hardware-level deals with the neural mechanisms that embody the computational and algorithmic functions specified at the other two levels, showing how their physiological properties and anatomical connectivities enable them to do so. Hardware-properties may vary between species even more than algorithmic ones do, and are very different in machines.

As his choice of labels for the three explanatory levels suggests, Marr saw computer-modelling as useful to psychologists. He had always approached neuroscience in the broadly computational spirit of W. S. McCulloch and W. H. Pitts. In the late 1960s he described the overall behavioural functions of the cerebellum and cerebral cortex in terms of the distinct but interrelated functions of different cells. He became aware of AI in the early 1970s, and in 1973 – passing from one Cambridge to the other – he moved to the AI laboratory at MIT, where he remained until his early death in 1980. His thinking was deeply influenced by AI ideas, and at MIT he worked on a number of computer models of vision.

Nevertheless, he came to see AI as largely irrelevant to psychology, irrespective of any psychological interests on the part of the AI programmer. The reason for this apparent paradox is that too little work in AI – Marr implied (unjustly) virtually none – follows the methodology that Marr tried to use in his own computer-modelling, and which he commended in his definition of psychological science.

Marr's methodology was centred on computational, top-level, understanding of the nature of the information-processing task being modelled. He insisted that only if psychology is grounded in such understanding can it be a systematic science, as opposed to a ragbag of empirical findings, theoretically unjustified hunches, and *ad hoc* assumptions introduced to compensate for inadequacies in so-called theory.

His own computer models, accordingly, were based on his top-level account of visual tasks and representations. They were intended as simulations of his theory rather than as programs that (somehow or other) managed to perform visual tasks. Success in implementing edge-finding, for example, would support his theory of edge-finding by adding an "existence-proof" to his abstract proofs, and would show that a particular algorithm (initially justified in terms of the abstract computational theory) was indeed efficient at performing the task of finding edges. Failure would suggest that a mistake had been made in the top-level "proof", or in the abstract justification of the algorithm—or of its efficiency. For Marr aimed to model vision in the most efficient way that was consistent with psychophysiology.

In line with his views on the relative autonomy of the three explanatory levels, he stressed that many different computational *processes* could carry out one and the same computational *task*. So he would compare the performance of various algorithms addressed to the same basic task, considering the different conditions under which they failed in the light of empirical evidence about the limits on human vision.

For instance, he developed two distinct algorithms for stereo-matching (comparing two images, one from each eye, to find corresponding parts of each image in which identical input is slightly shifted horizontally). As we shall see presently, the first was based on a purely iterative form of computation in which all the relevant information was already present at the first cycle. The second introduced new information (coded at different scales of spatial resolution) with successive stages in the stereo-matching process. But both types were based on his top-level analysis, and so qualify as potential candidates for a theory of stereopsis. Marr criticized previous psychological accounts of stereopsis (saying that "not one of them computed the right thing" [1980, p. 122]), irrespective of the form of computational process specified by the psychologists in question. He argued not only that their inadequacy would have been recognized if they had been tested in a computer implementation, but that they would not even have been suggested if his methodology had been followed.

This approach explains why Marr dismissed most work in AI as having nothing to contribute to a theoretical psychology, even though he admitted that AI has heightened psychologists' appreciation of rigour and of process. For *ad hoc* assumptions are often employed in AI to improve a program's performance. Even where there are relatively few obvious "kluges", or programming tricks, AI-programs are usually based on unarticulated and theoretically independent insights, rather than on a coherent understanding of the task and its fundamental constraints. In short, according to Marr, AI-workers typically do not know what it is that their program is doing, nor why – as opposed to how – it is able to do it.

"Typically", perhaps – but certainly not always. For instance, we have seen that scene-analysis models gradually evolved towards a deeper understanding of the nature of the task facing third-phase programs. Their emphasis on systematic 2D-to-3D mapping provided some crucial theoretical insights: Marr himself drew on A. K. Mackworth's work on gradient-space in his own theory of vision. Likewise, as we shall see in Chapter 6, the theoretical importance of abstract task-analysis had been stressed by Newell and Simon in the context of computer models of problem-solving. And the influential AI-work on logical "theorem-proving" was theoretically oriented also – so much so, indeed, that its relevance for both technological and psychological purposes was impaired (this point parallels the suggestion made below: that, *pace* Marr, brains often employ theoretically messy computational methods).

Moreover, from the undeniable fact that AI-workers often lack any deep theoretical insight into what they are doing, relying instead on *ad hoc* programming tricks, it does not follow that AI can produce little or nothing of interest to psychological science. For Marr's methodology, like most other rational reconstructions of science, does not accurately reflect the way science in general is done (nor even the way his own research was done). Ideally, there would be no false starts and no blindness to theoretical implications. But if angelic scientists might progress in this way, mere humans cannot. With hindsight, it is admittedly surprising that A. Guzman failed to understand why his vertex-classifying program succeeded, or failed, on specific pictures. But hindsight makes poor science: the full import of even the best work may not be recognized until later.

Outline of a theory of vision

On Marr's view, psychologists must start with an identification of the information-processing task that defines the class of phenomena concerned. The basic task of vision, he said, is a 2D-to-3D mapping. The incoming light is a 2D-array, describable in the vocabulary of physics. This is mapped onto reliable perceptions (descriptions) of the position, orientation, and depth of surfaces in the 3D-world – "reliable" in terms of the interests of the species concerned.

This abstract definition of vision does not mention the eyes, colour, or "visual experience". The retina is part of normal visual hardware, but since hardware is logically distinct from psychological competence, it does not enter into the definition of vision as such. A blind man (a man with no retinal function) could enjoy *vision* in this basic sense if he were to be equipped with a light-responsive tickling-pad on a patch of the skin of his back that enabled him effectively to map the 2D-array of skin-excitation onto the 3D-structure of objects in the world behind him. (Recent studies, in which a TV-camera was connected to tactile stimulators on the skin of blind people, suggest that this pseudo-visual input is not enough in practice, that voluntary movement also is necessary for "visual" perception. When the camera was fixed, or moved by someone else, the blind subjects reported touch-sensations; when they controlled the movement of the camera themselves, they referred to objects located in the space in front of them [Bach-y-Rita, 1984].) The prime reason why colour is excluded from Marr's definition of vision is not that our (and some animals') vision can be black-and-white, but that he regards colour as of interest to biological creatures only insofar as it helps them to compute the presence and nature of 3D-objects. As for "visual experience" in general, this term begs the question since it assumes we already have a way of telling what *visual* experience is.

Even if we grant that "vision" should be defined in terms of task rather than retina, colour, or experience, it is not obvious that Marr's characterization actually does identify the basic purpose for which the visual system has been evolved [Sloman, 1983]. One might, for instance, include the direct (as opposed to description-mediated) initiation of motor action as among the basic tasks of vision, especially in the lower animals. One might also say that, insofar as it produces descriptions, vision typically maps not from 2D to 3D but from 3D to 4D – so as to take time (and movement) into account. Marr does mention temporal change in the visual field, such as "optical flow"; but he considers this primarily in terms of its usefulness in effecting 2D-to-3D mapping. Or one might say that a *basic* purpose of vision is to map from 2D-input onto reliable descriptions of ecologically significant environmental features, including not only 3D-properties and movements but aggressiveness and sexual attractiveness too (and the variety of features classified by Gibson as "affordances").

Marr's answer would be that all these are indeed biologically useful capacities, in which vision plays a crucial part, but that 2D-to-3D mapping *of a particular kind* must take place before any of them can be successfully exercised. That is, he assumes that vision typically involves the bottom-up construction of a detailed object-description by abstractly justifiable general procedures, rather than the (speedier) reactivation of some previous percept (or action) by means of theoretically unreliable, or redundant, special-purpose rules. Although this assumption will be criticized below, the critique allows that vision often may involve constructive computations of a more general kind, such as he describes. For the present, then, let us accept Marr's identification of the task of vision as 2D-to-3D mapping, and ask how his methodology follows from it.

The first effect of the input-light on any visual system is the formation of an image. An *image* in this sense is not a phenomenal experience, or an internal representation such as those discussed in Chapter 2, but a pattern of excitation in a sensory receptor caused by light reflected from the environment. Normally, this is a retinal image; but in the visual tickling-pad it would be a pattern of cutaneous excitation. If vision is to be effective, seeing creatures must map from 2D-image to 3D-description in a way that is sensible with respect to the way the image was originally formed.

Since the image is the data-base for vision of the external world, the physical relations between light and surfaces are theoretically fundamental. Marr used Horn's studies of image-formation as essential groundwork. Having realized in the early 1970s that the visual system needs to be able to distinguish the optical factors responsible for specific properties of the image, Horn based his computer models on a general analysis of object-geometry, surface-reflectance, illumination, and viewpoint. (Roberts had considered these in relation to his prototypes for scene-analysis but did not attempt to develop a general theory.) Horn had realized also that pervasive regularities in the physical world might be used by visual systems as computational constraints enabling them to interpret images sensibly. Marr regarded the discovery of such constraints as basic to any visual *science,* and his theory relied on his identification of six very general features of real-world surfaces (some of which were to be criticized by other psychologists as insufficiently general, as we shall see).

The image cannot be immediately transformed into the final perception, because the mapping between raw light-intensities and 3D-information is too complex to be computed in one step. Marr therefore argued that there must be a *series* of visual representations, of increasing abstractness, between the image and the final perception. A theory of vision must specify distinct representational primitives at each stage, showing how they might be constructed from the primitives of the stage before and so, ultimately, from the image. And because information required for later computations must not be lost at earlier representational stages, the theorist should prove that specific sorts of information can be implicitly preserved at a given level, even if they are not explicitly coded by the primitives of that level. Marr's theory distinguished three representational stages, defined in terms of increasingly abstract visual symbols: the Primal Sketch, the 2½D Sketch, and the 3D-model representation.

According to this theory, the Primal Sketch is itself built up on three hierarchical levels, starting with the construction of the "raw" Primal Sketch. This stage (by processes more fully discussed below) detects the light-intensities present in the image and codes them in terms of (2D) shape, size, orientation, and discontinuities. That is, the primitives of this early representational level distinguish blobs and bars of varying widths and lengths, and mark the location of bar-terminations and points of curvature. The next level of coding makes explicit local geometrical relations within the image that are merely implicit in the raw Primal Sketch: *groups* of bars, or blobs, with a common shape, size, and orientation, are now distinguished from each other. Finally, the full Primal Sketch is reached with a representation of the overall disposition of these groups themselves. For example, a boundary is constructed between two *sets* of group-tokens sharing a common orientation. These successive stages in the construction of the Primal Sketch are outlined in Figure 3.1.

Marr's choice of primitives for the three stages within the construction of the full Primal Sketch was justified partly in theoretical terms. He specified them by using only topological and geometrical concepts (such as termination, width, length, and orientation) that are relatively simple to compute; and he related them to general properties of physical surfaces (such as smoothness) that are exploited at the second representational level, the 2½D Sketch. But he appealed also to empirical evidence, much of which had already been gained by Gibsonian psychologists (this provenance is not surprising, for Gibson's "environmental invariants" are very similar to Marr's "physical constraints"). For example, experiments on the perception of texture had shown that it does not depend on the recognition of familiar physical objects in the visual field [Julesz, 1975]. This suggests that relatively low-level processes are responsible (and that these are to a high degree autonomous with respect to central processing). Moreover, we easily distinguish textural differences that are defined in terms of the sorts of basic elements, groupings, and local spatial relations that are incorporated in Marr's representational theory of the Primal Sketch (see Figure 3.2).

Thus far, only (2D) properties of the retinal image have been explicitly coded: no representation of (3D) surfaces has yet emerged. Surfaces begin to make their appearance (*sic*) in the next stage of representation, the 2½D Sketch. This codes the information in the Primal Sketch so as to make explicit the orientation and relative depth of the visible surfaces and the contours of surface discontinuities. The primitives of this stage of representation symbolize the local orientation of surface elements, their relative distance from the viewer, and the location of discontinuities in these two features. Marr described this second stage as only 2½D, rather than 3D, because the co-ordinate frame is still centred on the viewer. The "depth" that is coded at this stage is not a position in 3D-space, but relative distance from the viewer's retina. Moreover, what is represented as being at that depth is not a 3D-object, but a portion of a visible 3D-surface. There is no representation of the fact that a physical object has a volume bounded by its visible and invisible surfaces.

This fact could not be represented at this level. Because the 2½D Sketch is constructed in a way that relates it relatively directly to the

Image

Raw
primal
sketch

Level 1
tokens

and

Level 2
boundary

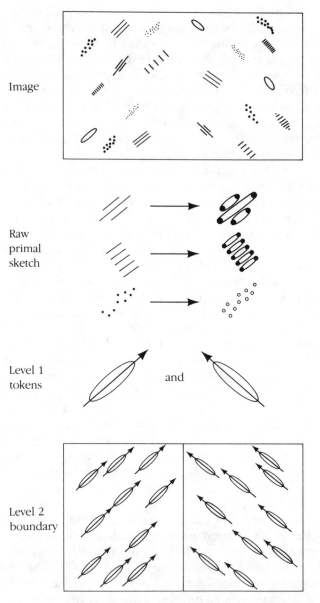

Fig. 3.1. A diagrammatic representation of the descriptions of an image at different scales which together constitute the Primal Sketch. At the lowest level, the raw Primal Sketch faithfully follows the intensity-changes and also represents terminations, denoted here by filled circles. At the next level, oriented tokens are formed for the groups in the image. At the next level, the difference in orientations of the groups in the two halves of the image causes a boundary to be constructed between them. The complexity of the Primal Sketch depends upon the degree to which the image is organized at the different scales. (From *Vision* by David Marr. Copyright © 1982 W. H. Freeman and Company. Reprinted with permission.)

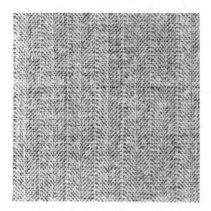 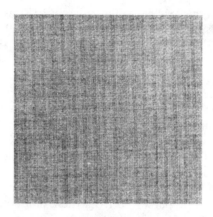

Fig. 3.2. In a herringbone-pattern such as this, a clear part of the spatial organization consists of the vertical stripes. These cannot be recovered by Fourier techniques such as band-pass filtering the images, but yield easily to grouping processes. (From P. Brodatz [1966], *Textures: A Photographic Album for Artists and Designers*. New York: Dover. Pls. 16, 17. Repr. in D. Marr [1982], *Vision*. San Francisco: Freeman. P. 46.)

image, different projections of the same pattern must be given distinct representations – different 2½D Sketches. (Similarly, property-list models, which were even more closely tied to the image, classified a pattern presented in different orientations and/or sizes as different patterns.) Admittedly, interpretations ordinarily included under the general term "object-perception" can occur in the earliest stages of representation. In the Primal Sketch, for instance, different sets of features within the same visual image can be grouped together (if they are caused by reflectance-gathering processes operating at different scales, or spatial frequencies, on a single physical object). And the 2½D Sketch records depth-discontinuities (the results of stereo-matching of the Primal Sketches of the two eyes), thus distinguishing those adjacent parts of the image which are caused by objects lying at different distances from the eye. But these interpretations do not suffice to construct viewpoint-independent spatial descriptions of an object.

Such descriptions are achieved in the final representational stage discussed by Marr: the construction of the 3D-model. The primitives of this stage code volumetric as well as surface-properties, both located by reference to an object-centred co-ordinate frame. The representation of 3D-shapes is based on the information about edge- and surface-contours coded in the 2½D Sketch. It is now possible to represent the fact that two different images depict a particular physical object whose shape, size, volume, and location are independent of the viewpoint.

In defining his 3D-models, Marr adapted previous work relating contour and shape, such as T. O. Binford's descriptions of varying 3D-shapes in terms of "generalized cones" [Binford, 1971; Agin & Binford, 1973; cf. Binford, 1981], and H. Blum's [1973] axis-based representations of the (2D) contours of biological shapes. With respect to the task of interpreting a silhouette in terms of 3D-shape, Marr argued that certain general constraints on the image-forming process can be exploited by, and only by, a representation based on generalized cones (sometimes called generalized cylinders). This is the class of volumes generated by moving a closed curve along an axis, where the curve may change its size (and, in a fully generalized cone, its shape). According to Marr, the ability to perceive this class of 3D-shapes is grounded in innate visual mechanisms, as is the ability to see the silhouettes themselves.

He even claimed that complex shapes such as animal and human bodies can be perceived from their silhouettes independently of prior experience (though his evidence was anecdotal rather than experimental). In Marr's third stage of representation, objects are described not only in terms of their overall shape and size but also in terms of their modular spatial organization. This description involves hierarchically structured models, which represent objects as made up of parts distinguishable on successive levels.

A mammalian body, for example, can be represented as one axis, or as a major axis with four minor axes representing the limbs. These, in turn, can be articulated in terms of the upper and lower limb, while the hand or foot can be described as an unanalysed unit or as a structure consisting of five jointed digits. Humans differ from horses in that the typical spatial orientation of their major body-axes are different, and a standing person can be distinguished from a rearing horse by the different spatial relations of the constituent axes (such as the angle between head and body, and the length of the neck). Marr allowed that the specific differential significance of these spatial relations has to be learnt, but claimed that they can be perceived by general mechanisms evolved by the visual system: *how* an elephant differs from a horse has to be learnt, but *that* the two body-shapes differ is evident to the untutored eye.

(Marr's critics have pointed out that many objects are not in practice economically describable in terms of hierarchies of generalized cones. An alternative representation has recently been suggested for the description of natural forms, which uses as its primitives deformable "lumps of clay" supposedly corresponding to naturally perceptible "parts", and which takes into account the possible *history of formation* of the object out of such parts [Pentland, 1986]. This representation relies neither on point-by-point construction of a detailed image nor on specific high-level object-models, but on primitives at a level intermediate between these two. Unlike Marr's, it can provide succinct 3D-descriptions of arbitrary new objects such as clouds, human faces, trees, and mountains. To what extent it tallies with our "commonsense perception" is still unclear, but the author reports that computer models based on it are more readily intelligible to people than are those using pointwise image-descriptions.)

Marr's theoretical appeals to hierarchically articulated 3D-models bring to mind the third-phase work described in Chapter 2. (And, as remarked above, even "data-driven" connectionist models of vision exploit very general knowledge of the world in searching for edges or surface-fragments.) Yet Marr's early writings on vision gave evidence of a strong reaction against this approach. There, his emphasis on the power of *general* processes in vision was so strong that he sometimes seemed to imply that knowledge-based top-down processing is irrelevant to vision.

Marr's main complaint against scene-analysis work was that it unrealistically, and inefficiently, ignored the vast informational potential that (in conditions of good visibility) is available in the ambient light. If the input was not actually a line-drawing, it was immediately massaged by quasi-intelligent line-finders whose output simulated line-drawings, and these were consequently used as the sole data for visual processing. The Gibson in Marr objected. This objection can be justifiably sustained even though 3D-models eventually crept back into Marr's theory, and even though he admitted that there must be many top-down visual processes besides those he outlined.

But if Marr was Gibsonian in his respect for the richness of the real-world stimulus, he was anti-Gibsonian in seeing low-level vision as an active process of construction. Gibson posited a direct informational pick-up of environmental "affordances", registering ecological properties likely to be of interest to the perceiver (such as shape, texture, motion, and even intent). Marr claimed instead that a series of distinct visual representations is built up by specifiable computational processes functioning on different levels.

Because his theory views the 2½D Sketch as the last stage of visual representation that is constructed bottom-up by autonomous (presumably innate) low-level mechanisms, without needing the influence of high-level schemata, Marr describes it as the last stage of "perception proper". Despite his use of the term "perception" in this context, Marr's description is reminiscent of the traditional philosophical distinction between sensation and perception – according to which the former is automatic and unthinking, and only the latter involves anything comparable to conceptual thought or rational judgment. However, most people who made this distinction (empiricists and rationalists alike) assumed that sensation was a simple, passive process. On Marr's view, by contrast, processes that are automatic and untouched by conceptual schemata may nevertheless be extremely complex, involving a series of active constructions whereby real-world (3D) significance is ascribed to the initial (2D) sensory data. This is why he uses the philosophically stronger term, *perception,* to characterize the early stages of vision – and why his approach qualifies as a Kantian hybrid of empiricism and rationalism.

Marr's methodology in practice: representation of the intensity-array

Having outlined Marr's account of the stages whereby successive representations of the image are constructed, let us turn to consider Marr's methodology. This is of interest with respect not only to the psychology of vision, but also to Marr's claim to have identified the explanatory functions of psychological science in general.

Marr's methodology is a combination of *a priori* argument and empirical study (including computer-modelling). His theoretical primitives for each representational stage were suggested in the light of abstract computational considerations, tested by being embodied in computer models, and also judged by psychological evidence. In general, Marr assumed that the less computationally demanding a method of representation is, the more likely it is that it may have evolved. Given this assumption (which will be queried later), the best strategy is to identify and compare – by mathematical means – the computationally optimal and near-optimal methods, to look for psychological and physiological evidence of their operation in living organisms, and to explore their potential for useful embodiment by computer-modelling.

But although he saw *a priori* argument as logically prior, Marr allowed that empirical work on organisms or artefacts can sometimes provide clues about first-level constraints and second-level mechanisms. Indeed, his view that visual computation requires parallelism was not arrived at in an empirical vacuum, but was grounded in known facts about the retina and visual cortex (similarly, his earlier work on cerebral and cerebellar cortex attempted to make functional sense of neuroanatomy). And we have already noted that his choice of primitives for the three representational stages within the construction of the full Primal Sketch was both theoretically and experimentally motivated. The possibility of a detailed coupling of, and a fruitful interplay between, the three levels promises what cognitive science too often seems to lack: a theoretically integrated interdisciplinarity.

An example that provides a good illustration of Marr's methodology is his approach (with E. Hildreth) to the problem of how the visual system represents the intensity-array in the image. This is the first stage in the construction of the Primal Sketch (the "raw" Primal Sketch).

In my subsequent discussion, the mathematics of this example is presented only in outline, and only insofar as it exhibits Marr's general strategy, which is first to derive psychological hypotheses from highly abstract (and optimal) mathematical criteria, and then to modify them by physiological or psychological knowledge. Readers interested in the mathematical details, wherein lies the full power of Marr's approach, should refer directly to his book (and to Ballard & Brown, 1982).

The first question Marr asks is "*What* is the visual system computing, and *why?*" Perhaps the visual system codes the absolute values of the intensity at every point, as a suitably programmed computer could do? Marr and Hildreth rejected this idea as biologically implausible, partly because it would require a high degree of quantitative precision, but primarily because top-level considerations suggest that the absolute intensities within the retinal image are not psychologically important. They have little or no significance in terms of object-properties likely to be of interest to the perceiver. It is *changes* in intensity which the visual system needs to compute, because these (rather than absolute intensities) carry information about physical edges, contours, texture, surface-markings, depth, shadows, and the like. For simplicity's sake, and to ease comparison with the scene-analysis tradition, I shall concentrate here on the computation of descriptions of physical edges in the real world.

The next question is *how* these changes could possibly be computed. Clearly, what the visual system needs to construct a meaningful representation of the changes in the intensity-array is some sort of *differential* operator (by definition, an operator sensitive to changes). But which particular operator is this likely to be?

It was remarked above, in reference to Roberts' line-finder, that we are sensitive to intensity-changes at different scales, being able to see edges that appear more or less blurred (see Figure 3.3). In Marr's view, it is in principle most unlikely that a single low-level operator would be computationally complex enough to respond to changes at arbitrary scales. Moreover, psychophysical experiments on visual habituation to spatial gratings (initiated by F. W. C. Campbell and J. Robson [1968]) suggest that independent physiological mechanisms, or psychological "channels", respond to different spatial frequencies. These two reasons each imply that there must be many different operators.

If, Marr argued, the only way to detect intensity-changes was the computationally demanding method of measuring and comparing absolute intensities, then visual systems (if any) would have to have evolved so as to be capable of doing this. However, the information that an intensity-change has occurred can be mathematically represented in at least two other – more economical – ways: one by reference to the first spatial derivative, the other by reference to the second spatial derivative. (The first spatial derivative plots *the rate of change in intensity* across the receptive field; the second spatial derivative plots *the rate of change in the first derivative*.) As Figure 3.4 illustrates, changes of light-intensity are represented in the first derivative as a peak (or trough), and in the second derivative as a zero-crossing. (A zero-crossing is a place where the value of a function passes from positive to negative, or vice versa.) So a mathematical operator computing one or other of these functions, were it to be embodied in a visual system, could in principle be used as the basis of edge-perception. That is,

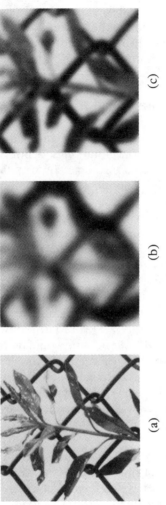

(a)   (b)   (c)

Fig. 3.3. Blurring images is the first step in detecting intensity-changes in them. (a) In the original image, intensity-changes can take place over a wide range of scales, and no single operator will be very efficient at detecting all of them. The problem is much simplified in an image that has been blurred with a Gaussian filter, because there is, in effect, an upper limit to the rate at which changes can take place. The first part of the edge-detection process can be thought of as decomposing the original image into a set of copies, each filtered with a different-sized Gaussian, and then detecting the intensity-changes separately in each. (b) the image filtered with a Gaussian having $\sigma = 8$ pixels; in (c), $\sigma = 4$. The image is 320 by 320 elements. (From D. Marr & E. Hildreth [1980], Theory of Edge Detection. *Proc. Royal Society, London*, B, 207, p. 190. Repr. in D. Marr [1982], *Vision*. San Francisco: Freeman. P. 56.)

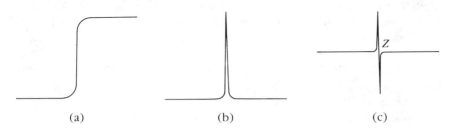

Fig. 3.4. The notion of a zero-crossing. The intensity-change (a) gives rise to a peak
(b) in its first derivative and to a (steep) zero-crossing Z (c) in its second derivative.
(From *Vision* by David Marr. Copyright © 1982 W. H. Freeman and Company.
Reprinted with permission.)

changes in light-intensity could be picked up by a receptor-mechanism
capable of responding either to peaks and troughs in the first derivative or
to zero-crossings in the second derivative.

Marr's next step was to ask what the *optimal* differential operator would
be. His general strategy, as remarked above, is to compare the computational power of distinct operators, each of which is theoretically capable of
performing the information-processing task, and to consider the optimal
operator first. This strategy is only partly due to Marr's predilection for
mathematically elegant theories. It rests also on his assumption that evolution has had so many opportunities to generate and test operators that it
has very likely produced the optimal one.

An alternative and not implausible assumption is that, since evolution
works by random mutations and selection pressures, it is not likely that
animal brains contain nothing but theoretically elegant solutions: more
probably, they contain a hodge-podge of theoretically unrelated methods
for doing the right thing quickly in normal circumstances. To the extent
that this is so, Marr's strategy of looking for computationally optimal methods is psychologically unrealistic. (Moreover, evolution or learning may
well have provided organisms with ways of reacting *quickly,* ways that do
not require the stage-by-stage construction of a complete object-representa-
tion – or, in the case of speech, a complete parse-tree. So even if such
computationally expensive construction can take place, it may occur less
often than Marr implied.)

Setting aside the comments in the previous paragraph, let us follow
through Marr's argument in answering the question "What would the optimal differential operator be?" Since this argument is largely mathematical,
our discussion must touch on mathematical issues. But for present purposes, the details of the mathematical formulae are not important. Rather,
our concern is to understand, in a general way, *how* Marr compares a
variety of differential operators so as to identify the optimal one.

The differential operators that first come to mind, Marr says, are the familiar first-order ($\delta/\delta x$, $\delta/\delta y$) and second-order ($\delta^2/\delta x^2$, $\delta^2/\delta y^2$) derivatives. But if these functions were used to detect edges (that is, contours of intensity-change) they would put an enormous computational load on the visual system. For they are functions involving specific directions or orientations, which would have to be taken into account. A distinct operator would be needed for every different edge-orientation (as was the case for the operators defined in property-list models). It would be computationally simpler if a single operator could respond to edges in any orientation.

(Since we can perceive orientations, the visual system must be able at some point to represent orientation. But this need not be done at the earliest stage. Intensity-changes might be computed first, and their orientation afterwards – provided, of course, that the relevant information was implicitly preserved within the first stage of representation.)

Given that the optimal differential operator would be insensitive to direction, Marr and Hildreth asked next which is the *simplest* of the orientation-independent differential operators that have been defined by mathematicians. The answer, they said, is the Laplacian operator (∇^2). Because this is a second-order operator, in the sense explained above (it is defined as $\delta^2/\delta x^2 + \delta^2/\delta y^2$), it is sensitive to zero-crossings. And because it is non-directional, its distribution or scope is in theory an infinite field. In practice, however, its distribution will not be infinite: if it were embodied in a physical mechanism, its receptive field would be circular. (This is the simplest case; special hardware could be designed to make it any shape; some computer-vision systems implement "square" operators because they make the mathematical calculations more convenient.) In short, a neural mechanism embodying a Laplacian operator, if such a mechanism were to exist, would be able to respond to bars of *any* orientation, provided that they lay within the receptive field.

We saw above that psychological evidence suggests that there must be a class of differential operators of the same general type, sensitive to different sizes. But, as Marr and Hildreth were quick to point out, a pure Laplacian cannot provide size-sensitivity. The reason is that its definition involves no size-variable. So Marr and Hildreth needed to define a class of *filters* that would blur the image at different spatial resolutions (by getting rid of all lower-scale detail).

Again, they drew on mathematics for theoretical inspiration. From the various mathematical functions that *could* be used to blur images, they chose the Gaussian distribution, G (defined as

$$G(x,y) = e - \frac{x^2 + y^2}{2\pi\sigma^2}$$

where σ is the standard deviation). The value of the size constant σ determines the *scale* of blurring, so that changing σ generates a range of Gaussians effective at different resolutions. They gave two reasons for choosing the Gaussian, rather than any other filtering operator. Each of these picks out a mathematical property of the Gaussian function that they felt was significant on psychological grounds.

First, a Gaussian distribution, although in principle it extends to infinity, is in effect localized to a specific (circular) part of the image. So a series of Gaussian operators allow different parts of the image to be blurred to different scales at the same time – which tallies with our ability to see fine detail in only *part* of the image. (They rejected Fourier transforms, which also are mathematical functions that can filter patterns of specific frequencies, because they are not localized: they mask the entire image. Moreover, not all visible patterns can be represented by a Fourier analysis. The transform of a herringbone-pattern like the one shown in Figure 3.2, for instance, has no power in the vertical dimension, and so cannot explain our ability to detect vertical stripes in a herringbone-pattern.)

Second, a Gaussian distribution is smooth at the edges, in the sense that its value does not fall suddenly at its limits of frequency (scale), nor at the bounds of its localized field. (Indeed, Marr and Hildreth described it as the only comparable distribution which is smoothly bounded in both these aspects.) This mathematical property is psychologically significant because it means that a Gaussian is least likely to introduce spurious intensity-changes that were not present in the original image.

So far, then, Marr and Hildreth had identified two useful mathematical functions: (1) a size-insensitive, orientation-independent (second-order) differential operator and (2) a class of filters that can be "set" at different scales (below which the finer detail is blurred).

Their next step was to combine them. Putting the differential operator (∇^2) together with the blurring operator (G), Marr and Hildreth defined a composite function $\nabla^2 G$, which is the second-order differential *of a Gaussian function*. If a specific value is given to the size-variable, σ, then it defines the second-order differential of a Gaussian *at a given scale*.

We saw earlier that both ∇^2 and G have a circular field. Their combination has a distribution that resembles a sombrero, so they are often called Mexican-hat operators (see Figure 3.5). In other words, the $\nabla^2 G$ function has a circularly symmetrical receptive field, with concentric circles corresponding to different intensities. Because of the contribution of the Gaussian (as described above), $\nabla^2 G$ functions can in principle be applied not only at a particular scale, but at a particular place in the image – and different ones can be simultaneously applied at different places. So a group of these mathematical functions, tuned to differing spatial frequencies, could be used to detect a rich variety of zero-crossings in an image. (It is sensitive to zero-crossings because it is a *second-order* differential operator.) Figure 3.6 shows an example: (a) is the image, (b) is the blurred image (produced by $\nabla^2 G$), (c) shows positive values in white and negative in black, and (d) shows only the zero-crossings in the (blurred) image.

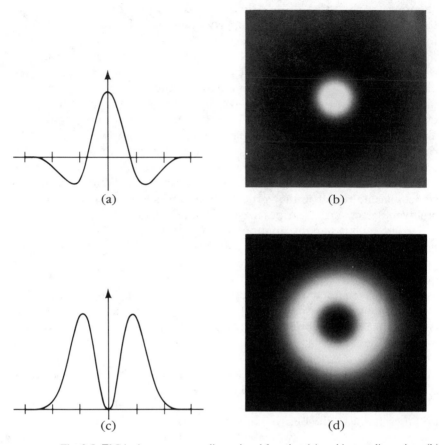

Fig. 3.5. $\nabla^2 G$ is shown as a one-dimensional function (a) and in two dimensions (b) using intensity to indicate the value of the function at each point. (c) and (d) show the Fourier transforms for the one- and two-dimensional cases respectively. (From D. Marr & E. Hildreth [1980], Theory of Edge Detection. *Proc. Royal Society, London*, B, 207, p. 191. Repr. in D. Marr [1982], *Vision*. San Francisco: Freeman. P. 55.)

The next question is how this newly defined differential operator could be embodied in a physical mechanism. Again, mathematical (top-level, computational) argument suggested an answer. Marr and Hildreth proved that the mathematical values of any $\nabla^2 G$ function are almost exactly equivalent to those of *a function that compares two Gaussians (one positive and one negative) at different scales*. The latter is called a DOG function, because it computes the Difference of Gaussians (one Gaussian being subtracted from another). The closest approximation of $\nabla^2 G$ to a DOG-function occurs when the two Gaussians that form the DOG have space-constants in the ratio of 1 : 1.6. In practice, therefore, $\nabla^2 G$ could

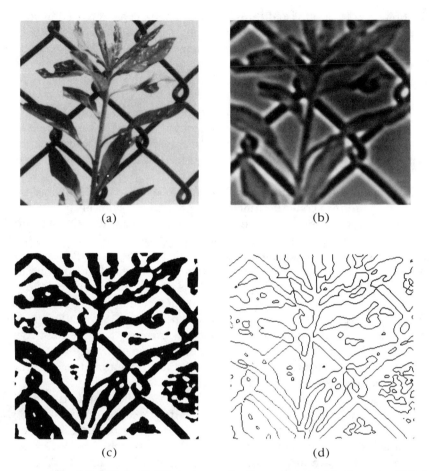

(a)

(b)

(c)

(d)

Fig. 3.6. This figure shows an example of zero-crossing detection using $\nabla^2 G$. (a) shows the image (320 × 320 pixels); (b) shows the image's convolution with $\nabla^2 G$, with $w_{2-D} = 8$ (zero is represented by grey); (c) shows the positive values in white and the negative in black; (d) shows only the zero-crossings. (From *Vision* by David Marr. Copyright © 1982 W. H. San Francisco: Freeman and Company. Reprinted with permission.)

be computed by mechanisms – either evolved or engineered – capable of computing DOG-functions at differing scales (the ratio between the scales being 1 : 1.6).

The idea that DOG-detecting mechanisms exist in the visual system did not originate with Marr and Hildreth. In 1966 the contrast-sensitivity of retinal ganglion-cells, known since the 1950s to have on-centre and off-centre circularly symmetric fields, was described by C. Enroth-Cugell and Robson in terms of two (excitatory and inhibitory) Gaussian domes centred on the same point. Since then, DOGs had featured in explanations of psychophysical data on visual thresholds, and had even been used in computer models of vision. But Marr, by proving their near-equivalence to the mathematically optimal $\nabla^2 G$, offered a computational (top-level) justification of a specific class of DOGs. (We shall see later that Marr's claim that the actual receptive field-sizes in the retina match the mathematically required ratio has been challenged.)

What of the neurophysiological embodiment of intensity-detectors? Given that (as argued above) we are concerned with detectors of *changes* in intensity, the theoretical question to be asked is: What type of neural mechanism could, in principle, perform the task of computing zero-crossings?

Marr argued that *on-centre* and *off-centre* receptive cells (probably the X-cells in the retina) could in principle give rise to mechanisms having this function. A zero-crossing is not (or not simply) a place where the absolute value is zero, but a place where the value changes from positive to negative (or vice versa) – with peak values on either side (see Figure 3.4, above). So an on-centre cell and an off-centre cell (with receptive fields of appropriate scale) would be firing strongly on either side of the zero-point. It follows that the existence of a zero-crossing could be detected if the two ("on" and "off") cells were connected to a third cell functioning as an AND-gate in the way described by McCulloch and Pitts. Moreover, because high-contrast intensity-changes would give stronger firing in the "on" and "off" cells, the sum of their firing would vary with the contrast, and so could be used to code this property of the image.

Further theoretical argument in the spirit of McCulloch and Pitts shows how these retinal mechanisms could underlie the detection of edges. Edges have both length and direction, and according to Marr both these properties are explicitly represented in the raw Primal Sketch. The $\nabla^2 G$ zero-crossing detectors are direction-insensitive, as we have seen. However, if "on" and "off" cells were arranged in neighbouring columns and connected to other cells functioning as AND-gates, we should have a mechanism capable of detecting an edge and of coding its length and orientation. (These edge-finders, in their turn, could in principle function as the computational basis of neural mechanisms for detecting motion in a specific direction: Marr suggested that selectional motion-detectors might be AND-NOT gates, in which unit 3 fires if and only if unit 1 is firing and unit 2 is not, that incorporate time-delay.)

(One might ask why having a combination of DOGs and AND-gates is better than having a set of orientation-operators in the first place, a question which Marr's emphasis on *optimal* information-processing appears to warrant. Both DOGs and AND-gates, given DOGs running before them, are relatively simple, and so perhaps more likely to have evolved. Sets of "first-pass" orientation-detectors would be computationally extremely complex.

And if the DOG data-base is useful for computing other features besides orientation, there would be additional pressure for its natural selection.)

More strictly, the AND-gate described above would function not as an edge-finder but as a mechanism capable of coding continuous intensity-changes in the image. Considered independently, these do not suffice for edge-detection, because some will correspond not to 3D-edges but to 2D-phenomena such as shadows. To compute edges, additional evidence about depth-changes is needed, derived from stereopsis or motion.

Mention of shadows reminds us of another potentially troublesome fact about images of the real world; distinct physical phenomena can produce intensity-changes in the same region of the image but at different scales. Examples include a shadow superimposed on a sharp reflectance-change, or a piece of milliner's net stretched tightly over a hat made of patterned fabric. In such cases, we can see clearly that the underlying surface and the superimposed phenomenon are different. But how do we manage this? How do we distinguish shadow from surface-pattern, or net from fabric? This cannot be done on the basis of depth-cues, for each member of the two pairs lies at the same distance from the eyes.

Marr argued that, provided the visual system is equipped with operators tuned to different scales, the existence of two distinct physical phenomena rather than one in such cases can be readily computed from information coded in the Primal Sketch. The basic strategy is to try to identify sets of intensity-change lines, whose members have the same orientation and are located at the same position in the image, but which are detected by zero-crossing operators of different frequencies. Any such set is assumed to be caused by one and the same physical phenomenon; if the zero-crossings at different scales do not coincide in location and orientation, they are taken to represent two distinct physical phenomena. Marr derived this computational strategy (called the spatial coincidence assumption) from a general property of physical surfaces, arguing that at least two different sizes of DOGs are therefore required – by Martians as by men – for the visual detection of physical reality.

Marr made an observation about zero-crossings that relates to a point of general psychological interest, mentioned above in the context of third-phase work. Zero-crossings, Marr said, provide a natural way of moving from an analogue or continuous representation to a discrete, symbolic, representation – *and this transformation probably incurs no loss of information.*

The latter claim is highly counterintuitive. Indeed, many people have opposed psychological theories based on artificial intelligence in general by arguing that continuous information (such as seems to inform human experience) cannot be represented in a digital form. And the idea that zero-crossings in particular could retain all the information in an image (including information about orientation, for example) seems highly implausible. Surely, much of the original information must be irretrievably lost?

There are several answers to this. Marr's *a priori* answer was to cite Logan's theorem: a proof that, in certain highly restrictive conditions, a signal can be completely reconstructed from its zero-crossings alone. (Logan was interested in zero-crossings from an abstract mathematical point of view, and radio-communication theorists had studied the transmission of signals as a sequence of zero-crossings; Marr was the first to use zero-crossings in the analysis of vision.) Marr admitted that the scope of Logan's theorem is mathematically problematic, and that in any case its conditions are not satisfied for vision. (It is concerned with uni-dimensional signals of only one octave.) He therefore suggested, though without outlining any possible mechanism, that the *slope* around the zero-crossings might also be used in visual coding. But a member of his research-group (H. K. Nishihara) found empirical evidence that an image can indeed be reconstructed from its zero-crossings. And G. D. Sullivan [1983] has shown that if an image is passed through a suitably chosen set of DOG-filters, it can be reconstituted by superimposing the results of all of these at once. The reason is that, since each of the DOG-filters subtracts a given band-width from the image, one will get the image in its original form when they are summed. Someone who has a clear understanding of the mathematical principle here will not be surprised by Sullivan's result, but many other people are.

In short, as I remarked with respect to Waltz's "filtering algorithm", even our very strong intuitions about the power and limitations of different forms of representation and computation may be unreliable. This is especially likely to be true of the intuitions of non-mathematicians; but mathematicians too can be surprised. Logan's theorem is counterintuitive, irrespective of whether it is applicable in the conditions of visual perception. And Fourier transforms (again, irrespective of their usefulness for visual psychology) exemplify a similarly counterintuitive fact, that *any* signal can be represented as a set (perhaps an infinite set) of sine-waves. In the absence of reliable intuitions about representational potential, both *a priori* mathematical-computational arguments and computerized tests or demonstrations are methodologically important in disputes about such matters.

Of course, the fact that a particular form of computation *could* process a given type of information does not prove that in human beings it actually does. Marr's *a priori* derivations of the usefulness and potential embodiment of DOG-functions were therefore complemented by attention to empirical research, including computer-modelling and experimental studies of human vision.

Marr's references to previous psychophysical and neurophysiological work, such as that on spatial-frequency *channels,* sometimes suggested a satisfying match between speculation and data. For example, H. R. Wilson in the late 1970s found psychophysical evidence for four different-sized filters having spatial receptive fields closely approximating that of a DOG. Marr argued that considerations of efficiency (the 1 : 1.6 ratio mentioned above) fitted well with the specific size-constants found by Wilson. (He also predicted the existence of a yet smaller channel, possibly corresponding to the midget ganglion-cells in the retina, whose receptive-field centres are driven by a single cone.)

Similarly, Marr claimed that his mathematical analyses were supported by records of electrical activity in visual neurones: his analyses of the responses of on- and off-centre receptors (presented with an isolated edge, a thin bar, or a thick bar) correlate well with some previous electrophysiological recordings of individual retinal X-cells (see Figure 3.7). (I say his "analyses" rather than his "predictions" here, for–unlike O. G. Selfridge when speculating about Pandemonium–Marr already knew of the existence of bar-receptors and had seen electrophysiological records of their action potentials.)

Later work (largely inspired by Marr's ideas) has provided further evidence for some of his claims. For example, recent psychophysical studies of visual location [Watt & Morgan, 1983a; Morgan *et al.*, 1984] have supported his view that zero-crossings are used in edge-perception–though apparently not in quite the way he thought. As this qualification suggests, however, there are grounds of various kinds for thinking that Marr's mathematically elegant account does not fit human vision as neatly as he hoped.

Some objections

Marr's claims about the primitive spatial code underlying human vision have been challenged in some recent psychophysical research. Thus the match between his theory and Wilson's data is now less close: since Marr's death, Wilson has modified his model to include *six* different-sized filters, and he argues that the receptive field is best approximated by a difference of three Gaussians, not two as specified by Marr [Wilson & Gelb, 1984]. Again, the work of M. J. Morgan and his colleagues suggests that if zero-crossings are involved, they are not employed in the mathematically pure form posited by Marr. (Admittedly, Marr himself suggested using the *slope* around zero-crossings, as noted above. But he offered no guidance as to potential mechanisms. His elaborated theory used zero-crossings alone.)

Morgan has pointed out (for example) that Marr's theory predicts that, if the contrast of an edge were changed with the positions of the zero-crossings remaining unchanged, there would be no perceived shift of edge-location. In fact, however, there is: the edge-location is shifted into its dark phase. Of course, Marr's simple theory of zero-crossings could be complicated to some extent. For instance, it could be altered so as to take into

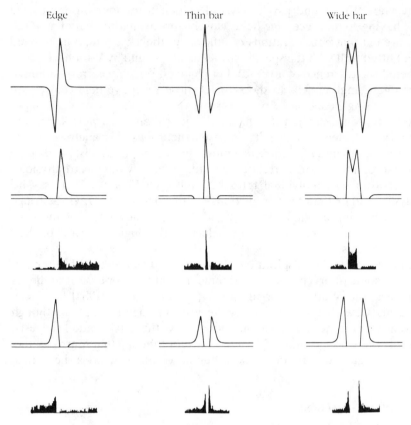

Fig. 3.7. Comparison of the predicted responses of on- and off-centre X-cells with electrophysiological recordings. The first row shows the response to $\nabla^2 G * I$ for an isolated edge, a thin bar, and a wide bar. The predicted traces are calculated by superimposing the positive (in the second row) or the negative (in the fourth row) parts of $\nabla^2 G * I$ on a small resting or background discharge. The corresponding physiological responses (third and fifth rows) are taken from B. Dreher & K. J. Sanderson [1973], Receptive Field Analysis: Responses to Moving Visual Contours by Single Lateral Geniculate Neurons in the Cat. *J. Physiology (London)*, 234, 95–118 (figs. 6d and 6e), for the responses to an edge and from R. W. Rodieck & J. Stone [1965], Analysis of Receptive Fields of Cat Retinal Ganglion Cells. *J. Neurophysiology*, 28, 833–849 (figs. 1 and 2). (From D. Marr & S. Ullman [1981], Directional Selectivity and Its Use in Early Visual Processing. *Phil. Trans. Royal Society, London*, B, 211, p. 165. Repr. in D. Marr [1982], *Vision*. San Francisco: Freeman. P. 65.)

account such factors as image-intensity; or it could be extended to use the value of the peaks and troughs that lie on either side of the zero-crossing itself (information which Marr ignored). As well as showing that some features of edge-perception can indeed be better accounted for in these ways, Morgan has questioned Marr's claim that orientation is not explicitly represented at the earliest stage of visual processing – citing psychophysical evidence that spatial frequency-selectivity and orientational selectivity occur together [Watt & Morgan, 1983b; Morgan *et al.*, 1984; Watt & Morgan, 1985]. Also, he has criticized Marr's reliance on the "spatial coincidence assumption" for leading to a complication of the logical rules relating filters of differing frequencies [Morgan, 1984].

Neurophysiological (as opposed to psychophysical) objections, too, have been raised against Marr's views on the first stages of visual processing. For example, Morgan [1984] argues that spatial frequency-tuning does not seem to arise until the cortex (by which point orientation-tuning has also appeared). But Marr claims that units of different scale (simultaneously processing the same point in the image) occur in the retina or lateral geniculate nucleus, and function before orientation is explicitly represented. Again, J. G. Robson [1983] holds that retinal processing cannot involve $\nabla^2 G$-functions, because the ratio of the radii of the centre and surround functions of the X-cells does not match $\nabla^2 G$ acceptably. (It is larger than the optimal DOG-ratio, 1 : 1.6.) And some recent work suggests that cortical simple cells are not AND-gates as defined by Marr, although this evidence is consistent with their computing a function weaker than, but similar to, AND [Movshon, Thompson & Tolhurst, 1978; Schumer & Movshon, 1984].

Notice, however, how detailed these varied objections are. A prime criterion of a fruitful psychological theory is its ability to generate specific, falsifiable, predictions. Indeed, this applies to scientific theories in general: they should lead to what I. Lakatos [1970] has called *progressive,* rather than *degenerative,* research-programmes. It is less important that a theory be true than that it lead to empirical work that advances scientific understanding. Should it turn out that zero-crossings are less important, or less pure, than Marr believed, his contribution will nonetheless have been valuable. For although some of the evidence for and against Marr's position already existed in the empirical literature, much of it has been (and more will be) culled from experimental studies generated by his ideas.

Marr's theory of the detection of light-intensity by zero-crossings was considered at length in the previous section because it illustrates his methodology especially clearly. It shows the sort of way in which his general aim of integrating all three explanatory levels might be satisfied. But other aspects of his theory, too, have encouraged psychologists to conceptualize low-level vision as a set of abstractly definable information-processing tasks and to design experiments accordingly.

As in the case of zero-crossings, work inspired by Marr and his colleagues has not necessarily ended in agreement with him. His views on stereopsis and motion-parallax, for instance, led to detailed empirical studies (for example by J. E. W. Mayhew and J. P. Frisby [1981]), to deeper mathematical analysis of the task (for example by C. H. Longuet-Higgins and K. Prazdny [1980]), and to significant theoretical disagreements: Mayhew [1983] has described his theory as "almost completely wrong".

This provocative remark reflects the fact that some of the disputes concern the most basic, computational, level of explanation, at which the abstract information-processing task concerned is specified.

This is the case, for instance, as regards stereopsis. B. Julesz [1960] showed that stereopsis can sometimes be independent of high-level processes. He did this by experiments using random-dot stereograms, produced as follows: first, an area is covered with randomly generated dots of varying shades (grey-scale or coloured); next, a nearly identical "copy" is made by arbitrarily choosing some sub-area of the first dot-pattern and shifting it very slightly sideways (deleting the dots on the right which have been newly covered up by the shifted sub-area, and filling in the empty space created to the left by the same dot-randomizing procedure). The two random-dot patterns, when viewed simultaneously by the left and right eyes, fuse to give the phenomenal appearance of a solid object at a depth different from that of the background-plane. Since both input-images were randomly generated, there is no question of any high-level, top-down, knowledge being responsible for this stereoscopic effect.

Julesz suggested that some sort of locally co-operative mechanism underlies the matching of those pairs of items, in the images of the two eyes, which correspond to one and the same environmental point. Various attempts were thereafter made to specify such a mechanism, but Marr (with Poggio) argued that such attempts did not correctly specify the nature of the task. They computed the wrong thing because they did not start from the discovery of the general, top-level, computational constraints on stereopsis.

One of these, according to Marr, is the "continuity"-constraint: because physical surfaces are smooth (so that distance to the surface varies continuously except at object-boundaries), ocular disparity varies smoothly almost everywhere in the two images to be matched. He used this constraint to determine some of the specific connections between individual computational units implemented in his computer model. For instance, he arranged the connectivities such that any two depth-coding cells that code the same depth or closely similar depths and lie on adjacent lines of sight from one eye will facilitate each other's activity.

But Marr's continuity-constraint has been criticized for assuming too much about the cognitive friendliness of the world. Some surfaces are not smooth, yet stereopsis is still possible. Mayhew [1983] suggested a theoretically more general alternative: an *ordering* constraint, based on the fact that stereo-projection normally preserves the ordering and adjacency relationships of intensity gradients in the two images. Thus those matches should be preferred which maintain the order and adjacencies of corresponding edge-descriptions. (This stereo-matching rule was used in an AI-model developed in 1981 by H. Baker and T. O. Binford, and Mayhew points out that there is experimental evidence that the human visual system uses it too.)

Mayhew and his colleague Frisby have raised additional objections to Marr's theory of stereopsis. Some are *a priori* in nature, like that concerning the continuity-constraint (though here, too, past and possible psychophysical experiments are discussed). Thus Mayhew has defined a simple method by which the quantitative 3D-structure of the scene can be computed using *only* retinal disparities. This method is based on Longuet-Higgins' mathematical analysis of stereopsis, which shows that, whereas horizontal disparities carry information about local depth-variations (as has long been known), vertical disparities could in principle be used to compute the actual distances involved. But Marr, in common with most psychologists, had assumed that one needs some scaling information about absolute distance (such as the convergence-angle of the eyes).

Other objections are based on experiments designed to test Marr's view that stereo-matching relies mainly on zero-crossings (as opposed to information that is coded only in the raw or full Primal Sketch). For example, Frisby and Mayhew dispute Marr's assumption that the image-points to be matched are intensity-coded but not yet orientation-coded; they show that although stereo-vision sometimes occurs before texture-discrimination (which accords with Marr's stress on zero-crossings), at other times it depends on eye-movements controlled by texture (which is computed in the Primal Sketch); and they cite stereopsis-experiments which prove that "pure" zero-crossings (without reference to the surrounding slopes or peaks) cannot be the sole computational primitives for vision.

Clearly, Marr's views on zero-crossings and stereopsis (as on other aspects of vision) cannot be uncritically accepted as gospel-truth. But Mayhew acknowledges "an immense intellectual debt" to him, even while saying his theory is "almost completely wrong". For it was Marr's overall conception of visual psychology, and his identification of key theoretical issues, that enabled these mathematical and empirical questions to be asked. We have here, then, the germ of what Lakatos called a "scientific research programme": a progressive body of hypothesis and experimentation, generated by a central theory that is amended as research proceeds.

This novel research-programme is complicated by being an interdisciplinary project, involving concepts and data drawn from psychophysics, physiology, psychology, and computation. It will take many years to show which of Marr's claims are wrong. Moreover, it is clear that his approach cannot solve all the important problems about vision.

For instance, it was suggested above that Marr's definition of vision as 2D-to-3D mapping is problematic. Quite apart from the fourth (temporal) dimension, it may be that to take ecological validity really seriously would bring many other mappings into consideration. Indeed, Gibsonian psychologists posit perceptual "affordances" that cover behavioural features of various sorts, not just physical properties like size, distance, and texture. A comprehensive definition of the *basic task* of vision might feature examples of an agent's intent, such as happiness, aggressiveness, hunger, and the like [Sloman, 1983]. In other words, the basic semantics of vision may not be purely three-dimensional, or even four-dimensional, but distinctly *animal* too. (If we allow learnt semantics, we must add all manner of things which, it seems, can be "immediately" seen – such as the causal connections within a piece of machinery, as seen by an engineer.)

Again, normal vision arguably requires high-level, top-down, processes – which do not figure prominently in Marr's approach. As remarked above, the nearest he got to analysing such schema-driven constructive processes was his discussion of hierarchically structured object-models. This neglect of top-down vision was primarily due to two questionable theoretical assumptions.

First, Marr's hope for an *axiomatic* visual science predisposed him to regard learnt "schemata" as theoretically messy. But it was suggested above, in discussing his optimalist account of intensity-perception, that evolution and learning may in fact be theoretically messy. This is not a question merely of the randomness of the genetic mutations involved in evolution. Time-constraints may lead the visual system to use fallible top-down methods rather than mathematically justifiable processes, *even when the latter are in principle available to it.* Several people have argued that essentially contingent learnt high-level schemata, or pattern-matching rules, are used to effect quick decisions, even in situations where we could arrive more slowly at the same (or a better) decision by a "general" generative process. For instance, J. D. Becker's [1973; 1975] concepts of "experiential encoding" and the "phrasal lexicon" apply this idea to visual experience and language respectively, and A. Sloman [1983] has specifically challenged Marr's work along these lines.

The second, and related, point is that Marr was a *modularity* theorist. This term, which will be explored further in later chapters, involves a theoretical preference for dealing with psychological capacities that are not only relatively *encapsulated* (the procedures for computing stereo-depth being essentially isolated from those which compute motion, for instance), but also *innate*. However, much visual recognition involves concepts that are not innate: we are not born knowing how to recognize telephones. The schemata we learn may function in significantly different ways from the visual processes that have been built in by evolution. Indeed, it is not impossible that evolution itself has provided us with visual processes that are sub-optimal from the purist's point of view (as it has done for many other species). In short, Marr's methodological stress on mathematically proven optimality may be less psychologically realistic than he assumed.

(Very little is known about how our visual schemata actually function: What visual cues do we use, and how do we access distinct schemata from the information in the retinal image? The answer would presumably preserve the best insights of Marr's work and of the scene-analysis against which he initially reacted. A recent attempt to integrate these two approaches is a computer model that describes the position and movement of a human body, whether wholly visible or partially occluded; it uses DOG-functions to preprocess the camera-input, and a high-level human-body schema based on some early ideas of M. B. Clowes [Oatley, Sullivan & Hogg, in press].)

Even if one restricts discussion to *low-level* visual mechanisms, it is not clear how much of Marr's work is well grounded. Certainly, he was not strongly committed to his suggestions about neural embodiment. He noted, for instance, that cortical neurones are more complex than was thought by McCulloch and Pitts: individual dendrites may be distinct functional units, capable of embodying logic-gates. Psychophysics will have to become more precise to address all his ideas, and to rule out alternative explanations as well as confirming the empirical plausibility of his theories. Nor is it yet evident which of Marr's hypotheses could be saved by added qualifications (such as peaks or other "impurities" in zero-crossings) without leading to a degenerative research-programme of no scientific value.

The general assumptions on which his recommended methodology is based are also open to question. Marr's specification of *three* levels has been criticized as simplistic [Sloman, 1983], for it ignores the concept (explained in Chapter 6, below) of the *virtual* machine (although Marr does allow for several levels of representation in the formation of the Primal Sketch). Critics have argued also that the first two of his three explanatory levels are not so clearly separable as he implied, because the concept of *representation* cannot be defined without positing some interpretative processes (or algorithms) in virtue of which the representation has meaning [Morgan, 1984]. Marr himself admits this, in defining a representation as "a formal system for making explicit certain entities or types of information, *together with a specification of how the system does this*" [1980, p. 20; italics added].

Moreover, even the axiomatic core of Marr's theory is not beyond question, as we have seen. His arguments at the abstract computational level are reminiscent of what Kant called a transcendental deduction. They make universal claims about what the world must be like, and what see-ers must be like, if vision is to be possible. The world must have certain kinds of cognitive friendliness (for instance, it must not consist merely of sliced cakes or mosaic pavements, where all objects are equidistant from the viewer). And seeing creatures have evolved accordingly, having a built-in epistemological bias towards the perception of worlds having the requisite general properties. But even if one accepts the project of founding an axiomatic science of vision, there is room for dispute about just which general properties are required (as the examples of continuity and vertical disparities show).

So, while there is little question that Marr's work is leading psychologists to a deeper understanding of vision, this is not because he has solved all the basic problems. Rather, he has integrated a number of pre-existing ideas from work on visual psychology and computer-modelling, weaving them into a novel methodological pattern for the investigation of low-level vision. Whether his approach promises to be equally well suited to other areas of theoretical psychology will be considered in later chapters.

Further examples of connectionism

The type of connectionism represented by Marr's theory is the most elaborate and psychologically relevant example that exists as yet. But the basic connectionist scheme outlined earlier (at the beginnings of Chapter 2 and of this chapter) allows for wide variation.

There are already several types of connectionism (and potentially many more) which differ significantly about the way in which a decision is computed. For example, there may or may not be more than one (hierarchical) level of decision-making. If there is, there may be a feedback of information from some or all higher levels, or there may be a one-way flow only. And a single processing unit may always code one and the same decision (with more or less confidence), or it may code different decisions at different times.

As an indication of this theoretical diversity, let us consider two further points on the connectionist spectrum (one more will be described in Chapter 7). These can be illustrated, as was done above in explaining *relaxation,* by the analogy of a classroom of schoolchildren required to make a communal decision. Like Classroom A, which was described at the outset of this chapter, each child in these two classrooms (Classroom B and Classroom C) thinks only about a particular aspect of the overall decision. Nevertheless, Classroom B and Classroom C form their communal judgment in ways different from each other (and from Classroom A).

Consider Classroom B: Every child has enough information and processing-power to choose among a range of opinions on a certain question. (The child need not have *intelligence:* the individual units of connectionist systems are very limited; intelligence is supposed to emerge as a global property of the whole system.) Each child forms a provisional opinion on the aspect of interest to her. She talks briefly to her immediate neighbours, and amends her opinion in the light of what they say. She then passes on her amended opinion to a low-grade class-prefect, who in addition to receiving suggestions from several different children already possesses extra knowledge relevant to the decision that has to be made. (In Classroom A, by contrast, there were no prefects: there was only one level of decision-making.) The prefects do not report back to the non-prefects, who therefore have no further role to play. This talk–amend–pass-on procedure is repeated within each grade of prefect, the developing decision being further refined at each stage. Finally, the top-grade prefects agree among themselves, and their decision is reported as the class-decision.

Now, consider Classroom C: This class consists of highly opinionated, simple-minded schoolchildren. They are divided into several groups, each group being concerned with a different aspect of the problem (a different problem-part). Within each group, every individual child is prejudiced so as to make only one judgment within the range of opinion that is possible. (Classroom A was different: there each child could have *more than one* opinion.) No child in Classroom C is capable of choosing between alternative beliefs. The groups thus have to be large enough for every discriminable opinion to be held by some child. However, although each child can say only one thing, she can say it loudly or quietly – depending on her confidence in its truth at the time of speaking. The desks are systematically allocated so that children with opinions relevant to each other are near each other; the opinions of neighbours are thus either confirmatory or contradictory.

Immediately a class-decision is asked for, each child in Classroom C states her opinion on the aspect which concerns her. She then listens continuously to her immediate neighbours, adjusting the loudness of her voice slightly with every interchange in the light of what she hears. That is, if some inconsistency is implied by having two (or more) neighbours shouting together – as opposed to both whispering, or one shouting and one whispering – then each of them modifies her vocalization accordingly. This interaction goes on for some time, so that the confidence-level of the child at one end of the back row will indirectly influence the confidence-level of every other child. Eventually (if the process is convergent), all the children will be shouting or whispering their individual prejudices in such a way that the noisiest opinions are mutually consistent. At this stage the opinion-forming process has stabilized, and this is taken to be the class-decision.

The communal decisions in both Classroom B and Classroom C are based on local communications, which have global effects through propagation from one child to another. But there is continuous mutual two-way adjustment only in Classroom C; in Classroom B, there is mutual adjustment between peers, but no feedback from the prefects to the lesser children. Moreover, in Classroom B each non-prefect's decision can be influenced only by her immediate neighbours; and her opinion may later be discounted by the prefects, who have greater responsibility for making the decision. By contrast, each child in Classroom C may (if there is no differential weighting) contribute just as much as any other child through the entire process of stabilization. That is, there is not only local communication but also mutual *co-operation*. Moreover, in Classroom C (again, assuming there is no differential weighting) no one child or elite group has special responsibility for the decision, which is *distributed* – as a pattern of mutually consistent part-opinions – over the entire class.

Both these classrooms will necessarily be large and will involve an enormous amount of talking. A small classroom would suffice if each child, like the elements of a general-purpose computer, were able to think about an indefinite variety of problems (and knew which classmates were thinking about the same problem at the same time). But these connectionist children are very narrow-minded: each is confined to a tiny range of opinions, like the units of a dedicated machine. Indeed, Classroom C will contain a child for every possible variable-value that can contribute to any possible answer to a question. (Because computer models based on this approach require a dedicated processing unit for each possible value of a variable, they are sometimes called "unit value" machines.)

Marr would be more at home in Classroom B. For his theory specifies a series of consecutive representations, where the descriptions coded at one level function as the primitives for constructing the next. These are the three stages within the construction of the full Primal Sketch, the 2½D Sketch, and the 3D-model representation. Even though everything depends on the information implicit in the zero-crossings, aspects are coded at one level which were not explicitly represented at the levels below. The role of the hierarchically articulated 3D-models (which are equivalent to the most senior prefects) is to furnish a high-level description, not to control edge-finding by feedback. The non-prefect children are the on-centre and off-centre retinal cells, and the zero-crossing detectors are the lowest grade of prefect. In general, a given representation is primarily carried by activity in a specific group of cells (hence Marr's many suggestions about which cortical cells might implement which function).

Hinton, by contrast, is a connectionist who would find Classroom C more congenial than Classroom B. Hinton's work on connectionism is not all of the same type: his earliest research, on relaxation, was closer to Classroom A; and a more recent model (the so-called Boltzmann machine) fits Classroom D, described in Chapter 7 below. Here, however, let us consider that part of Hinton's contribution which fits Classroom C.

In this model of Hinton's [1981a], a given representation is embodied by the stabilized pattern of activity over the whole network, some mutually reinforcing cells being active while others are suppressed. Or, rather, it is embodied by a stable state in a *sub-network,* or module. Any network comparable to the brain in its computational power will consist of many smaller networks, and a stabilized pattern in one of these modules may provide the input to others.

Hinton's system thus involves distributed, co-operative processing. Each unit can be activated or deactivated by an influence from outside the system (a certain light-stimulus, for instance), or by the combined influence of other cells. Although the units are classifiable into several broad groups, having different interests and influence, each is indirectly linked to the entire network. The stable pattern is arrived at by a relaxation-process involving repeated cycles of excitatory and inhibitory communication between the individual units. No new information is introduced at successive cycles. Co-operation and competition between the units continue in an iterative process until an overall equilibrium is reached.

Iterative models of computational processing had been considered too by Marr. Indeed, the first of his two stereo-matching algorithms was of this type, using a form of relaxation in which the units oscillated over a narrow range of opinions. But he later rejected this approach, as both neurophysiologically implausible and computationally inefficient.

For instance, Marr argued that repeated cycles of neural communication would take too long: the speed of nervous conduction is relatively slow, yet we can achieve stereo-fusion very quickly.

The question of time per iteration is indeed crucial to the plausibility of Hinton's model. But this question is a difficult one, because it depends on what the neural code is taken to be. Mammalian cortical neurones appear to be rather noisy, in the sense that they emit action-potentials at irregular intervals even when receiving constant input. Because of the stochastic nature of individual action-potentials, it has been conventional to assume that the real signal is the firing rate – that is, the number of action-potentials per unit time. Neural models that assume that the firing rate is communicated on each iteration are much too slow to allow co-operative computation. As Marr pointed out, the output of a neurone must be observed for about 100 milliseconds to decide whether it is emitting 100 pulses per second or 90. Yet, as already noted, we achieve stereo-fusion very quickly. Virtually the whole time that is allowed for stereo-fusion is thus equal to the time needed for one neurone to communicate its firing rate to its neighbour.

Recently, however, Hinton (with T. J. Sejnowski) has described a form of co-operative computation that could allow many iterations within 100 milliseconds [Hinton & Sejnowski, 1983]. The neurones are treated as stochastic *binary* variables, so that all that needs to be communicated in one iteration is whether the neurone is on or off (whether or not it emits an action-potential). The stochastic nature of the action-potentials is no longer treated as a problem which must be eliminated by averaging over time. Instead, it is a positive advantage. For (as we shall see in Chapter 7) it allows a co-operative network of binary units to break out of states that constitute locally optimal but rather poor interpretations of the input, and to settle on much better interpretations.

A second reason why Marr rejected iterative models was that he had an *a priori* objection to computational methods in which a decision, once made, may have to be changed. This "principle of least commitment" condemns not only the hypothesize-and-test methods of scene-analysis models (which involve backtracking) but also iteration in which decisions are amended even in the absence of new information. Marr preferred his second stereo-algorithm, since it involved successive stages at which information of increasingly fine detail was introduced (using spatial filters of decreasing scale). However, Marr's critique of iteration was confessedly tentative, and Hinton's approach cannot be ruled out of court by Marr's scepticism.

A degree of scepticism is nonetheless in order. Hinton's work is largely speculative (though to some degree based on mathematical argument). Although it can be related in broad terms to empirical data, it is not yet open to detailed experimental study. It has been tested by computer-modelling only in a highly simplified way (by simulating a tiny network on a serial computer), because the necessary parallel machines are still being designed. In short, his model exemplifies a new form of computational system, whose properties have only just begun to be explored.

Hinton's [1981a] account of shape representation, for example, is significantly different from Marr's. For his system can, in principle, discriminate arbitrary 3D-shapes without using high-level interpretative schemata. ("In principle", because Hinton does not have a working program that can interpret images: rather, he has an abstract theory that has been modelled only in toy systems.) A shape is represented as a stable overall pattern of activity, different shapes leading the system to settle into different equilibria. Veridical representations are favoured by the system because, in setting the appropriate excitatory and inhibitory connections between the units, Hinton (like Marr) suggests the exploitation of constraints on the image-formation process. These connections influence the processing by encouraging plausible interpretations and suppressing implausible ones. The system can also in principle allow for top-down guidance, if desired, since models of familiar 3D-shapes can be incorporated in a way that is consistent with the overall approach.

The stable patterns derive ultimately from activity in retinotopic units (equivalent to cells in the visual cortex, not the retina), which interpret the light-intensities within their own receptive fields in 3D-terms. These units detect local features, and like all other low-level image-descriptions (such as Marr's 2½D Sketch) are viewer-centred rather than object-centred; so Hinton's retinotopic units alone could not compute real-world shape independent of the viewpoint.

For suppose that, somewhere in the 2D-image, there is a continuous line, or intensity-gradient. In the retinotopic representation this will be registered as a 3D-edge having a specific orientation relative to the retina (lying horizontally across the eye, perhaps). But the object-edge this corresponds to may or may not be really horizontal, depending on whether and how much the retina is tilted. (Even if it is, it may be an object-edge that is normally vertical, like the side of a drinking-tumbler; but this should not

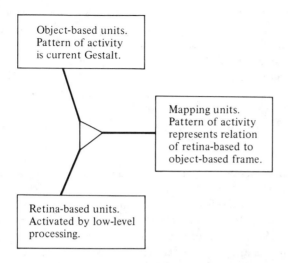

Fig. 3.8. Schematic network for computing object-constancy. (From G. E. Hinton [1981a], Shape Representations in Parallel Systems. *Proc. Seventh Int. Joint Conf. Artificial Intelligence,* Vancouver, p. 1092.)

prevent its being recognized as such.) In short, the retinotopic units do not suffice to compute shape-constancy.

To enable his system to recognize objects as having the same shape irrespective of viewpoint, Hinton distinguishes three groups of cells within the network (see Figure 3.8). One registers retina-based features, in the way described above. Another registers object-based features, which are independent of viewpoint and make up the description of the object's real shape. The third does not register features at all. Rather, it controls the specific way in which the previous two groups interact with (map onto) each other, depending on the current viewpoint. That is, the third cell-group imposes a canonical frame of reference, which mediates the conversion of retina-based into object-based representations.

Different canonical frames can be specified by activating different units within the third cell-group. Alternative interpretations of a given object are possible because different frames generate distinct object-representations, the object's constituent parts always being described with reference to the current frame. This is reminiscent of the fact we noted in discussing the picture-grammar approach, that the different ways in which one can experience the ambiguous sail or stingray figure may depend on the assignment to it of different implicit axes.

In general, the specific mapping between a given retina-based description and the corresponding object-based feature depends upon the viewpoint. To specify the inter-group connections appropriately, Hinton relies on the constraint that objects can be perceived from only one position at a time (a fact ignored in Cubist painting). For any given viewpoint, there will be only one physically consistent way of pairing retina-based with object-based features. So if each possible viewpoint is distinguished, all the appropriate pairwise mappings can be specified.

Since a shape is represented as a stable overall pattern in a population of cells, in which some units are simultaneously active and the others are suppressed, only one shape can be represented at a time. This raises some basic difficulties for distributed connectionist models.

How can one representation be stored so as to influence another? How, for example, can successively perceived shapes be integrated into larger wholes (as when one sees a large animal passing behind a fence with a narrow vertical gap in it)? And how is top-down guidance possible (so that recognizing a horse's leg leads one to look for the horse's head in the appropriate region)? Since distinct shapes – legs, heads, tails – are implemented by different patterns of activity within the same cell-network, it would appear that the first representation has to be destroyed to allow the generation of the next.

Hinton therefore specifies two further groups of cells. The units of one of these represent a set of scene-based features, while the units of the other specify the mapping between scene-based and object-based features. Each unit within the scene-based-feature group is activated by the combination of a particular object-based representation with specific values of its various properties with respect to the scenic reference-frame (such as position, orientation, and size). So one unit in the scene-buffer might be maximally activated by the head of a pony grazing at bottom right, and another by the head of a Shire rearing at top left.

This fivefold organization (including the three cell-groups previously described) gives the network some powerful computational properties. It enables an object-edge, such as the edge of a tumbler lying on its side, to be recognized as really horizontal but normally vertical (even if it is diagonal to the retina). It provides for contextual effects and top-down influence, since an object's representation in the scene-buffer can feed back into the activity of the object-based (and thence the retina-based) units. It enables many objects to be simultaneously represented within the same scene. And the multi-dimensional units can bind distinct properties to individual objects in the scene, identifying the pony's head as small and the Shire's as large. This could not be done by the pure representational method of simultaneous excitation within the network, because *pony, Shire, small,* and *large* would all co-exist. Like McCulloch and Pitts, then, Hinton tries to show how basic logical distinctions could be implemented in neuronelike mechanisms.

In view of the multi-dimensional units just mentioned, and the rich mappings required to allow for viewpoint, it might seem that Hinton's model needs an impossibly large number of units. The mapping computations require that each slight variation in size, position, or orientation be separately registered. The number of discriminable features is literally astronomical. If at least one, precisely tuned, unit were required to register each of them (which is what one might expect *prima facie*), the size of the system would be neurophysiologically implausible as well as technologically impracticable. Admittedly, Hinton (like all connectionists) posits a massively parallel system, taking the human brain as his exemplar. But even the brain has its limits.

In this context, Hinton has made an interesting – and, to many people, counterintuitive – suggestion. He claims that many fewer (and less finely tuned) computational units are needed for the efficient parallel computation of shape than one might suppose. Moreover, their coarseness is not a tolerable flaw, but a positive computational advantage.

These claims are justified by Hinton in terms of a mathematical proof. With respect to the computation of shape, he demonstrates that overlapping groups of coarsely tuned receptive units, within specified size-constraints, are capable of computing spatial properties with specifiable gains in efficiency. (So the fact that biological neurones do not respond to a perfectly defined narrow class of stimuli may be a strength rather than a weakness.) It follows that there are many more discriminable features than there are units needed to compute them (though it may not be possible to achieve a reduction on a scale that will make the model usable). Indeed, this mathematical result applies to PDP-models in general: in any domain, not just vision, a relatively small number of coarsely tuned units will be more efficient than a larger number of finely tuned ones.

Hinton relates his model to psychological phenomena in general terms. For example, he suggests that many of the visual phenomena stressed (though not satisfactorily explained) by the Gestalt psychologists are intelligible in terms of his model. Ambiguous images can be perceived in either of two ways (as a sail or as a stingray) but cannot be simultaneously perceived as both. The way in which one structures a visual image determines one's ability to describe and transform it. One can (according to the Gestaltists) perceive a whole without analysing it, even unconsciously, into its parts. And seeing an image as a part or as a whole are subjectively different experiences.

Analogously, in Hinton's system different object-based frames can be assigned to the input, but only one at a time. The way the object is described, and the way it relates to its context, depends on the canonical frame of reference assigned to it. A shape can be represented as a whole without its constituent parts being explicitly coded as such. And a shape is represented in a very different way according to whether it is seen as a part (coded by a multi-dimensional unit) or as a whole (coded by an overall pattern).

In addition, Hinton's system shares with us the ability to perceive a whole given only a part–where this is achieved by holistic reconstitution rather than by piecemeal inference. In the scene-analysis tradition, a set of schema-driven *inferences* led to descriptions of the hidden parts of a partially occluded object. Hinton's approach allows for a small part of a (familiar) equilibrium-state to seed the reconstitution of that entire state (for a recent discussion, see [Hinton & Sejnowski, 1986]). Introspectively, it seems that we do not usually *infer* that a cat part-hidden by an open door has a tail, but somehow "just see" it as having a tail. Although the computational approach will not allow that there is any such process as "*just* seeing", the contrast between Hinton's work and scene-analysis shows that it allows debate about what sorts of computation are involved.

Suggestive though such analogies are, however, they should be treated with caution. Hinton's views on vision have not yet been brought into correspondence with detailed experimental data. Nor can this be done for his work on learning or motor-control (some of which will be discussed in later chapters). Indeed, ideas about neural networks in general are still in their formative stages, and in most cases have not even been fully implemented in a suitable computer model (because massively parallel hardware has not been available). Their psychological interest is that they suggest novel ways of thinking about mental processing, some of which hold a promise of explaining phenomena–such as perceptual recognition, reminding, and multiply determined flashes of insight–that are intransigent to a conventional computer-modelling approach.

Furthermore, the conventional von Neumann approach seems better suited than the connectionist approach to the implementation of logical, symbolic thinking. Serial thought-processes often take place in conscious thought (and some theories of problem-solving, as we shall see, posit strictly sequential processes at subconscious levels also). If no psychological theory is acceptable which treats all thinking (not to mention perception) as a process of formal-symbolic reasoning, it is equally true that no theory is acceptable which cannot explain the fact that people do, sometimes, do logic and mathematics. Some suggestions about how a connectionist theory might address such matters are discussed in Chapter 6.

In sum, the fourth phase of vision-research has not only raised detailed questions about the psychology of seeing but has also highlighted several basic methodological issues. These include: the extent to which psychologists should aim for an axiomatic science based on abstract task-analyses; the relevance or otherwise of physiological considerations in psychology; the psychological plausibility of the serial general-purpose computer, as contrasted with dedicated connectionist machines; the sense in which connectionist computation is really *computation* (it does not fit Z. W. Pylyshyn's definition, for example); and the extent to which built-in low-level processes function independently of high-level knowledge (or the extent to which low-level image-processing requires compiled low-level models, for instance of intensity-gradients). All these issues are problematic, and all will arise again in the following chapters.

4   Parsing natural language

Understanding our native language is a task performed effortlessly by us all every day, yet in psychological terms it is highly complex – and still largely mysterious. Psycholinguists disagree about even the broad outlines (never mind the details) of what is being done, or how, when people interpret everyday remarks.

Consider, for instance, the deceptively simple utterance "Just off to buy Ruskin's birthday card!" Even to ask whether this word-string is a grammatical sentence will involve disagreements about which account of English grammar is correct. Are syntactic transformations necessarily involved or not?

Moreover, agreement on what the syntactic structure of a sentence is does not solve the problem of how that structure is used or recognized. Does the speaker generate sentences by taking syntactic structure into account, and if so, how? Does the hearer assign a syntactic structure to every sentence, marking such features as the absence of subject and verb: *who* is off to buy Ruskin's card, and where is the verb that goes with "off"? If so, is this done word by word, or only after the whole sentence has been heard? Is the syntactic analysis completed before, and so independently of, the interpretation of each and every word in terms of its meaning, as seems to be the case for " 'Twas brillig, and the slithy toves Did gyre and gimble in the wabe"? Or are syntax and semantics employed simultaneously, from the very first word of the sentence? Suppose we had started out by assuming that the sentence was going to be like "Just off King's Road lies Chelsea College": on reaching the word "to", would we have to backtrack and undo our past decisions about the grammar of "Just off"? Certainly, this example is unlikely to lead to *conscious* backtracking – such as might happen on hearing the last word of "The horse raced past the barn fell." (If you have difficulty in interpreting the last sentence even with the help of conscious backtracking, try comparing it with "The dog locked in the kitchen barked.") But why the difference? Each sentence has the same number of words.

Further, what more does one understand about the speaker in understanding her words? Does one know what she is up to, what sort of personal relations she has with Ruskin, what she might do if the nearest stationer's turns out to be shut? And what psychological processes mediate one's knowledge of these things or of what might be an appropriate conversational response to her remark?

Historical background

Questions like those listed above inform current psycholinguistics. Psycholinguists study syntax (the topic of this chapter), semantics, text-analysis, and conversational pragmatics (all discussed in Chapter 5), seeking to specify the mental processing that brings these matters to bear in the generation and understanding of language. Each of the debates suggested by the preceding questions has been sharpened, if not initiated, by work in computer-modelling.

Psychologists had little to learn, however, from the first computer models of language (though with hindsight one might say that these anticipated the notion of the "phrasal lexicon": a collection of stock-phrases normally recognized entire, without syntactic analysis). The machine-translators of the 1950s and the keyword-recognizers of the early 1960s (such as ELIZA, PARRY, and STUDENT) did not reflect the structural complexities of language [Boden, 1987, chap. 5]). The dialogue-program ELIZA (which, to be fair, was intended as a programming exercise rather than an investigation of language) responded to sentences of the form "I———you" by producing "Why do you———me?" but this was effected by a simple rule of pattern-matching rather than by a systematic representation of the syntax or semantics of pronouns. Moreover, sentences were considered as isolated units: although ELIZA could (in the absence of a keyword) revert to a previously mentioned topic, this performance did not rest on any understanding of the semantic structure of connected texts. Nor did these early programs include representations of the intentions and presuppositions underlying conversation.

The seminal influence encouraging the computer-modelling of language in a more realistic fashion was N. Chomsky's transformational grammar, the first version of which was published in 1957. This grammar distinguished between the "surface structure" of a sentence (a linear string of words) and its "deep structure" (described in terms of hierarchical grammatical categories like *noun-phrase, verb-phrase, determiner, noun,* and so on). Although Chomsky's work was not presented as a computer model, four aspects of it encouraged psychologists to consider a computational methodology in studying language.

First, Chomsky depicted language as a formally specifiable generative system – which a computer language, considered as an abstract mathematical entity, is also. Second, he used the powerful mathematical concept of *recursion* (in which a function is defined in terms of itself) to describe language, at a time when early computer models of problem-solving (the Logic Theorist and GPS) were showing that recursive procedures could be applied in practice to generate structures on distinct hierarchical levels. Third, he posited the autonomy of syntax: not only did he (in his early theorizing) ignore semantics, but he seemed to assume that syntactic interpretation is normally carried out independently of semantic considerations. Like all assumptions of psychological *modularity* (a concept which includes that of *encapsulation,* or computational autonomy), this could be used to justify a programme of research that promises some advance. (Recently, he has explicitly endorsed a modular approach to psychology in general, recommending the identification and study of "mental organs" comparable to the functionally distinct, though interdependent, bodily organs [Chomsky, 1980].) Fourth, his work alerted psychologists to the possibility of specifying the nature and order of the processes by which sentences are actually generated and/or understood.

The last of these influences is a matter of historical fact rather than primary intent. As remarked in Chapter 1, Chomsky himself was not interested in the processes of language-use, but in the abstract mathematical structures (and mathematical transformations) of language. His distinction between *competence* and *performance* was intended to avoid consideration not only of errors and memory-limitations but also of psychological processing in general. He was no more concerned with successful language-processing than with the unsuccessful variety.

Admittedly, Chomsky did not disown those who suggested that his grammatical transformations might have psychological reality. He even co-authored a paper [Miller & Chomsky, 1963] that was an influential source of the "derivational theory of complexity". This theory postulated that the abstract transformations which, in Chomsky's (early) theory, derive the surface-structure from the deep kernel-string correspond to the psychological processes involved in understanding a sentence. The idea that transformational grammar is directly exploited during sentence-processing appeared, at first, to be confirmed by experimenal results. But it was eventually falsified, for example, by experiments showing that syntactic complexity as measured by transformational grammar does not predict difficulty in understanding or remembering [Fodor & Garrett, 1966; Fodor, Bever & Garrett, 1974]). Despite this empirical falsification, Chomsky did not feel any need to abandon his own theory.

He justified his indifference to psycholinguistic evidence on the ground that he was a linguist, not a psychologist. Adopting the terminology of the previous chapter, however, one might say that Chomsky was doing pioneering *psychological* work all along, though at the computational rather than the algorithmic level. D. Marr has said just this, and has approved Chomsky's disdain for computer models of language that are not based on theoretical analysis of the information-processing task. The task Chomsky concentrated on is the assignment of syntactic structure to input word-strings. Unlike Marr, he was content to leave the development of theories at the algorithmic level to others. (We shall see later that a recent computer model of parsing has been constructed by asking what sort of processing system could embody the syntactic constraints defined by Chomsky [Marcus, 1980].)

Chomsky's claim that the human mind contains a mental representation of grammatical rules (whether transformational or not) is still controversial [Stabler, 1983], but it has prompted both computational and experimental work of great interest. His influence naturally led to an emphasis on syntax in the early computer-modelling of language, semantics and pragmatics being stressed later. A decade after the publication of Chomsky's *Syntactic Structures* (which had been supplanted in 1965 by his *Aspects of the Theory of Syntax*), the first psychologically influential computer models of parsing appeared [Thorne, Bratley & Dewar, 1968; Woods, 1970]. They were soon followed by T. Winograd's [1972] model, wherein parsing was supplemented by (or even partly dependent on) semantics and world-knowledge. This program was considered so significant as to have an entire issue of *Cognitive Psychology* devoted to it. Simultaneously, models of language-understanding – hardly of *parsing* – were described wherein syntax took decidedly second place to semantics [Schank, 1972]. The late 1970s saw computer models of the interpretation not only of single sentences but also of connected text [Schank & Abelson, 1977], and by the 1980s there was an interest in pragmatic issues such as speech-act recognition and conversation [Power, 1979; Allen & Perrault, 1980; Gazdar, 1981a]. Concurrently, psychological interest in these models of natural language grew (although some psycholinguists remained sceptical of their relevance [Dresher & Hornstein, 1976]).

Augmented transition-networks

Psychological reality was a major motivation behind the first computer model based on augmented transition-networks, or ATNs, whose authors declared, "We have, as far as possible, treated the task of constructing an automatic parser as being itself a psycholinguistic experiment" [Thorne *et al.*, 1968, p. 281]. Their claim (based on hunch rather than experimentation) was not merely that Chomsky's [1965] grammar, on which their parser was based, identified syntactic generalizations that are somehow taken account of by the mind, but also that *the way in which this grammar was used* by their program parallelled mental processing to some degree.

Their program parsed sentences in only one pass: word by word, from left to right across the input-string. Introspection suggests that (except in the case of some jokes) we understand language without needing to backtrack at the end of the sentence. In effect, they claimed, we simultaneously consider all possible syntactic analyses of the sentence – or, rather, of that part of it which we have heard so far.

(I say "in effect" here, because their program not only ran on a serial-processing computer but like most ATN-parsers used depth-first rather than breadth-first search. In depth-first search, the successive implications of the first alternative at a given choice-point are followed through to the bitter end before the next alternative is considered at all. In breadth-first search, the immediate implications of every possible alternative are examined in turn before consideration of the immediate implications of the alternatives at the next level down [Boden, 1987, chap. 12]. For a first approximation, then, one can describe breadth-first search as considering all the alternatives at a given level "simultaneously". In parallel-processing systems, given some form of relaxation-technique as described in Chapter 3, a set of alternative options really could be considered simultaneously.)

The conclusion drawn by Thorne and his colleagues was that a representation of the (deep and surface) syntactic structure is incrementally built up by means of a continuous process of making and testing predictions about grammatical form.

ATNs were introduced as a way of doing this, and were soon developed further by W. A. Woods, whose work (though technological in aim) attracted attention from experimental psycholinguists. Woods did not use transformational grammar as such (and neither did Winograd, after him). The basic reason for this is that transformational rules map between entire syntactic structures (the deep and surface-forms of the sentence as a whole); the computational load involved is much less if the surface-structure being examined is a single word or syntactic constituent. Since their inception in the early 1970s, ATNs have been used in varying forms, including one based on a psychologically grounded reformulation by R. M. Kaplan [1975]. However, the core idea remains the same [Winograd, 1983].

An ATN is a left-to-right parser, which interprets the syntactic structure of a sentence by looking at one word at a time. Or, more strictly, an ATN – and an RTN, discussed below – is a particular *formalism* for representing a grammar. But ATN-representations are often referred to as "parsers", because they so readily suggest a certain parsing process. The typical ATN-parser works top-down, in the sense that it first thinks of a syntactic rule or category, and then looks to see whether the input-word fits that category. (A bottom-up parser looks first at the input-word and then tries to decide its syntactic category. Some ATNs designed for speech-understanding function in this way.)

ATNs are based on a class of computational systems known as recursive transition-networks (RTNs), with respect to which they are "augmented" by the addition of extra features. To understand what an ATN does, we must first consider what transition-networks in general can do.

A simple *non-recursive* transition-network consists of a set of nodes connected by labelled arcs, where one node may have several arcs leading from it. The arcs in effect state the rules allowing transition from one node

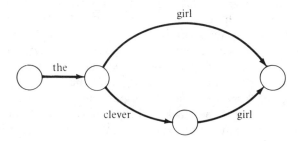

Fig. 4.1. A non-recursive transition-network.

to the next, each transition corresponding to the acceptance of one word in the sentence. For example, let us assume that the processor has already reached a node corresponding to prior recognition of the word "the", and that there are two alternative arcs leading from this node, one demanding "girl" and the other demanding "clever". Clearly, both "the girl" and "the clever . . ." would match the arc-rule and so enable the processor to leave the node, whereas "the pretty . . ." would bring the process to a halt with only the first word ("the") accepted. If the node reached by traversing the arc labelled "clever" happened to have an arc labelled "girl" leaving it, then "the clever girl" would be accepted by the network – but "the clever boy" would not (see Figure 4.1).

Clearly, non-recursive networks, in which specific words have to be associated with the arcs, are very limited. True, they can generate (and accept) an infinite set of strings, because they are allowed to contain loops and so can handle iteration (the repetition of a constituent). But the constituent in question has to be a word: iteration can generate "the very very very clever girl" but not "the clever generous witty girl", which would require iteration to be defined over lexical categories, such as adjectives. And non-recursive networks embody no explicit syntactic knowledge, being innocent of such concepts as noun-phrase and verb-phrase.

In an RTN, by contrast, the arc-labels can lead the processor recursively to pass to *another network* rather than to a word-recognition node. Indeed (as we shall see shortly), an RTN may be multiply recursive, in the sense that it is made up of RTNs nested within RTNs. Accordingly, an RTN (whether considered as an abstract mathematical structure or as an implemented processor) can embody knowledge of hierarchical grammatical structures. An RTN for handling sentences can thus incorporate phrase-structure rules, such as: S → NP + VP; NP → Det (Determiner) + Noun; NP → Noun; NP → Adj* + Noun; NP → Det + Adj* + Noun (the asterisk means that the constituent may be repeated, or absent).

The initial node of a recursive sentence-network (an S-network) will normally have an arc leading from it that is labelled NP. This arc, in effect, allows the mechanism to forget (for the moment) about the VP and concentrate on the NP, by creating a new network (the NP-network) whose first node it now treats as though it were the initial node. In computational terms (which reflect the use of a push-down stack to effect this recursion), the original S-network is *pushed* down a level by the newly created NP-network. If and when traversal of the NP-network has been completed (which assumes that the input-sentence starts with a noun-phrase), it is *popped* off the stack and the S-network automatically appears at the top again. Since the processor has by now succeeded in finding an NP, it can pass on to the next node (on the original level), from which there will be an arc demanding a VP. When this too has been found (by means of a VP-network at a lower level), the system has reached the terminal node. This means that, if no words remain, the input has been recognized as a grammatical sentence. (Notice that this is a binary decision. No structural description of the sentence has been built by this RTN, which has been used as a *discriminator* of some grammatical sentences, not as a *parser* – which by definition builds a structural description.) If the input-sentence has no initial noun-phrase, so that the terminal node of the NP-network cannot be reached, the NP-network is popped and the system now looks for an initial verb-phrase, by means of an arc leading to a VP-network on a lower-level.

Most nodes of an RTN have several arcs leading out of them. For example, since the phrase-structure rules given above provide for four different ways of starting an NP, there could be four arcs leading from the first node of the NP-network defined by these rules (see Figure 4.2a). Given a dictionary in which input-words are labelled by syntactic category, this NP-network will accept noun-phrases like "Polly", "The girl", "The black kitten", "Wise virgins", and "The dear sad little puppy". But it will not accept "The black and white kitten", because of the conjunction occurring between the two adjectives. Rules marking a constituent (such as an adjective) as *optional* can be represented by a special JUMP arc, which allows access to the next node even if the optional-constituent arc cannot be matched.

There is in general more than one way of representing a network so as to embody a given set of phrase-structure rules. Some of these network-representations will be more elegant than others, but each defines the same range of structures. For instance, Figures 4.2a and 4.2b, despite their superficial differences, represent equivalent networks. Figure 4.2a is highly redundant, in that two (the top two) of its four main arcs are unnecessary. The second-from-top arc labelled "Noun" is unnecessary given the third-from-top arc, which allows one to accept either a noun or an adjective as the first word; likewise, the top arc (demanding first a determiner and then a noun) is not needed because the bottom arc represents interposed adjectives as merely optional. By contrast, Figure 4.2b is a minimally complex

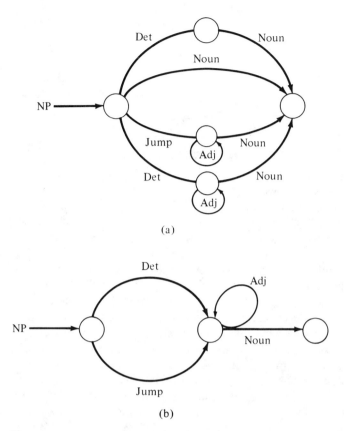

(a)

(b)

Fig. 4.2. Two equivalent (non-recursive) NP-networks.

representation of the relevant rule-set. If these two networks were to be implemented in computer-processors, each would accept/reject precisely the same word-strings as the other. But the processor corresponding to Figure 4.2a would be the less efficient of the two, because it would repeat some tests unnecessarily.

The NP-networks shown in Figure 4.2 are actually non-recursive fragments of possible RTNs (defining entire sentences) rather than RTNs in themselves. They cannot accept any noun-phrase with another noun-phrase embeded in it, such as "The mother of the bride". The reason is that my list of four phrase-structure rules defining NPs, which the network of Figure 4.2a represents, did not include any recursive rule. If the rule "NP → NP + Preposition + NP" were to be added to the list, any equivalent NP-network would itself be an RTN (capable of accepting as a single noun-phrase "The dear sad little puppy under the moth-eaten sofa behind the mahogany table in the small octagonal bedroom in the upper East wing"). Even such a

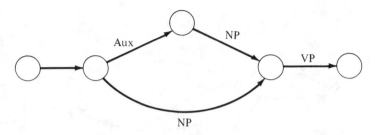

Fig. 4.3. An RTN that would accept initial auxiliary verbs.

network, of course, would in practice be a mere fragment of a larger RTN, namely a sentence-network.

Although RTNs are more powerful than non-recursive transition-networks, they are less powerful than ATNs. These are derived from RTNs by adding *conditions* and *actions,* of which the former allow for context-sensitivity and the latter enable syntactic structures to be built, saved, and output. Thanks to the structure-building actions, ATNs (unlike RTNs) can be used as parsers, as opposed to mere grammaticality-testers.

Before considering the conditions and actions of ATNs in general terms, let us look at a very simple (and unrealistic) example that illustrates the difference between RTNs and ATNs. Suppose we defined a sentence-network (representing the rule: S → NP + VP) in which Figure 4.2a or 4.2b was used as the NP-network. Suppose also that the VP-network could be accessed only *after* the terminal node of the NP-network had been reached (there being no JUMP-arc allowing access to the VP-network in the absence of an initial noun-phrase). Such a sentence-network would not be able to accept any sentences having a verb as their first word, such as "Has Anita left?" One way of enabling the S-network to accept this sentence (though not "Pass the salt!") would be to modify the NP-network so as to allow the processor to search for an auxiliary verb in the initial position (see Figure 4.3). (This example is given for illustrative purposes only; in practice, no one with any sense would attempt to deal with verb-initiality in this way.)

However, the RTN in Figure 4.3 will accept not only "Has Anita left?" but also "Has Anita leaves?" – a word-string which, if "Has" is an auxiliary verb, is ungrammatical. (This network does not allow for the possibility that "Has" is the main verb, as it would be were the speaker enquiring whether Anita possesses any foliage.) One way of preventing this ungrammaticality is to *augment* the RTN shown in Figure 4.3 so as to convert it into the ATN schematically indicated in Figure 4.4. The augmentation has two aspects. A structure-building *action* is added to the Aux-arc, so that the parser stores the information that the specific auxiliary verb in question is "Has". Also, a grammatically constrained *condition* is added to the VP-arc, so that the parser will accept only a main verb which is grammatically

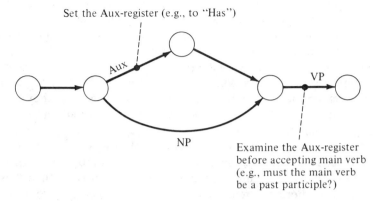

Set the Aux-register (e.g., to "Has")

Aux

NP

VP

Examine the Aux-register
before accepting main verb
(e.g., must the main verb
be a past participle?)

Fig. 4.4. Fragment of an ATN that would accept initial auxiliary verbs.

consistent with the auxiliary verb (if any) in the preceding context. The
auxiliary "Has" is consistent with a past participle but not with a present-
tense main verb. So this augmented network will accept both "Anita has
left" and "Has Anita left?" but it will justifiably reject "Has Anita leaves?"

The simple example just given illustrates a general point of theoretical
importance. An unaugmented RTN is formally equivalent to a context-free
grammar, which is a grammar whose rewrite-rules apply (or not) to a
syntactic category irrespective of its context. Chomsky claimed to have
proved that context-free phrase-structure grammars are not a descriptively
adequate mechanism for characterizing natural language, and he introduced transformational rules accordingly. It was to allow for context-
sensitivity that *conditions* were included in ATNs (though most ATNs did
not attempt to model Chomsky's grammar as such).

Conditions are attached to specific arcs, and given that the input-word
matches the arc in question they allow an arc to be selected only in circumstances where it is appropriate in context. For instance, selection may be
conditional on the system's already having found a particular syntactic
feature or sub-structure (such as an auxiliary verb or a plural noun). This
requires the system to test for more than one symbol at a time, which
cannot be done by unaugmented RTNs because they can only look at the
current input-word. Since the ATN network therefore needs a form of
memory, a set of *registers* is added to each level of the network, to record
the syntactic features and structures that have already been recognized by
the parser. Transitions from a given node are then controlled by tests on
the node-register as well as on the current input.

The *actions* are the operations which build the growing syntactic interpretations, and set the values of the registers accordingly. Sometimes, a special
register is used for "the story so far": the parse-tree of that part of the
sentence which has been examined. When the terminal node of the net-

work is reached, the structure in this register is output as the final interpretation of the sentence. (More usually, intermediate results are assembled in different registers and then put together at the end.) Actions would be needed even if conditions were not, because (as noted above) a parser should be able to decide not merely whether or not a word-string is a grammatical sentence, but what sort of sentence it is. It is the structure-building actions which enable ATNs to do the latter (so they would be needed even were it to turn out, *pace* Chomsky, that the syntax of natural language is context-free).

So far, we have been considering ATNs as abstract structures of computational logic. This is not the same thing as an ATN embodied as a processing algorithm. Even assuming that the choice of syntactic theory is non-controversial, there are many different ATN-parsers that could embody the same grammar (many distinct psychological hypotheses about parsing processes). For example, given a serial processor, one has to decide which of the alternative arcs is to be inspected first by the parser. Should the S-network lead first to a search for a noun-phrase, or an auxiliary verb, or an adverbial phrase . . .? Different choices will lead to different patterns of processing by the parser. Some of these will be more efficient than others, much as one stereopsis-algorithm is more efficient than another. (If all the possibilities relevant to a given word were explored in parallel, then this particular issue of efficiency would not arise – although there might be problems of using space efficiently, or of minimizing the number of currently active processes.)

But whatever the specific order of search may be, the parsing procedure of ATNs is typically (though perhaps not necessarily) *non-deterministic*. This term does not imply any randomness in the parser's software or hardware. Rather, it means that there are many points within the parsing process at which a number of alternative decisions are possible, and that on average more than one of these will have to be considered.

Non-deterministic parsing is computationally wasteful, effort being spent on alternatives that eventually are rejected. Sometimes many successive transitions, creating nodes on several levels, will occur which later have to be undone (or in a breadth-first search, left unused) when they reach a dead-end. When this happens, a lot of structure that had been built up is destroyed, as when one has to unravel a whole knitted sleeve in order to correct an error made in the cuff. Within-sentence backtracking can be reduced to some extent, but cannot be got rid of entirely. Thus the order of search can be made to reflect the relative frequency of the different syntactic structures, and recent ATNs can save partial interpretations that might need to be used again (so given the sentence "Is the doctor investigating the epidemic your sister?" the noun-phrase "the epidemic" is stored as a parsed sub-structure and re-used if the system has to backtrack on finding the last two words). The *time* wasted could be reduced by parallel-processing, all of a node's arcs being explored simultaneously; but even so there would be much wasted *effort*. We shall see later that some recent work has modelled a deterministic parser, in which this wastage is minimized.

Not surprisingly, psychologists soon became interested in ATNs [Kaplan, 1972; 1975; Stevens & Rumelhart, 1975; Wanner, Kaplan & Shiner, 1976; Wanner, 1980]. On the one hand, ATNs can be regarded as *procedural* models of parsing. (Better: they are an abstract class of procedural model originally developed to do parsing; as we shall see in Chapter 5, they have also been used for non-syntactic purposes.) On the other hand, they can be regarded as mostly *declarative,* with all the procedural information in the interpreter or compiler that processes them. They provide both an abstract (in Marr's sense, "computational") analysis of the task and a way of expressing detailed algorithms about how the task might be done. They are models in which the order, criteria, and effects of the individual processes can be represented in a relatively perspicuous way. (In this, ATNs resemble *production systems,* to be discussed in a later chapter.) The content of the grammar can be clearly distinguished from the schedule for applying that knowledge. Thus a given arc (representing a certain syntactic possibility) can be included in the system *or not;* and if included, it can be traversed *before* or *after* other arcs leading from the same node. And the use of node-registers holding partial interpretations means that hypotheses can be stated about the intermediate stages of parsing, not merely about the final parse of the whole sentence. This explicitness regarding both the content and the utilization of syntactical knowledge can prompt detailed studies of people's "on-line" language-understanding in real time, provided that experimental techniques can be devised to address the relevant theoretical questions.

On-line language-processing had either been experimentally ignored before, or had been inferred in broad outline from studies of whole-sentence parsing. For instance, consider the experiments designed to test whether people perceive sentences as being syntactically segmented [Fodor & Bever, 1965; Bever, Lackner & Kirk, 1969]. Subjects listened to spoken sentences (both with and without intonation) during each of which a brief click was presented; their task was to say when the click had occurred. The clicks were perceptually shifted to a point corresponding to a boundary between major grammatical constituents, at the level of surface-structure or even of deep-structure (this was one of the early results seeming to confirm the psychological reality of Chomsky's transformational grammar). But even if we assume that syntactic (as opposed to semantic) processing was responsible, this tells us little about how the segmented perception was constructed. At most, it suggests that moments at which clicks are relatively difficult to perceive are moments at which many other tasks (presumably pertaining to syntactic analysis) are being tackled – but which tasks?

Similarly, the theory of "heuristic strategies" for parsing (which replaced the derivational theory of complexity when that was shown to be false) identified distinct parsing strategies, and their relative priorities, only in the broadest terms. To say that people tend to look for noun-phrases first does little to specify the computations actually involved in interpreting the initial word of "Have the students who failed the exam take the makeup today" as an imperative verb.

In consequence, a number of psychologists welcomed ATNs as a way of expressing detailed empirical hypotheses about the nature, order, and even time-relations of sentence-interpretation. For instance, E. Wanner and M. P. Maratsos [1978] used ATNs to formulate a hypothesis about relative-clause comprehension. According to many linguists, every relative clause contains a syntactic gap, which signals the within-clause function of the head-NP (that is, the NP that precedes the relative clause). In each of the following examples, the asterisk denotes the location of a "missing" noun-phrase, and the head-NP is printed in capitals: ". . . THE GIRL who * talked to the teacher about the problem", ". . . THE TEACHER whom the girl talked to * about the problem", and ". . . THE PROBLEM that the girl talked to the teacher about *". As these examples illustrate, the gap always comes after the head-NP, but is not always close to it. In effect, then, a relative clause is a syntactic category that requires a parsing decision to be postponed. But there are other such categories: if we understood how this is done for relative clauses, we might be able to adapt the solution to them too.

Bearing in mind the description of ATNs given above, the "obvious" way of parsing relative clauses is to complicate the NP-network by adding a set of independently specified arc-sequences, one corresponding to each possible gappy form of relative clause. The parser would follow these arcs in turn (or simultaneously in a parallel system), backtracking (or killing processes, in a parallel system) until one of them, which in a serial system might be the last one, resulted in a successful parse. But since there is an infinite set of admissible forms here, such a piecemeal approach would not be theoretically adequate. And even as a purely practical measure, this would be a highly inefficient method.

Wanner and Maratsos used an ATN-model to specify a theoretically adequate, and more efficient, mechanism: the HOLD-function. This enables the parser to continue parsing without backtracking, since instead of requiring a (provisional) decision about the within-clause function of the head-noun to be made immediately, it postpones any such decision until after the gap has been found. The HOLD-function allowing relative clauses requires only three new arcs to be added to the NP-network. The first tests for the presence of a relative pronoun at the end of the head-NP, and if it succeeds it places the head-NP on the HOLD-list. The second finds the gap: it leads the parser to try to parse the relative clause as though it were an ordinary declarative clause, which attempt will come to a halt when the system reaches the gap. When this happens, the third arc retrieves the NP currently stored on the HOLD-list, and this NP is used to fill the gap. Parsing then proceeds in the normal way.

In order to test their ATN-model for its psychological reality, Wanner and Maratsos pointed out that the HOLD-mechanism requires the parser to store the head-NP until the gap is found. Accordingly, they devised an experimental method for tracking fluctuations in memory-load during comprehension. In essence, they presented their subjects with a comprehension-task and a memory-task (remembering lists of names) simultaneously. Assuming that working memory is limited, these tasks should interfere; and the more memory is needed for one, the less will be available for the other. The HOLD-hypothesis predicts not merely that the parsing of sentences with relative clauses will put an extra demand on the subject's transient memory, but that the memory-load will be increased at the moment when the relative pronoun is identified and decreased at the point where the gap is filled. For example, consider the pair of sentences "THE WITCH who * despised sorcerers frightened little children" and "THE WITCH whom sorcerers despised * frightened little children." These are the same length, contain the same content-words, and have very similar meanings. They also have the same head-NP, in identical positions. But the gap is located near the beginning of the first sentence and near the end of the second. Clearly, the HOLD-hypothesis predicts different patterns of task-interference in the two cases.

The results of Wanner and Maratsos' experiments were consistent with the HOLD-hypothesis and inconsistent with the notion that (as in a "basic" ATN) the hearer tries all possible analyses in turn until one succeeds. They pointed out, however, that a more "active" ATN could be specified, such that the parser forms and tests predictive hypotheses while following the various possible arcs; in such a case, memory-load would be increased. (They report follow-up studies that suggest that people do not actually do this.)

This raises a methodological point mentioned in Chapter 3 with respect to Marr's theory: to show that one's own hypothesis is consistent with the facts (and even that someone else's is not) is not to show that one's own is correct. There may be other possibilities. Scientific theories in general are under-determined by the evidence. Worse, because any effective procedure is Turing-computable, computer-based systems in principle have sufficient power to express any conceivable algorithm, including those which people do not employ. Unless there is only one (practicable) effective procedure for a certain task, there are bound to be non-human ways of performing that task.

For this reason, B. E. Dresher and N. Hornstein [1976] criticized Wanner and Maratsos' work considered as psychology. They added that the HOLD-hypothesis made no contribution to theoretical linguistics. ATNs as such are a *general* computational tool, while the HOLD-hypothesis is a specific application that was given no principled (as opposed to pragmatic) justification by its authors. Dresher and Hornstein claimed that the HOLD-hypothesis is a special case of a general linguistic principle already noted by Chomsky and Miller. If it had been presented as such, it would have been of some interest as a way of implementing this principle (though problems of validation would remain). But it cannot be regarded as having contributed to linguistic theory as such, for it identified no syntactic phenomenon that had not previously been noted by linguists. (They made similar criticisms of Winograd and other AI-modellers: these people might or might not be able to produce technologically useful systems, but they used – and sometimes ignored – linguistic theory rather than contributing to it.)

The autonomy of syntax

As we have seen, early psycholinguistics and computer-modelling of natural language were heavily skewed towards syntactic problems. This was due largely to the influence of Chomsky, in particular to his assumption of the *autonomy of syntax*. In principle, syntax could be autonomous in at least two senses. First, syntactic structure might be definable independently of all (or all but the most general) semantic considerations. And second, syntactic interpretations might actually be assigned by hearers to sentences independently of semantic and contextual information – irrespective of whether the parsing is done on the fly or only after completion of the sentence. (Two more senses of syntactic autonomy will be mentioned in Chapter 5.)

A Marrian approach to syntax requires that Chomsky be right about the autonomy of syntax in the first sense: it must be possible for syntactic interpretation *as an abstract information-processing task* to be considered in isolation. (It does not follow that one can always recognize syntactic interpretation when one sees it. In other words, the extension of the natural kind "syntactic" phenomena may not be intuitively obvious. For example, sentences showing VP-deletion – such as "Ruth smoked but Mary didn't" – were accounted for in Chomsky's standard theory by a syntactic transformation, whereas some linguists see VP-deletion as an essentially semantic phenomenon.) But it allows that there may be only limited autonomy in the second sense. Analogously, when Marr considered edge-detection and depth-detection separately, as distinct mathematical problems, this left open the question whether, and when, the perceptual algorithm for edge-detection makes use of stereoscopic information. The notion that syntax and semantics are procedurally separated in humans is in fact controversial.

(It is also controversial, from an engineering point of view, whether they *should* be separated in computer systems.)

Largely because of Chomsky's influence, the first language-using programs took a strong position on syntactic autonomy. That is, parsing was totally separated from semantic interpretation (if any). In Woods' question-answering program, for instance, the sentence was first parsed and then translated into a semantic representation. (This was not due to any incapacity of ATNs to model semantic influences: ATNs are an abstractly defined class of computational system, whose specific rule-content may be indefinitely various.) Admittedly, Winograd's work in computer-modelling challenged this approach, arguing that sentence-understanding involves interaction among syntax, semantics, and contextual knowledge [Winograd, 1972; Boden, 1987, chap. 6]. But even Winograd's program involved a clear separation between processing stages, sentence-constituents being provisionally parsed before the parsing was subjected to semantic test.

This early assumption of syntactic autonomy in the second, processing, sense is now widely believed to have been mistaken. (It may have been correct, for all that – as we shall see.)

Precisely timed studies of speech-perception have been widely taken to show that syntactic assignment happens very rapidly, and relies throughout on semantic and contextual information [Marslen-Wilson, 1980; Marslen-Wilson & Tyler, 1981]. Thus speech-shadowing tasks suggest that shadowing, which happens extremely fast, involves the understanding of the words, not just their repetition. And another experiment suggested that people predict distinct pronouns according to the syntactic and semantic context. Subjects heard the sentences "As Philip was walking back from the shop he saw an old woman trip and fall flat on her face. She seemed unable to get up again" followed by one of three continuation-fragments: "Philip ran towards . . .", "He ran towards . . .", or "Running towards . . ." Their task was to identify a word presented *visually* immediately at the end of the fragment. W. D. Marslen-Wilson found that people are relatively quick to recognize pronouns that are consistent with the context (specifically, "her" is more quickly identified than "him"). These experiments are generally regarded (perhaps wrongly) as proof that co-operative interactions between stored vocabulary, syntactic structure, and semantic context are initiated right from the beginning of the sentence. They are cited not only by psycholinguists, but also by programmers of computer models that use semantic information to guide parsing [Dyer, 1983].

Marslen-Wilson sees his experiments as having three important computational implications. First, psycholinguistic theories, or computer simulations, in which semantic or contextual interpretations are computed only *after* parsing are inappropriate. Even word-recognition cannot properly be regarded as a separate (initial) stage, for it makes use of syntactic and semantic information. (This applies to normal language-processing; in abnormal cases, such as the poem "Jabberwocky", we can apparently parse sentences containing nonsense-words – as Thorne and his colleagues' parsing program could too.) Second, connectionist models are more neurophysiologically realistic than sequential ones; the relevant computations happen so fast, and are so various, that (given the slow speeds of nervous conducton) they suggest parallel computations distributed over a huge processing machine. And last, top-down influences (according to Marslen-Wilson) do not normally enter into speech-perception, despite appearances to the contrary that result from co-operative interactions wherein low-level syntactic and semantic constraints are propagated through the network (in the sort of way discussed in Chapter 3).

The similarity to the way in which Marr describes low-level vision is evident. For in Marslen-Wilson's view, parsing involves psychological operations that are both obligatory and automatic. Much as low-level vision enables 3D-interpretation to occur early in the construction of the perceptual representation, so speech-perception appears to have evolved so as to allow mesage-level interpretation to start as soon as possible. This is normally done, according to this hypothesis, by a bottom-up rather than a top-down process.

(It might nevertheless be the case that some input-phrases are not parsed word by word in this way. Much as high-level vision may need to be understood in terms that do not fit the Marrian paradigm, so normal language-understanding may involve mechanisms that cannot be derived in a principled way from theories of syntax, semantics, or phonetics. One example might be the *phrasal lexicon*, mentioned above: a store of stock-phrases normally recognized without any syntactic analysis. This recognition might be computed by processes analogous to programming *demons*. A demon is a rule that lies latent in the system until it recognizes the occurrence of its cue-condition, at which point it triggers a predetermined action. Perhaps language-users learn many independent phrasal demons, each of which treats the early part of a stock-phrase as a cue that automatically triggers recognition of the whole.)

However, Marslen-Wilson's approach has been criticized by some psycholinguists for (as one might put it) not being Marrian enough. Thus J. A. Fodor argues that syntax is isolated from extra-syntactic processes to a significant degree: it is one example of the mental modularity that Chomsky endorses too [Chomsky, 1980; Fodor, 1983]. According to Fodor [personal communication], Marslen-Wilson's results are due to faulty experimental design, and his own (ongoing) experiments bear out his predictions but not Marslen-Wilson's.

Fodor bases his experiment on the type of context cited above, about Philip and the old lady who slipped and fell, but concentrates on the third fragment, "Running towards . . ." He points out that not only "her" but also "them" would be a sensible continuation. Given that this plural pronoun (the object of "Running towards") refers to both the people already identified, the agent of the verb "Running towards" must be some third person yet to be named. Fodor uses this fact as the ground of a crucial experiment to decide between the two hypotheses.

Marslen-Wilson's claim is that parsing is predictively influenced by semantics. If so, the word "Running" should trigger the creation of an NP-structure in which the agent-label is assigned to "Philip" (for the old lady cannot run, and no other agent has been mentioned). On reaching "them", the parser would have to undo this assignment, because "them" must include Philip, who therefore cannot be the subject of the verb. It follows, Fodor argues, that "them" should (like "him") take longer to recognize than "her"–which indeed it does. But there is no reason why "them" should take longer than "him" does, for both are equally incompatible with Philip's being the subject of the verb.

Fodor's contrary hypothesis is that parsing is not predictively guided by semantic processes, whose role instead is to test the parser's independently arived-at output for semantic acceptability. He assumes that the semantic module always tries to assign pronouns to referents that have already been introduced into the discourse, and that only if this strategy fails does it consider the possibility of new referents. This assumption is not only intuitively plausible, but is also what one might expect if the hearer is building *mental models* of the speaker's domain of reference [Johnson-Laird, 1983]. In this case, "them" should take longer to recognize than "him" (though both should be longer than "her"), because "him" can be assigned to the already named Philip without absurdity (this is true whether it is the old lady or a third party who is doing the running).

Fodor's preliminary results suggest that "them" does indeed take longer to recognize than "him", which is evidence against Marslen-Wilson's theory.

Of course, since different amounts of time are needed for recognizing "her", "him", and "them", these experimental results do suggest (though they do not prove) that semantics influences parsing at some time prior to the end of the entire sentence. Indeed, Fodor assumes that the parser outputs structural descriptions of sentence-constituents (such as are stored in the non-terminal node-registers of ATNs), and that the semantic module then tests the semantic acceptability of these syntactic descriptions. But since the syntactic module (on his view) is procedurally isolated from the semantics, this test merely delivers a binary decision. *Yea* allows the parser to assume the correctness of its analysis so far, and to proceed to the next sentence-constituent. *Nay* instructs the parser to think again–but it is not advised by the semantics on *how* to think again. The situation thus seems to be broadly comparable to that within Winograd's program, which allowed semantics to influence parsing on-line by checking the semantic acceptability of already parsed sentence-constituents.

Winograd's program (SHRDLU), published in 1972, was an impressive programming achievement which significantly advanced the state of the art in AI. The details of this program are not relevant here (it is discussed at length in [Boden, 1987, chap. 6]), for Winograd neither claimed nor attempted to achieve a precise computer simulation of psychological reality. But its general nature is important. Despite Winograd's warning that it was not intended as a model of actual mental processing, it caused a great deal of excitement in psychological circles.

One reason for this excitement was that the program offered an existence proof that it is indeed possible to formulate precise rules for handling natural language. Admittedly, the semantics involved was very limited: the program could converse only about a table-top world containing a few coloured blocks and a box. But its syntactic power (though not unlimited) was prodigious. It could parse syntactically complex sentences, such as "How many eggs would you have been going to use in the cake if you hadn't learned your mother's recipe was wrong?" And it could cope with logical quantifiers and comparatives, as in "Is at least one of them narrower than the one which I told you to pick up?" No previous language-using program had approached this level of syntactic subtlety, though Woods' early ATN-system came closest. Indeed, many of them ignored syntax entirely: ELIZA's transformation of the personal pronouns in replying to "I———you" with "Why do you———me" was based on a simplistic pattern-matching rule, and the programmer's syntactic insight here was implicit rather than explicit in the program.

But over and above its mere existence, Winograd's program offered psychologists two ideas about language-processing which were to become highly influential.

First, Winograd saw language-understanding as a procedural matter: lexical and syntactic items were defined as procedures, there being no representation of a word's meaning independently of how the system actually processes it. To be sure, language had already been treated as procedural by Thorne and his colleagues, as we have seen; but Winograd's proceduralism was both more explicit and more detailed. It influenced many psycholinguists, leading them for example to describe utterances as programs [Davies & Isard, 1972; Longuet-Higgins, 1972], and to assimilate the development of word-meanings to the learning of perceptually based procedures for establishing reference [Miller & Johnson-Laird, 1976]. Winograd's emphasis on procedural (as opposed to declarative) knowledge is now generally agreed to have been exaggerated: we saw above, for instance, that ATNs can be seen both as declarative representations of the content of a grammar and as procedural representations of parsing. But the general idea that lexical and syntactic aspects of language are associated with specific mini-programs in the mind remains influential – as the discussion above of the psychological applications of ATNs, for example, showed.

Second, SHRDLU achieved a fruitful integration of its knowledge of syntax, semantics, and world-knowledge. That is, it did not merely solve these different sorts of problem, but solved one by making use (if necessary) of the others. This strategy is a form of constraint-propagation, essentially comparable to the Waltz filter discussed in earlier chapters. For instance, the program's semantics and world-knowledge influenced the parsing process so that it was able to construct a *sensible* syntactic representation of the structurally ambiguous "Put the blue pyramid on the block in the box." This could mean either "Put the blue pyramid which is on the block into the box" or "Put the blue pyramid onto the block which is inside the box." Winograd's program always handed control over from the parser to the semantic specialists whenever a main sentence-constituent, such as a noun-phrase, had been (provisionally) identified. Hence it interrupted its parsing of the sentence above at the point where it had identified the noun-phrase "the blue pyramid on the block". Its semantic specialist knew that the word "on" can be used to refer either to the current location of a thing or to the place towards which it may be moved. Accordingly, the semantic specialist asked the world-knowledge ("perceptual") module to see whether or not there was one and only one blue pyramid sitting on top of a block. If so, the provisional parse was accepted. If not, the alternative role of "on" was assumed to be relevant – and was later checked, likewise, by seeing whether there was indeed a block inside the box. The likeness to Fodor's view of parsing has already been remarked.

How our minds might determine our syntax

Winograd was forced to address procedural matters, since he was building a parser. But he did not attempt a psychological simulation: it was difficult enough to construct a functioning system, and in any event virtually nothing was known about how humans parse sentences. Chomsky ignores both procedural and psychological details, and refuses to be discomfited by experimental evidence about human language-use on the ground that his interest is in abstract syntactic structures rather than actual parsing processes.

However, the question obviously arises as to what the mental operations are which compute the syntactic structures posited by Chomsky. This question has recently been addressed by M. P. Marcus [1980], who uses computer-modelling in the attempt to specify what sort of parsing algorithm would provide an explanation for the existence of certain language-universal constraints (whose precise nature need not concern us) postulated in Chomskian grammatical theory. He uses the "trace" version of Chomsky's later theory, in which the number and complexity of transformations involved in parsing a sentence are less than in the standard theory. In trace-theory, a sentence is represented by an *annotated surface-structure,* in which there are *traces* reflecting its deep structure and derivation.

From the psychological point of view, annotated surface-structures have the advantage that they are less computationally complex than sets of tree-structures. Moreover, they allow for the phonological form of a sentence to be determined not only by its surface-structure but by its deep structure too [Winograd 1983]. It seems intuitively obvious that the definition of phonological forms must be based primarily on surface-structures, for these are what we say when we speak. Yet many examples show that phonology reflects deep structure also. Thus in uttering the two sentences "This is the sauce my mother used to make" and "This is the sauce my mother used to make Boeuf Stroganoff", one can contract the words "used to" (giving "useta") in the first case but not in the second. Psycholinguists need some theory of syntax that can be integrated with a processing theory explaining phonological evidence such as this (which is not to say that Chomsky's trace-theory is the best one).

Marcus' project is not just to start with Chomsky's grammar and implement it, nor even to do this in a psychologically plausible way. Rather, he is seeking to discover what are the general features of a parsing procedure, or grammar-interpreter, which are necessary to enable language to have (or which necessarily result in its having) the syntactic structure posited by Chomsky. In other words, how do the processing properties of the mind affect the abstract nature of language?

In Marr's terminology, Marcus is trying to go from the algorithmic level to the computational level, rather than vice versa (though admittedly he starts with a knowledge of trace-theory). If this sounds as though the algorithmic cart is being put before the computational horse, one should remember that whereas physical objects with their optical properties exist independently of human minds, language does not. Since language exists only in and through the mind, it is not absurd to suggest that its abstract structure may depend on mental properties.

Indeed, Chomsky said just this. As well as claiming that syntax is genetically given, he said that putative, highly abstract, syntactic universals common to all languages result from properties of the "mental organ" responsible for human language. But he did not say just what these properties are. Marcus aims to specify them and to show that the universal constraints are universal not because they are necessary features of any conceivable grammar but because sentences that violate them cannot in fact be parsed by the human language-processor. (It may be, though Marcus does not discuss the issue in these terms, that these constraints are not specifically human, but can be derived from general requirements for designing intelligent systems whose central processors have ample space but limited speed.)

The basic hypothesis to which Marcus is committed is that the parser inside our heads is *deterministic*. That is, it allows only one choice at every point during the parsing process: namely (in nearly all cases), the right one.

In his view, this fact accounts for the introspective ease, and the speed, with which we typically understand speech. It explains why garden-path sentences lead us up the garden-path, and predicts which sentences will do so ("The horse raced past the barn fell" is a garden-path sentence: it is more difficult to understand than the equally short "Just off to buy Ruskin's birthday card", and also many sentences of a Proustian length). And, what is even more surprising, the hypothesis of determinism accounts for some of the grammatical rules and "linguistic universals" that Chomsky described but could not explain.

The obvious attraction of deterministic parsing is that it minimizes wasted computational effort. As explained above, most computer-parsers and psychological theories associated with them are non-deterministic. For instance, ATNs allow many different choices at a given node, and sometimes all but one of these have to be traversed (and their computations at least partly undone) before the correct analysis is found. Similarly, Winograd's program offered great flexibility of choice, at the cost of extensive backtracking to recover from incorrect analyses made early in a sentence (though Winograd tried to counteract this by using semantics and world-knowledge to prune the syntactic search-space). These wasteful methods can hardly be regarded as optimal solutions to the parsing problem.

Moreover, non-deterministic parsers do not support any principled distinction between those sentences that are understood without any conscious difficulty and those that are not. At most (assuming limited resources of space or time), they might lead us to expect that deeply embedded sentences will be more troublesome than sentences involving fewer levels of recursion – but *how many* levels are readily intelligible? Provided that a sentence can be shown (by however complex a process) to satisfy the rules of syntax, it is in theory as acceptable as any other. This was true also of Chomsky's competence-theory. Chomsky admitted that multiply embedded sentences (such as "This is the dog that the cat the rat the fly tickled fled scratched") are in practice almost unintelligible. But he was unable to explain why this is so, referring vaguely to "performance factors" and "memory limitations". Similarly, garden-path sentences will all be accepted by a non-deterministic parser. It may take longer than usual for this to happen, if (in a serial processor) the order of arcs leaving a node leads to the wrong choice's being made at first. Thus having parsed "The horse" as an NP, the first arc tried will probably be the one searching for a VP – which "raced past the barn" appears to be; only when the parser encounters another word, "fell", instead of the terminal node does it realize that its VP-assignment was mistaken. But this approach cannot explain why sentences of even a Proustian length may be easier to understand than the seven-word "The horse raced past the barn fell."

But is deterministic parsing possible? The notion that we are allowed only one choice at any given point in parsing appears absurd if we consider sentence-pairs like "Have the boys taken the exam today?" and "Have the boys take the exam today!" The initial "Have" in these sentences should be interpreted as an interrogative (auxiliary) and imperative (main) verb respectively. But there is no way of knowing how one should parse this first word until one has considered the fourth, either "taken" or "take". And to be confident that one has parsed the first word in the following example correctly, one needs to consider the sixteenth: "Have the cruel boys who threw stinking rotten apples at the farmer's big ginger cat taken/take the exam today?/!" How, then, can parsing be deterministic?

Marcus' answer is that since (as these examples show) a deterministic parser cannot rely on a simple left-to-right pass through the word-string, it requires some degree of lookahead. That is, it must somehow be able to inspect the future context. If it could inspect the whole sentence, the determinism-hypothesis would clearly be vacuous. Unbounded lookahead would give deterministic parsers indefinitely great computational power. This high degree of flexibility, while useful in a general computational tool (such as ATNs), would undermine the claim that determinism is an empirical principle of psycholinguistics. For no grammatical sentence would be unparsable by such a parser: there need be no mismatch between theoretical competence and actual performance. Deterministic parsing is a substantive – and testable – hypothesis only if the size of the lookahead is specified, and strictly limited.

This leads Marcus to posit a data-structure he describes as the "heart" of his grammar-interpreter, the central feature that distinguishes it from all its predecessors: namely, the *constituent buffer*. This is a left-to-right sequence (not a push-down stack) of three "boxes", or nodes, each of which at any given time is either empty or holds only one item. Each item in the buffer is one which is seeking a higher-level syntactic attachment – where S is higher than NP, NP is higher than Det, and Det is higher than "the." The basic idea embodied in the buffer is that the parser can look at up to three such items in applying its syntactic rules. Marcus' substantive hypothesis is that a deterministic parser whose flexibility is strictly limited to a *three-item lookahead* will suffice to parse all those sentences that human beings parse without conscious difficulty. (Note the assumption that all human beings share the same difficulties in parsing.)

"Item" here cannot mean "word". For even the brief "Have the boys taken the exam today" would require four words to be looked at simultaneously, as we have seen; and the similar sentence mentioning the ginger cat would require the inspection of sixteen words. Rather, "item" means *any grammatical constituent,* including not only words but also syntactic sub-structures that the parser has already built. (These sub-structures are comparable to the intermediate results stored in the node-registers of an ATN; but because Marcus' program PARSIFAL is deterministic, they cannot be unravelled or rejected as ATN-sub-structures can.)

Given that the parser can recognize a complex noun-phrase and place its parse-tree in the buffer, it is clear that a three-place buffer enables "Have" to be inspected simultaneously with "taken/take" in both of our problem-strings. For there are three bracketings in each of them: "[Have] [the boys] [take/taken]" and [Have] [the cruel boys who threw rotten stinking apples at the farmer's big ginger cat] [take/taken]". Notice that the noun-phrases in these examples are unattached at their higher level – which is why they are in the buffer. Neither "[the boys]" nor "[the cruel boys who . . . ginger cat]" can be confidently (that is, deterministically) hooked onto other sentence-constituents until the inspection of "taken/take" has enabled "Have" to be parsed as an interrogative or an imperative verb. Until this time, the parser does not know whether "the boys" is going to be the subject or the object of the sentence, because the main verb has yet to be established. While it is still unclear whether "Have" is the main verb or not, the parse-tree of the NP in question must exist as an unattached item, seeking attachment at a higher level.

In addition to the buffer, Marcus' parser PARSIFAL has another modifi-able data-structure. This is a push-down stack called the *active node-stack*. At any given moment, this contains a set of tree-structures representing the syntactic analysis that has been done so far, and the current goals associ-ated with it. All the trees on the active node-stack are unattached at their lower levels. Some of them will have *gaps* at their lower levels demanding some other item as gap-filler (for instance, the fragment "The cruel boys who" will be represented as an NP including a relative clause, where the content of the relative clause has yet to be found). Others will have points at their lower levels where further items might perhaps be attached (for instance, "The boys" is an NP which may or may not turn out to include a relative pronoun).

The topmost node on the push-down stack is called the *current* node. It remains as the current node until one of three things happens: once it has been supplied with a complete set of higher-level and lower-level syntactic attachments, it is popped off the stack; if it has received all its lower-level attachments but is still unattached at its top level, it is popped off and transferred into the leftmost place in the buffer (see below); or it may be pushed down by the creation of a new current node. A node gets to be the current node either by being newly created and placed on top of the stack, or by surfacing when the (previously current) node immediately above it is popped off the stack.

The way in which nodes get onto the stack and off again is reminiscent of the recursive transition-networks discussed above: the parsing of a constitu-ent can be temporarily interrupted and resumed only when some other constituent has been parsed. This is hardly surprising, for a push-down stack (which is also embodied in ATNs) is a computational mechanism well suited to capture recursion in general. It is therefore likely to be used in the modelling of any psychological phenomenon with this feature (the General

Problem Solver mentioned in Chapter 1 used this technique to effect means–end analysis). One strength of the computational approach in general is that it has given psychologists a way of implementing the mathematical concept of recursion, one which (since it provides working models) can be used to map the dynamics of recursive systems.

Each node in the active node-stack is associated with particular "packets" of grammatical rules (based on Chomsky's trace-theory). When a node becomes the current node, its own rules are activated; otherwise they are latent. So what goes on depends directly on the node currently on top of the active node-stack.

The grammatical rules are expressed as condition–action pairs which look to see whether a certain condition is satisfied, and if so perform a certain action (PARSIFAL is thus a form of *production system*). Broadly, a rule asks what words are visible and what partial parsing decisions have already been made, and accordingly recommends a further parsing-step or a search for another word. The *conditions* are defined in terms of the contents of five places: the three nodes in the buffer and two of the nodes in the active node-stack (the current node and one other, as explained below). That is, the rules can in effect look at up to five different items – but no more than three of these can be in the buffer.

If the only node in the active node-stack that the rules could look at were the current node, the parser would not be able to cope with natural language. For when a rule looks at a node it cannot see its higher-level syntactic attachment: what it sees is the node itself, together with all the lower levels of the parse-tree hanging from it. For example, if the parser looks at the current node it may see a well-developed parse-tree representing the structure of the noun-phrase "the cruel boys who threw rotten stinking apples at the farmer's big ginger cat" (notice that this NP is potentially incomplete, since the next word that has yet to be inspected may be "yesterday", "in", "which", "because" . . .). But it does not know whether the boys are the subject or the object of the sentence. For this it needs to look "upwards" in the overall developing parse-tree, to some node on a higher level than the current node.

In accordance with his aim of making his parser as inflexible (and therefore testable) as possible, Marcus insists that upwards-looking should not be unlimited. He therefore stipulates that the rules can inspect only one node in the stack besides the current node, and that this is the S-node which is nearest in the stack to the current node. So, given the sentence "Mary told Jemima that Ann believed Pamela cooked the dinner today" and assuming that the current node is the NP dominated by "dinner", the parser could inspect only the S-node headed by "Pamela"; the S-nodes headed by "Mary", "Jemima", and "Ann" would be invisible to it even though they are still present in the stack. (So although an S-node is – by definition – a Sentence-node, *one* sentence may have *several* S-nodes associated with it on various recursive levels.)

One must not confuse "upper" and "lower" in the syntactic-dependency sense with "above" and "below" in the sense of different places within the push-down stack. In fact, "upper" goes with "below" and "lower" with "above". For example, let us assume that the sentence being dealt with is "The farmer's wife scolded the boys who threw stinking rotten apples at the farmer's big ginger cat" and that the parser has reached as far as the word "big", with the NP referring to the boys being the current node. The parser has already decided that this NP is hanging as a direct object from the main verb, "scolded", and that this in turn is hanging from the highest node of all, the S-node. And since neither the VP nor the S is yet completed, both will still be present in the active node-stack. But because it is a push-down stack these previously created, syntactically higher, nodes will actually be situated *below* the current node in the stack (with the S-node at the bottom).

The buffer is the heart of the parser. It is conceptualized as a left-to-right row of three nodes. There are two ways in which items can enter the buffer, depending on whether these items are words or partially parsed constituents. Words enter from the right and constituents from the left. Although an item can be pushed rightwards in the buffer (provided there is an empty buffer-place to receive it), it cannot be pushed out of the buffer at the rightmost end. Items can leave the buffer only at the left end. (An item leaves the buffer after it has been attached to some higher-level constituent by one of the rules whose condition it matches.)

Words are not read in to fill all the available buffer-places. A word can enter the buffer only if some rule has asked to see the contents of a buffer-place which happens to be empty. For example, the main S-node (which is always the first node to be placed on the active node-stack) activates rules asking about the syntactic category of the initial word. The reason why words are not freely welcomed into all the empty buffer-slots is that this would cause buffer-overflow (see below).

Constituents enter the buffer at the left, and come from the top of the active node-stack. This happens when the grammar-rules find that the current node needs no further attachments at its lower levels but has not yet been attached at its highest level (this requires "upwards-inspection"). When the current node is popped off the stack in this way, the node immediately below it automatically becomes the new current node. The old one is now sitting in the leftmost buffer-place, and any items that were already in the buffer are shunted along one place. If this would cause any item to fall out of the buffer at the right, the parse fails forthwith. (Marcus uses this buffer-overflow to predict garden-path sentences.)

To take an informal example, consider the sentence "Have the boys taken the exam?" Let us assume that parsing has proceeded to the point at which the current node is an NP-node holding "the boys" and that a rule has just been fired seeking a verb in the empty leftmost buffer-place. The word "taken" is read in and matches the rule's condition. The discovery of a verb in this position shows the current node ("the boys") to have been completed at its lower level (this would be true irrespective of whether the verb-form were "taken" or "take"). But the NP in the current node has not yet been attached at its higher level, because – given what the parser knows so far – "the boys" might be the object of an imperative "Have" functioning as the main verb, or alternatively the subject of some other verb with respect to which "Have" is functioning as an interrogative auxiliary. In such a case, the NP would be transferred from the top of the node-stack to the leftmost position in the buffer. Accordingly, "taken" will be shifted along to the middle buffer-box. The S-node with unattached "Have" becomes the new current node. It will activate its associated rule-packets, just as it did when it was first placed on the stack.

One of its rules asks whether there is an auxiliary verb in the current node, an NP in the first buffer-place, and a verb-participle in the second buffer-place. When this condition was considered before (when the S-node was the current node for the first time), it did not find a match, since there was at that time no NP in the buffer. Now, there is. Accordingly, the NP in the buffer can be attached at its top level (labelled as the subject of the main verb "taken"). As noted above, every item in the buffer is seeking a higher-level syntactic attachment. Once it has been attached to some higher-level constituent, an item can leave the buffer. The high-level constituent (with the newly attached item hanging from it) is now placed on the top of the active node-stack. This causes its rule-packets to be activated, and so the parsing proceeds. When there are no more words in the input-string, the highest-level S-node (which will be the current node at this point) is popped off the stack, to be output as the final analysis of the whole sentence.

(Because it is deterministic, PARSIFAL cannot produce two alternative parsings of a globally ambiguous sentence, such as "Put the blue pyramid on the block in the box." But it can recognize global ambiguity, in which case it attaches an ambiguity-flag to its output. This allows for the possibility that another system might force the parser to produce the alternative parse-tree and decide between the two in light of extra-syntactic factors.)

Marcus makes much of the claim that his parser is bottom-up, whereas ATN-parsers (such as Woods') are usually top-down. He insists that deterministic parsers make no predictions. Sceptics have pointed out that, whereas an ATN-arc represents one specific hypothesis, rule-packets in effect represent a disjunctive hypothesis. Moreover, since rule-packets are sometimes de-activated or ignored while they are active, Marcus' parser might be said to do what ATNs were criticized for doing, namely, building structure which is later discarded. However, one might equally say that unit-value machines for visual perception (such as Hinton's connectionist system discussed in Chapter 3) make multiply disjunctive predictions, since they have a separate computational unit for every possible decision. And insofar as they involve excitatory and inhibitory connections whose influence varies up to the point of equilibrium, they too might be said to make provisional decisions that are unmade later. There has to be some flexibility in a powerful perceptual system, whether this is provided by backtracking or otherwise. The fact that PARSIFAL changes the activation-state of its rules as parsing proceeds does not mean that it is building structure which later has to be discarded. The parsers designed by Woods and Winograd, by contrast, do precisely this.

Considered as a psychological theory, Marcus' model predicts that those sentences which cannot be parsed by using a three-item lookahead will cause difficulty for us, whereas others of equal length will not. Psycholinguists already knew of the existence of garden-path sentences, but had no principled explanation of them. They could not predict what is highly counterintuitive, that a short sentence such as "Have the packages delivered tomorrow" would mislead its hearers. Not only does Marcus' model make this prediction, but he reports that twenty out of forty people questioned by him were fooled by the sentence.

The other twenty, of course, require explanation. Doubtless some picked the right path initially by chance. Some may have picked it because of intonation cues. Some may have been less conscious of backtracking than others. And some may have learnt to extend their buffer so as to allow four places (Marcus reports that a few people appear to be "five-item" parsers).

The latter suggestion goes against the spirit of the original theory. Marcus' central claim is that the genetically given (presumably neurophysiologically based) constraint on the buffer is three, no more and no less. Perhaps "four-buffer" subjects are like people with six fingers, genetic anomalies? But then learning is not in question. Or perhaps they are people who have learnt extra, "abnormal" processing techniques, whose results make it look as though the buffer is increased even though it is not? Indeed, "abnormal" is perhaps out of place here, since we learn new representation-strategies all the time. Just as Marr allows that high-level vision can achieve perceptual feats which low-level mechanisms cannot, so Marcus could allow that learnt modifications of the basic parser enable us to cope with speech-signals that would otherwise be incomprehensible. For example, we can and do backtrack if necessary. And given paper and pencil, or exaggerated prosodic cues, we can even work out the meaning of multiply nested sentences like "This is the dog that the cat the rat the fly tickled fled scratched." (Marcus' model does not explain why centre-embedded sentences are difficult to parse, but he refers to an account that is consistent with his approach [Cowper, 1976].) However, the idea that the buffer itself is actually extended by learning (as opposed to having its small size compensated for by newly learnt, additional, parsing processes) does not sit happily with Marcus' account. (In Chapter 6 we shall consider the concept of *virtual machine;* it may be that newly learnt representational strategies can change the virtual machine involved in parsing.)

Marcus sees it as a prime strength of his model that it predicts interesting features of natural language as such. For example, he claims that the passive construction follows naturally from the rules provided for parsing active sentences. And he argues that his parser constrains parsable languages in the same way that certain linguistic universals identified by Chomsky do. (The linguistic universals mentioned by Marcus are the "complex noun phrase", "subjacency", and "specified subject" constraints; thankfully, their highly abstract nature is irrelevant to the present discussion.) Linguists differ as to whether this is so, and if so whether the relevant features of PARSIFAL are *ad hoc* rather than essential to its deterministic nature [Sampson, 1983].

But in enabling such questions to be asked at all, Marcus has broken new ground in the pursuit of a scientific (explanatory) psycholinguistics. His work can be seen as a case-study of how to investigate the processing implications of *any* syntactic theory. Its significance is the greater if Chomsky was right about syntax, but is not destroyed if he was not. Likewise, Marr's discussion of optimal algorithms for computing 2D-to-3D constraints is instructive irrespective of whether his putative constraints (smoothness, for example) are acceptable. This is worth remarking because Chomsky's most basic theoretical assumptions have recently been challenged.

Grammar liberated from context

As noted above, Chomsky argued that context-free phrase-structure (CFPS) grammars are not powerful enough to generate natural language – hence his use of transformations, which are theoretically inelegant as compared with CFPS-grammars. (Since transformational grammars considered as a general class have unlimited computational power, natural languages are computable by some such grammar if they are computable at all; an empirical theory must therefore specify which transformations it takes to be involved.) It follows that any parser, whether natural or artificial, must have greater computational power than would be needed for interpreting CFPS-grammars. Although this has been the received view ever since, it has recently been denied by G. J. M. Gazdar [1981b; Gazdar *et al.*, 1985].

The syntactic theory developed by Gazdar and his associates considers only the surface-string, and so does not need transformations (which were introduced to derive surface-level from deep-level structures). It characterizes a set of phrase-structure rules, formally equivalent to a CFPS-grammar. Gazdar claims that it not only captures all the true significant generalizations expressed by Chomskian grammar, but also explains a number of syntactic phenomena that are otherwise unexplained (for example, the behaviour of co-ordinate constructions). In addition to the familiar syntactic categories of phrase-structure grammar (S, NP, VP, PP, Det, and so on), he uses two new formal devices: "derived (or slash) categories" and "meta-rules".

A derived category labels a constituent with a syntactic gap, and is represented by the slash-symbol: thus "S/NP" represents a sentence with a noun-phrase missing. Obviously, the range of possible slash-categories is determined by the basic phrase-structure rules from which they are derived (a constituent can only have something missing if that something is normally present in that constituent).

Having introduced slash-categories into his set of grammatical symbols, Gazdar needs to provide rules for dealing with them. These are the meta-rules, and they operate on the basic phrase-structure rules. For instance, he points out that the derived category S/NP must consist either of an NP-missing-an-NP followed by an ordinary VP, or of an ordinary NP followed by a VP-missing-an-NP. Given that the basic grammar prescribes that S $\rightarrow$ NP + VP, these are the only two possibilities for "rewriting", or interpreting, the expression "S/NP". One might expect Gazdar's grammar to include a proliferation of such rules, several being needed for each distinguishable slash-category. However, a meta-rule provides a single definition of the entire set of relevant rules ("The set of derived rules with respect to a set of basic rules R and a category B is {A/B $\rightarrow$ . . . C/B . . . : where A $\rightarrow$ . . . C . . . is a rule in R, and C is a category that can dominate B, given R}.") Besides these rules for analysing derived categories (into other derived categories as well as basic ones), Gazdar provides a number of "linking" rules to introduce and eliminate the derived categories. These too are context-free rewrite-rules.

The fact that Gazdar's grammar is formally equivalent to a CFPS-grammar is psychologically interesting not only because it is an alternative to Chomsky's view, but because the computational power needed to parse context-free grammars is less than that needed (in general) to compute transformations between deep and surface-structures. That is, the basic information-processing task, defined at what Marr termed the computational level, is simpler in the CFPS-case. Consequently, context-free parsing rules could be embodied in algorithms that are relatively easy to run, and less evolutionarily improbable than parsing algorithms with greater computational power. (To say that the syntactic rules are context-free is to make a remark at the computational level. It does not follow that syntactic or semantic contexts do not actually influence parsing: we have already seen that they do.)

Moreover, Gazdar points out that much computational-level work has already been done on the mathematical properties of these systems, including their parsability and learnability. One such result is a proof that some CFPS-grammars are parsable in linear time. This provides a reason for expecting what is the case, that increasing the length of a sentence does not necessarily make it very much more difficult to understand (remember "The House That Jack Built"?). Mathematical work like this might play a role in psycholinguistics analogous to that played by psychological optics in visual psychology. And – again, as with vision – the account at the computational level could affect what are regarded as optimal algorithms. Thus the fact that parsing is very fast, starting right at the beginning of the sentence, fits well with a CFPS-grammar. (The general principles embodied in "compiler" programs might be relevant also, for these parse context-free high-level programming languages in order to translate them into machine-code [Johnson-Laird, 1983].)

The generation of syntax

Before we turn from syntax to semantics, one more computer model must be mentioned. All those discussed in this chapter so far have been parsers, but there is more to syntax than parsing. People produce grammatical sentences, as well as interpreting them, and they are not produced by magic. Very little work has been done on generation, however. *Speech-*generation has been studied, and computer models are helping psycholinguists to a better understanding of the function of intonation and prosody. But the syntactic aspects of speech-production are widely ignored. Even Winograd's program relied on essentially trivial programming tricks to produce its side of the conversation. It could not produce remarks of any syntactic complexity, still less of a complexity subtly suited to the specific meaning being expressed.

This has been achieved, however, by A. C. Davey's [1978] model of how one might make appropriate syntactic (and lexical) choices in the production of language. Syntactic decisions have to be made, for instance, about clause subordination: When is it in order, and which event should be expressed by the subordinate clause? One has to decide whether to produce two separate sentences or conjoin two clauses in a single sentence: Can a principled decision be made? And when and how should one make use of subjunctive and conditional constructions?

Davey takes noughts and crosses (tick-tack-toe) as his illustrative problem-domain. He provides rules for generating English sentences describing an indefinite number of games, such that the progress and strategy of each game are expressed by a range of syntactic variations. His program can either play a game (with a human or with itself) and then describe it, or describe a game presented to it as a *fait accompli*. For example, it was given the task of describing the game shown in Figure 4.5. Its response was

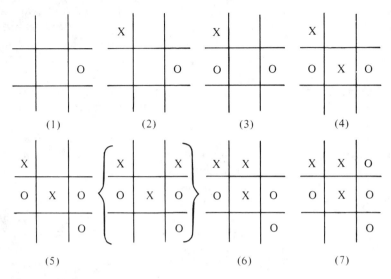

Fig. 4.5. Game of noughts and crosses (tick-tack-toe). The move in brackets was not actually made. (From M. A. Boden [1982b], Implications of Language Studies for Human Nature. In R. J. Scholes & T. W. Simon (eds.), *Language, Mind, and Brain.* Hillsdale, N.J.: Erlbaum. P. 139. Based on an example in A. C. Davey [1978], *Discourse Production: A Computer Model of Some Aspects of a Speaker.* Edinburgh: Edinburgh University Press. P. 18.)

impressive, for the following text is the program's actual output (no editing having been done by Davey):

I started the game by taking the middle of an edge, and you took an end of the opposite one. I threatened you by taking the square opposite the one I had just taken, but you blocked my line and threatened me. However, I blocked your diagonal and threatened you. If you had blocked my edge, you would have forked me, but you took the middle of the one opposite the corner I had just taken and adjacent to mine and so I won by completing the edge.

The syntactic structure of these sentences is not merely complex, but well suited to reflect the strategy and tactics of the game being described. Consider how much less felicitous the second sentence would have been if the order of the last two ideas had been reversed: "I threatened you by taking the square opposite the one I had just taken, but you threatened me and blocked my line." The order actually chosen by the program reflects in a natural fashion its understanding of the structure of attack, defence, and counterattack informing this game. Similarly, it would have been less happy to render the first conjunct of the sentence thus: "I took the square opposite the one I had just taken and so threatened you." This is because the syntax of subordinate and subordinating expressions actually chosen by the program corresponds to the strategic importance of the ideas involved:

that I suddenly threatened you is more important than *how* I did so, and should be the main focus of the sentence. This rule is apparently broken in the next (third) sentence of the game-description: "However, I blocked your diagonal and threatened you," because the blocking of the diagonal was the necessary defensive response to the previous threat from the opponent, and the fact that it also constituted a new threat *to* the opponent was a fortunate side-effect. (Similar remarks apply to the second conjunct of the second sentence.)

Part of the program's linguistic work of course is done in deciding just what to say; never mind how to say it. It takes into account pragmatic issues such as what the hearer can reasonably be assumed to know, what she does not need to know, and what she can be expected to work out for herself. These issues will be considered further in the following chapter.

But, given that it knows what it wants to say, myriad decisions remain as to whether, and how, to make use of linguistic devices such as referring expressions, determiners, modifiers, pronouns, tense, aspect, and modal verbs. As the discourse-snippet quoted above suggests, Davey has provided rules for making sensible choices about all these matters. His model also integrates these choices within an appropriate syntactic structure (so that the pronoun "I" is transformed into "me" when it appears in a context requiring it to be in the accusative form).

Although Davey did not attempt a detailed psychological simulation, he was aiming to illuminate the human language-facility. One reason why he did not use *transformational* grammar was that it had been shown experimentally to lack psychological credibility. Another was that it is designed to deal only with single sentences, a most unnatural constraint if one considers language in its normal use. Davey used instead a type of grammar known as "systemic functional grammar", which is in principle capable of being defined over contexts much larger than single sentences (although he did not actually use it in this extended way).

Moreover, transformational grammar has nothing to say about anomalous sentences (unless they are merely semantically anomalous, like "Colourless green ideas sleep furiously"). But Davey saw a potential in systemic grammar for showing how certain sorts of syntactically anomalous sentences arise in conversation (for example, clarificatory self-interruptions caused by the speaker's realization that he has embarked on a relative clause of too great a complexity to be easily understood). Systemic grammar (unlike its transformational cousin) is especially suitable, he said, because it allows the structure of each grammatical constituent to be determined only when (not before) it is actually constructed. Consequently, last-minute changes of plan can be incorporated at the local level without making the sentence as a whole unintelligible. (Recent work on speech-errors has classified them in terms of processing considerations [Cutler, 1982].)

Davey was not interested in syntax for its own sake, but for its role in communication: "The objective is to show how discourse is constructed to convey information" [1978, p. 6]. Grammatical rules can of course be used by grammarians to spin elegant syntactical spider's webs, but this is not their evolutionary importance. Conveying information is the purpose of natural language, much as gaining information about the environment is the purpose of vision. In the following chapter we shall look at how computational models have influenced psychologists' thinking about semantics and communication in general.

5   Meaning and messages

Natural languages have evolved for the communication of meanings. But what meanings?: How can messages be represented and distinguished? What are the relations between the messages expressed by single sentences, discursive texts, and interactive conversations? And just how are they communicated from one mind to another? These questions have formed the focus of various computer models of language-understanding, some of which have prompted experimental work.

Psychologists and AI-workers in this area are typically committed to some form of *procedural semantics*. A procedural semantics represents the meaning of a word or sentence in terms of how the system actually processes it. Utterances are thought of as mini-programs, as sets of instructions to the hearer to search for or set up certain representations in his or her mind and to perform certain operations on them; these operations include the making of inferences to conclusions that were not explicitly stated in the input.

T. Winograd [1972] was one of the first to recommend such an approach, but as we have seen, his own specific suggestions were not psychologically realistic. The psycholinguist has to consider these questions about communication in the light of psychological evidence.

Moreover, if they are to be answered at what we have been calling the *computational level,* some principled way of answering them must be found. However, it is not clear what sort of systematic answer it would be sensible to seek. Since the basic task facing the language-user is to communicate and interpret meanings, the psycholinguist needs a theory of semantics, or meaning, in general. But it is not universally agreed that such a theory is even possible, and among those who believe it to be possible there is much dispute over what it might be like.

Semantic primitives, and compounds thereof

Some people have sought to analyse meanings into *semantic primitives* of various types. This project has an ancient pedigree, having been recommended by Locke in the seventeenth century. The basic primitives are sometimes (as in Locke's case) conceived of as single concepts, and sometimes (as in the computer model developed by Y. A. Wilks [1972; 1975]) as abstract actor–action–object patterns. If it is indeed possible to analyse meaning into semantic primitives, then the basic information-processing task of language is to combine and communicate these primitives in ways appropriate to the interests of the persons concerned. If it is not, then some other account of semantics must be given and integrated with empirical evidence on linguistic communication. (Ideally, non-linguistic communication should be included too; for a discussion of the non-verbal actions contributing to conversation, see Goodwin, 1979.)

But many linguists doubt that it is in principle possible to analyse meaning into semantic primitives [Kempson, 1977; Wilks, 1978]. Indeed, J. A. Fodor has abandoned his psychologically motivated theory of "primitivist" *semantic markers* and *selectional restrictions* [Katz & Fodor, 1963], because of his doubts about the possibility of componential analysis in general. An account of semantic primitives must assume that each natural-language utterance could, in principle, be translated into one canonical form. This is denied by those who argue for the essential *indeterminacy* of translation [Quine, 1960]. Moreover, it is difficult to decide which concepts are basic – a difficulty that has both a semantic and a psychological aspect. It is not obvious what the semantic analysis should be, even in apparently simple cases – such as the concept of *cousin*. If one analyses family relationships into the "obvious" constituents of *mother, father, son, daughter* (and perhaps *brother, sister*), one cannot represent someone's being a cousin without committing oneself as to the sex of the various people involved (unless one expresses an explicit disjunction by using the word "or"). This problem disappears if the primitives are taken to be *parent, child, sibling, male, female;* but then one can only accept blood-cousins, not cousins by marriage (which would require the primitive *spouse*). Again, the suggestion has been made (see below) that *ingest* is a semantic primitive, contributing to both *eat* and *drink*. But it seems implausible to suggest that the abstract concept of ingesting is more *psychologically* basic, or salient, than either eating or drinking. (J. A. Fodor [1983] makes some interesting suggestions, based on the work of E. Rosch [1978], about how certain psychologically salient concepts may be the semantic focus of language.)

If these criticisms are correct, they undermine any psychological theory that grounds meaning in semantic primitives, however these are defined. Even if they are not correct, a "primitivist" psychology faces extra problems. It is highly implausible, on grounds of computational overload, that radical translation (that is: translation into purely *primitive* terms) is actually effected every time someone uses language. So the psychologist must specify when – and how – translation does occur, and when it is computationally unnecessary.

Despite these reasons for suspecting that componential analysis may be in principle impossible, there are a number of computer models based on putative semantic primitives, and on sentence-representations and/or text-representations defined in terms of them.

One of the earliest of such models was due to the AI-worker Wilks (who has discussed some of the arguments for and against primitives); we shall not examine Wilks' work in detail here, because he makes no claim to be doing psychology and refers to no psychological data other than his own introspective intuitions [1972; 1975; 1978]. A set of "primitivist" models which is psychologically motivated, and which takes into account extensive empirical data, has been developed by P. N. Johnson-Laird; his theories of *psycholexicology* and *mental models* are introduced in the following section and discussed further in Chapters 6 and 7 [Miller & Johnson-Laird, 1976; Johnson-Laird, 1983]. In addition, there is an extended family (still proliferating) of computer models generated by the work of R. C. Schank and R. P. Abelson, who see their work as having specifically psychological relevance (Abelson was already a well-known social psychologist before turning to computer-modelling) and who encourage experimentation designed to investigate their psychological claims [Schank, 1972; Abelson, 1973; Schank, 1975; Schank & Abelson, 1977; Lehnert & Ringle, 1982; Schank, 1983, 1986].

Schank posits a set of *primitive actions*, said to be language-neutral meanings that underlie all natural-language verbs. Their number has varied at different times, from fourteen to twelve to eleven. The current set includes items such as PTRANS (physical movement from one location to another), MTRANS (any sort of movement or transformation of a mental representation), ATRANS (transmission of ownership), and INGEST (the concept supposedly basic to eating and drinking). In addition, he posits unanalysable semantic relations such as POSS-BY (possession) and CAUSE, and quasi-syntactic relations such as "object" and (various) "cases".

These primitives are used to build semantic networks called *conceptual dependencies* (CDs), which support inferences to concepts and beliefs that were not explicitly mentioned in the text (for a detailed account, see [Boden, 1987, chaps. 7, 10, and 11]). CD-networks were initially embodied in the MARGIE program, using a form of ATN based primarily on semantic rather than syntactic features [Schank, 1975]. Schank's CD-diagrams for the sentences "Mary hit the dog" and "Jane punched Mary" are shown in Figure 5.1. His translation of the third diagram is "At some time past, Jane applied a force to the object Jane's fist, in the direction from-Jane-to-Mary; she did this by simply moving her fist in the direction from-Jane-to-Mary; her action of applying force to the fist caused Jane's fist to be in contact with Mary." (This example is clearly problematic. If "caused" is understood to mean *caused,* then this formulation does not distinguish between a punch, albeit a very tame one, and a situation in which Jane was exercising her muscles and happened to touch Mary. Even if "caused" is understood to mean *intentionally caused,* this formulation covers the case where Jane is experimenting, perhaps after an injury, to see whether or not she can control her arm well enough to touch, though not to hurt, Mary.)

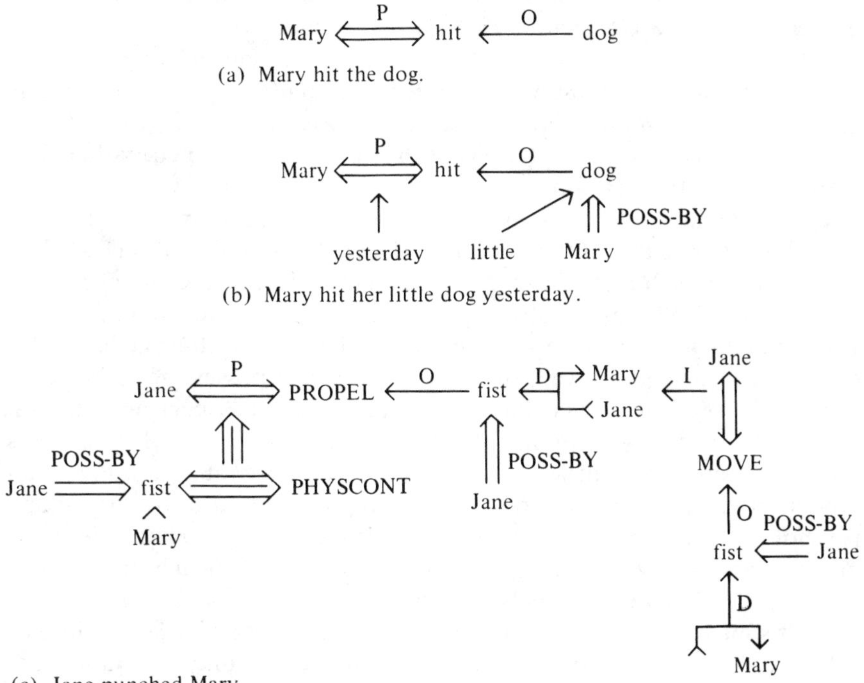

Mary $\overset{P}{\Longleftrightarrow}$ hit $\overset{O}{\longleftarrow}$ dog

(a) Mary hit the dog.

Mary $\overset{P}{\Longleftrightarrow}$ hit $\overset{O}{\longleftarrow}$ dog

$\uparrow$ $\nearrow$ $\Uparrow$ POSS-BY

yesterday   little   Mary

(b) Mary hit her little dog yesterday.

Jane $\overset{P}{\Longleftrightarrow}$ PROPEL $\overset{O}{\longleftarrow}$ fist $\overset{D}{\longleftarrow}$ $\overset{\text{Mary}}{\underset{\text{Jane}}{}}$ $\overset{I}{\longleftarrow}$ $\overset{\text{Jane}}{\Updownarrow}$

POSS-BY $\quad\Uparrow$ $\Uparrow$ POSS-BY   MOVE

Jane $\Longrightarrow$ fist $\Longleftrightarrow$ PHYSCONT   Jane

$\wedge$ $\uparrow$ O POSS-BY

Mary   fist $\Longleftarrow$ Jane

$\uparrow$ D

Mary

(c) Jane punched Mary.

Fig. 5.1. Conceptual-dependency diagrams for (a) Mary hit the dog, (b) Mary hit her little dog yesterday, and (c) Jane punched Mary. See text for a translation of (c). (Adapted with permission from *Computer Models of Thought and Language* by Roger C. Schank and Kenneth Mark Colby. Copyright © 1973 W. H. Freeman Company.)

In addition to the basic CD-theory, Schank and Abelson suggested a number of higher-level concepts that might be used in the interpretation of connected text (and the organization of memory). These include *scripts, plans, what-ifs, MOPs* (memory organization packets), and *TOPs* (thematic organization points). These concepts have been embodied in a range of computer programs whose task is to "understand" stories about the relevant subject-matter. Their understanding is evinced as answers to questions that were not explicitly answered in the narrative, including questions about things that might have happened but did not [Lehnert, 1978].

For instance, a script is a schematic representation of stereotyped behaviour (such as that appropriate in a restaurant). It includes definitions of different roles (customer, waitress, pay clerk) and of stereotyped ways of recovering from deviations. (What-if the waitress does not bring the menu? One can ask for it or borrow someone else's copy.) A MOP is a higher-level concept, denoting the central features – details being omitted – of a large number of episodes or scripts unified by a common theme (such as *requesting service from people whose profession is to provide that service*) [Schank, 1982]. TOPs, too, are high-level schemata that organize memories and generate predictions about events unified by a common goal-related theme (such as *unrequited love* and *revenge against teachers*). But, unlike MOPs, they store detailed representations of the episodes concerned, rather than their thematic structure alone.

The most impressive example of a functioning program written by Schank's group is the BORIS program [Dyer, 1983]. BORIS's knowledge-base concerns such matters as adultery and divorce, and the emotional and legal tangles they may involve. Given the sentence "Paul wanted the divorce, but he didn't want to see Mary walk off with everything he had", this enables it to interpret "walk off with" as meaning possession rather than perambulation, and to see Paul's distaste for this prospect as a natural reaction to his discovery of his wife's infidelity. Moreover, BORIS assumes that Paul's emotion will lead him to adopt certain strategies rather than others, in virtue of the program's stored representation of the origin and psychological functions of various affects. It also has general knowledge of planning and of some stereotyped behaviours, defined much as in the *plans* and *scripts* of Schank and Abelson's work.

Dyer's most novel theoretical concept is the *thematic abstraction unit,* or TAU. TAUs organize memory, direct the process of understanding, support analogical reasoning, and enable one story to remind the system of another superficially very different one. They are defined as abstract patterns of planning and plan-adjustment, capable of multiple instantiations. The aspects of planning Dyer considers include enablement-conditions, cost and efficacy, risk, co-ordination, availability, legitimacy, affect, skill, vulnerability, and liability. These planning metrics are used by the program to recognize individual episodes as examples of one TAU or another. Most TAUs are named by common adages, phrases, or concepts: *a stitch in time saves nine, too many cooks spoil the broth, many hands make light work, red-handed, hidden blessing,* and *hypocrisy.* Others are given new names by Dyer, such as *incompetent agent.*

All this heterogeneous knowledge is integrated in BORIS's processing (including its parsing) so as to make sense of the event-sequences mentioned in the text. For instance, it can give sensible answers to questions about a story in which a careless waitress, spilling soup on Paul's clothes, leads to his discovery of his wife *in flagrante delicto* in the conjugal bed.

Dyer's program is interesting as an existence proof of a system able to integrate many different data-bases, so that commonsense reasoning about planning and affect influences the syntactic and semantic interpretation of language. This is true irrespective of its psychological plausibility. A similar point was made above about Winograd's program (whose syntactic power was far superior but whose knowledge-base was less diverse). Unlike

Winograd's program, however, conceptual-dependency models are intended as computer *simulations*. Although they are being used in technological applications, their prime interest from their authors' point of view is as models of psychological reality.

Indeed, a significant number of experiments have been prompted by these ideas, and by similar computer-modelling work on the representation of knowledge – such as M. L. Minsky's [1975] concept of *frames,* which he compared not only with Abelson's early notion of *scripts* but also with F. C. Bartlett's *schemata* [Bartlett, 1932; Boden, 1987, chap. 11]. Some were isolated studies, more or less directly inspired by AI-work, while others formed part of an ongoing psychological research-programme based not only on experiments but also on large-scale computer-modelling [Norman & Rumelhart, 1975; Anderson, 1983]. Bartlett's work was re-examined sympathetically by psychologists drawn to it by work in the computer representation of knowledge [Brewer & Nakamura, 1984; Rumelhart, 1984]. These AI-influenced experimental studies are prominent in current textbooks of cognitive psychology [e.g. Lindsay & Norman, 1977; Anderson, 1980; 1983], and appear in texts on motivation [Bower, 1983; Brewer & Pani, 1983] and even social psychology [Hewstone, 1983; Wyer & Srull, 1984]. Many were at least partly inspired by Schank and Abelson's models of language-processing.

For instance, some psychologists have investigated the spontaneous inferences (about cause, intention, or spatial location) made in interpreting single sentences or brief texts [Bransford & Johnson, 1973]. Others studied hesitations and speech-errors as a function of the CD-representation involved [Kempen, 1977]. Still others asked whether people's understanding of and memory for stories are grounded in high-level concepts like plans, goals, scripts, MOPs, and TOPS and TAUs, how these are accessed by specific cues, and how they relate to so-called semantic and episodic memory [Mandler & Johnson, 1976; Thorndyke, 1977; Bower, 1978; Black & Bower, 1980; Lichtenstein & Brewer, 1980; Abelson, 1981; Mandler, 1984a]. Studies of story-understanding included some which asked how one's imagined role in the story affects one's memory for it [Pichert & Anderson, 1977], how one's emotional mood determines memory-storage and retrieval [Bower, 1983], and how the structure of the story-characters' goal-hierarchies influences the time needed for comprehension [Bower, n.d.]. Work on story-grammars, intended as representations of "sensible" plots, is related to computer models of text-interpretation [Van Dijk, 1972; Rumelhart, 1975; Black & Wilensky, 1979; Mandler, 1984a]. And developmental psychologists have studied the ways in which children's comprehension changes as they acquire high-level organizational concepts such as scripts [Mandler, 1984b].

Experiments like these are useful contributions to the "natural history" of the mind. Similarly, experiments on conversation (prompted by computer models of discourse and/or by speech-act theory) aid the description of everyday discourse. But descriptions of the natural phenomena may be more or less detailed and more or less distanced from the familiar, observable level. Experimental studies of text-understanding are currently much less precise than studies of single-sentence parsing. And CD-prompted experiments do not show that CD-theory is psychologically valid at a detailed level. For instance, they do not involve tests referring to precise temporal relations (which the ACT-system, mentioned later, does). Again, the fact that stories are classified by people as similar with respect to their thematic nature (not their specific content) is a result that shows only that something *broadly* like TAUs functions in human memory. Since TAUs were intuitively identified in the first place, and most were even named by clichés, it would be surprising if this were not so (this assumes what will be further discussed in Chapter 8, that our everyday psychological vocabulary corresponds to mental reality at *some* level). Indeed, CD-models in general are based on plausible intuitions, and do not generate counterintuitive predictions.

As natural history, this does not matter (and it is only fair to point out that similar remarks could be made about much empirical psychology). But for theoretical purposes, intuitions must be replaced by systematic explanation (based on task-analysis), which will very likely involve some surprises.

This is why some psychologists have dismissed the theory of conceptual dependency (and also Minsky's account of frames) as being no theory at all but merely a vague restatement of the problem [Dresher & Hornstein, 1976]. In particular, it appears to assume that to write a familiar English word (or even a neologism like PTRANS) in capital letters is thereby to transform it into an unproblematic language-neutral category. Schank offers no principled way of identifying semantic primitives, no systematic rules for constructing and interpreting CD-diagrams, and no general way of deciding when and how processing should pass from one representational level to another. Certainly, he is not alone in speaking of semantic networks in an intuitive and unsystematic fashion: other psychologists and computer modellers have been criticized for using this concept (and procedural technique) in a theoretically unconstrained way [Woods, 1975; Johnson-Laird, 1977]. But since a scientific psycholinguistics should distinguish semantic structures and linkages in a principled fashion, conceptual dependency cannot form the abstract computational base of a Marrian psychology of meaning (one based on a systematic analysis of the computational task).

If one criticizes Schank's failure to give a principled derivation of his primitive actions, one should note that Abelson [1973] tried to give a systematic account of a certain range of interpersonal relationships, based on the abstract notion of *plan*. He defined a plan as a means–end series of goals, with the logical possibility of obstruction or facilitation for each subgoal (the same notion of plans underlies Dyer's TAUs). Each of the two actors involved was thought of as having one plan. And each actor's relation to the other's plan was defined in terms of three logically independent dimensions: role, attitude, and facilitative ability. The *role* was itself three-fold: one actor can act as the other's agent (in respect of the whole plan or only certain parts of it); one may be involved in the other's goal (if the latter plans to change or to maintain the former's current situation); and one may be an interested party in the effecting of the other's goal (if the latter's success would influence the former's opportunities to achieve his own goals). The *attitude* was defined by the extent to which one actor approved or disapproved of the other's plan (in whole or in part) and of his own role in it. And *facilitative ability* was defined in terms of one actor's potential for helping or hindering the other's plan (in whole or in part).

Using these abstract dimensions, Abelson defined a matrix of distinct types of interpersonal relation. Each cell in the matrix identified a different structure of possible actor–plan mapping, and each was named by Abelson with a word (or words) denoting a familiar psychological phenomenon: betrayal, co-operation, dominance, and so on. Some cells had two or more words assigned to them, marking the non-reciprocal nature of the relation in that cell (victory and humiliation) or the strength of the attitude involved (devotion and appreciation).

The interest of this scheme (which I have discussed in detail elsewhere [Boden, 1987, chap. 4]) is that Abelson was attempting a systematic definition (though not yet an implementation) of some of the interpersonal relations that are in principle possible for plan-following and evaluating creatures. (Dyer's work on BORIS was much influenced by Abelson's thinking.) A social psychologist himself, Abelson hopes to base the psychological study of social life in a computational understanding of phenomena such as roles and personal interaction.

A powerful deontic logic would help in developing a better classification of plans (and potential plan-failures) than Dyer's, and would provide grounds for a better account of interpersonal relations than Abelson's. As yet, no such logic exists. J. Doyle [1983] has made an interesting preliminary attempt to formalize a "rational psychology" in terms of which examples of commonsense reasoning might be understood, and economists have developed a theory of so-called rational choice. But neither of these matches the complexity of the apparently sensible choices that are made by people. Nor have philosophers managed to agree on a formal account of the "practical syllogisms" used to decide or justify actions in daily life.

Indeed, as we shall see in Chapter 6, it is a point of philosophical dispute whether a formal account of everyday reasoning about actions and intentions is even in principle possible. If it is not, then social psychology cannot meet the challenge – posed by D. Marr, for example – that it be grounded in a systematic theory of the computational tasks concerned.

Psychological semantics

A complete formal theory of semantics (were such a theory possible) would involve a principled way of conceptualizing action in general and personal interaction in particular. But there is no consensus about what a general theory of meaning (including personal interaction as a special case) might be like.

Semantics is more problematic than the theory of image-formation, or even of syntax. It is a controversial matter whether a formal, or scientific, theory of meaning is possible at all. And those who believe that it is do not agree on what the specific nature of such a theory should be. Some writers favour semantic primitives; others, meaning postulates; and yet others, truth-conditions. (These three categories are not mutually incompatible, though some people use only one or two of them.) While some of this theorizing has been done in the contexts of psycholinguistics [Katz & Fodor, 1963] and (recently) computational linguistics [Woods, 1981], most arises in philosophical work on logic and formal semantics.

The work of the cognitive psychologist Johnson-Laird is interesting in this regard [Miller & Johnson-Laird, 1976; Johnson-Laird, 1983]. He has outlined a procedural semantics that is integrated with a wide-ranging programme of experimental research on language, memory, and problem-solving, and which is based on a general theory of meaning drawn from formal semantics.

Specifically, Johnson-Laird adapts R. Montague's [1974] recent technical work in philosophical semantics, which defines meaning in terms of logical *model-theory* and *possible worlds* semantics. From the computer modeller's point of view, this model-theoretic approach is of interest because it not only assimilates natural language to a formal logical system, but attempts to provide rigorous rules for translating English sentences into expressions of the predicate-calculus. In principle, such rules could be incorporated in a computational model of language-use. (Johnson-Laird also uses some ideas from situation semantics, which stresses the *contextual* interpretation of a specific utterance, rather than the meaning of a sentence detached from any of the various real-world situations in which it might be uttered [Barwise & Perry, 1984].) That is, much as Marr used physics and mathematics in formulating his visual theory, so Johnson-Laird grounds his psychology of language in an abstract account of semantics as such. Since semantics (unlike physical optics) is still controversial, however, Johnson-Laird has to justify his particular choice of semantic theory.

One reason why he favours this model-theoretic approach, he says, is because of its account of truth: it defines truth as a relation between language and the world. Some accounts of semantics define truth in terms of implicative relations between linguistic expressions (a notion sometimes associated with the definition of meaning in terms of "meaning postulates", which

specify the relations between *words* – such as "spinster" and "unmarried").
This potential contact with the real world reflects Johnson-Laird's intuition
that philosophical semantics – and empirical psychology too – needs a *correspondence* rather than a *coherence* theory of truth.

But whether, and how, this correspondence can be established by us is
no concern of logical semantics as such (though it is the concern of *causal*
semantics, as we shall see in Chapter 8). Although it imposes certain very
general logical – epistemological constraints, it is neutral with respect to
empirical psychology. No specific limit is put on the sorts of truth-conditions that are allowed. And *a fortiori* nothing is said about how any particular truth-condition can actually be computed. Analogously, the physics of
image-formation does not tell us which organisms are colour-blind, nor
how stereopsis is to be computed; and a theory of syntax says nothing about
how to go about parsing. It is the job of a psychologically plausible procedural semantics to complement the abstract "computational" (first-level)
analysis of meaning by providing answers at the algorithmic level, which
ideally would connect with the physiological level also.

Model-theory deals with how meaning can be assigned to an uninterpreted formal system. Broadly, it says that such a system can be interpreted as
being *about* a given domain if that domain can be systematically mapped
onto it. If there are two such domains, the formal system in itself is about
the one just as much as it is about the other. Thus a purely symbolic
computer program could be used by us as a specification of a dance-routine, or of tapestry-work, or of anything else isomorphic with it. (An
excellent illustration of the difference between an uninterpreted formal
system and a model in terms of which it can – or cannot – sensibly be interpreted is given by D. R. Hofstadter [1979]. He provides a set of rules for
manipulating meaningless symbols: the letters M and U. The reader gradually realizes that these rules are isomorphic with some, but not all, of the
rules of arithmetic. To the extent that they map onto arithmetic – for example, onto addition but not onto subtraction – they can be regarded as *about*
the natural numbers. And these, in turn, can to that extent be regarded as a
model satisfying the computational constraints specified by the formal rules
of the MU-game.)

Montague's model-theory assumes the logical principle of *compositionality,* according to which the meaning of a complex expression is a function
of the meaning of its parts and of the way in which they are arranged. So in
specifying how meanings are determined, model-theory cannot treat sentence-parts as marbles jostling in a bag, but must take account of sentential
structure. That is, it has to give logical rules (not procedural algorithms,
although these must be provided by the psychologist) stating how specific
constituents, in specific structural relations, give one sentence-meaning
rather than another.

In those cases where the component and resulting expressions are all declarative sentences (and so have truth-values), the truth-value of the complex expression depends entirely on the truth-values of its constituent parts together with their syntactic interrelations. Likewise, the truth-value of a compound expression constructed by Boolean connectives is a function of the truth-values of the parts and the connectives used. In the propositional calculus, for example, the complex expression $(p.q)$ is true if and only if both p and q are true. Once the truth-values of these two parts is known, and given the truth-table defining the connective "." (*conjunction*), nothing more is needed to establish the truth or falsity of the whole expression. In this case, the order of the parts does not matter; in other cases (such as "If p then q"), it does – but even here, the truth of the members of the ordered pair $< p,q >$ suffices to determine the truth of the whole expression.

Montague's version of model-theory offers a theoretically elegant account of what the syntax–semantics relation may be. This is relevant to the psychologist, for an adequate psycholinguistics would relate syntax to semantics in a theoretically coherent way. (It was remarked in Chapter 4 that, although syntactic interpretation can fruitfully be treated as a task in its own right, one of the purposes of syntax is to aid the communication of meaning.) According to Montague, the semantically significant syntactic structures concerned are the very structures identified by grammarians. For example, a noun-phrase, in virtue of being a noun-phrase, has a specific role in the semantic mapping between the linguistic expression and its model. At a certain level of theoretical description, not only is the content of the noun-phrase irrelevant (cabbages will do as well as kings), but its nature too. A proper name, a common noun, and a definite description (a noun-phrase beginning with the word "the") are all identical in their semantic significance, or function.

This proposition is not quite so counterintuitive as it may seem. For "semantic" here is being used in a highly technical sense, which does not imply that there is no interesting linguistic difference between a proper name and a definite description. Indeed, lower-level syntactic distinctions applicable within a noun-phrase (such as Determiner, Adjective, and Subject) are recognized, and each of these is assigned its own semantics. But the proposition is surprising in that it makes a strong claim against the *autonomy of syntax* (considered here in a third sense, two others having been defined in Chapter 4). It claims that all semantic rules for mapping expressions onto models are twinned by syntactic rules. (N. Chomsky favours the autonomy of syntax in this third sense as well as the other two, for he gives no semantics for his grammar; by contrast, G. J. M. Gazdar gives a semantics that can be interpreted in model-theoretic terms.)

However, model-theory as such is not an adequate theoretical base for psycholinguistics. For natural languages contain many compound expressions (having other expressions as constituent parts) whose truth-conditions are not a function, however complex, of the truth-conditions of the constituents. Notoriously, sentences containing verbs of propositional attitude – like "believe" and "desire" – do not have truth-conditions that can be defined in this way. For instance, the truth (or falsity) of "Jasia is generous" does not, in general, have any bearing on the truth (or falsity) of "Joyce believes Jasia is generous." Similar difficulties arise in defining the truth-conditions of sentences containing modal qualifiers such as "possible", "impossible", "probable", and "necessary".

Possible-worlds semantics is a version of model-theory that was introduced by logicians to deal with these (non-extensional) expressions. In this semantic theory, truth (which is still defined in terms of sets of models) in a world may depend on truth in other possible worlds. Specifically, the theory says that the truth-conditions of a sentence are determined by the set of all possible worlds that can be taken as models of that sentence. This is always an infinite set. Dance-routines, tapestry . . . anything that can be systematically mapped onto the linguistic expression is a model of it. Admittedly, the more we complicate the expression (for instance, to describe the dance-routine more faithfully), the more possible worlds are excluded (your tapestry-work will be excluded if it contains nothing corresponding to pirouettes). But the exclusion of tapestry-worlds does not get rid of the infinity: if you subtract infinities from infinities you may still be left with infinities.

This appeal to infinite sets does not mean that possible-worlds semantics must be psychologically useless. Similarly, DOG-functions are not made irrelevant to visual psychology by the fact that, in principle, they have infinite receptive fields. But it does mean that we need some account of how the infinite possible worlds of formal semantics, like DOGs of potentially infinite scope, can function in the finite human mind.

In developing a psycholinguistics grounded in semantic theory, then, Johnson-Laird's theoretical problem is threefold. First, he has to specify the truth-conditions (meanings) of the various parts of natural-language sentences. Second, he has to specify the algorithms which compute the meaning of an entire sentence from its constituent words in their given syntactic relations. And third, he has to account for our ability to recognize and reason about truth and falsity by showing, so to speak, how to get the possible worlds into the head, given that our finite minds cannot contain an infinite number of representations for every meaningful expression. Moreover, he has to do all this in a way which not only fits the psychological data but also allows for those aspects of natural language which seem to suggest that it is not properly thought of as an approximation to formal logic.

These three questions are approached by Johnson-Laird both experimentally and computationally. He models the semantic interpretation of words and sentences by way of condition–action tables implemented in a form of ATN which he calls a *semantic transition network*. The condition-tables enable the network to engage in breadth-first search, and in this sense to simulate parallelism, so there is no need to backtrack or to destroy previously built structure. As in the case of syntactic ATNs, these procedural models specify the content, the conditions, and the order of the various interpretative processes that enable the hearer to understand the spoken message. And they are used by Johnson-Laird and his colleagues in designing experimental tests of specific hypotheses about what meanings we can compute, and how.

Johnson-Laird's procedural models raise a question about *syntactic autonomy* in a fourth sense: whether we make use of a separate mental representation of syntactic structure as such. In Chapter 4 I discussed a number of psychological theories that assumed that an independent syntactic representation (of constituent or sentence) is constructed and then passed on to the semantic processor. But Johnson-Laird argues that no such syntactic representation is needed, or suggested by the psychological evidence. Syntax is psychologically important not for its own sake, but as a way of constraining meaning. All things being equal (with respect to computational efficiency), then, one would not expect the language-user to build a detailed parse-tree for a sentence before computing its semantic content. Accordingly, his networks incorporate syntactic judgments as crucial clues to the final semantic representation, but they do not build any separate representation of grammatical structure as such.

The first of the three theoretical problems just identified was the specification of the truth-conditions (meanings) of the various parts of natural-language sentences. A sentence's parts may include other sentences, but at base these are constructed out of words (or morphemes). What is required, then, is a theory of word-meaning – which, *qua* psychological, should provide some account of how specific word-meanings can be computed by the language-user.

Johnson-Laird's response (with G. A. Miller) to this problem is to posit a set of semantic primitives. But these are not the sort of primitives on which componential lexical classifications are normally based. He allows that some words are *linguistic* primitives, in the sense that they are undefinable by other *words*. But he denies that they are unanalysable psychologically. Their meaning is carried by underlying logical–procedural concepts that do not correspond exactly with any natural-language words.

Rather than relying on purely intuitive analyses of lexical concepts, Miller and Johnson-Laird try to give precise rules for identifying semantic primitives and their interconnections. The everyday verb "hand", for instance, is analysed in terms of *use, cause, travel,* and *get,* which in turn reduce to *allow, act, intend, possible, before, do, happen, at,* and *region.* The logical–semantic properties of each of these "ultra-primitives" are examined, and putative analyses of lexical concepts are judged with respect to these abstract criteria. Because the operators *possible* and *intend* are accepted as semantically basic, general issues in modal and deontic logic are discussed too. Partly because these issues are so problematic, this account of semantic primitives is speculative rather than definitive. But it is an intriguing attempt to use philosophical logic and semantics in defining a systematic theoretical base for psycholinguistics.

In identifying semantic primitives and defining word-meanings, Miller and Johnson-Laird bear in mind the fact that an adequate psychological explanation of word-use must specify algorithms whereby the meaning of each word can be computed. That is to say, their definitions of primitives and compound meanings take account of specific perceptual and motor capacities. These capacities are crucial to their computational analyses of prepositions like "in", "on", and "at" and of deictic words such as "left", "right", "here", and "there". Perceptuomotor capacities contribute also to their definitions of content-words like "red", "table", and "water" – although they allow that what counts as a table is largely a matter of cultural convention, and that the meaning of "water" is largely determined by physicochemical facts about the environment.

Johnson-Laird's account of language does not treat it as an uninterpreted formal system. That is, he is not a "methodological solipsist" (a term explained in Chapter 8). For the semantics of those words which derive their meanings from aspects of our material embodiment is biologically plugged in, much as the semantics of low-level descriptions in vision is plugged in – although the phonetic form of the word used to express the concept obviously is not. (My term "plugged in" should not be taken to mean that he treats indefinable concepts as innate, for he does not; his account of how infants learn lexical meanings will be discussed in Chapter 7.)

For example, Johnson-Laird's account of the meaning of the word "in" takes for granted various facts about our material embodiment, such as: we have hands; we develop motor-routines by which those hands can put things into enclosed spaces; we have a visual apparatus capable of seeing a space as enclosed, and as containing something; and we can see movement of an object from one location to another. Indeed, he even attempts (as Marr does too) to relate his computational-level and algorithmic-level ideas to the "hardware"-level of bodily mechanisms: his procedural definitions of the lexical items learnt in early infancy take account of physiological (not just behavioural) evidence wherever possible. The truth-conditions of utterances involving those words are partially determined by the perceptuomotor tests specified in his analyses of them. (He has accordingly been criticized as a crypto-verificationist, as someone who adopts the untenable philosophical position championed by the logical positivists in the 1930s that the meaning of a sentence is its method of verification [Fodor, 1978; 1979; Johnson-Laird, 1978].)

The second of the three theoretical problems listed above is specifying algorithms by which sentence-meanings can be constructed from the individual words in specific syntactic relations. Johnson-Laird attacks this problem by defining *semantic* ATNs for the interpretation of various linguistic features – for instance, the tense and aspect of verbs, and the use of definite descriptions (such as "The blue pyramid on the block"). As these examples suggest, he concentrates on features which are very general (within one language, or even across many), which are clearly defined in syntactic terms, and whose meaning (and truth-conditions) is relatively clear. He studies not restaurants (as Schank does), but tensed verbs and temporal reference. For a candidate theoretical analysis of these is both more reliably evaluated and (if successful) more generalizable than is knowledge about restaurants.

This is not to say that restaurant-scripts and the like play no part in our psychological processing. Clearly, they do. But what is not clear is how, if at all, they can be brought within a systematic psychological science. In general, familiarization with certain inputs may lead to the development of computational short-cuts (such as the *production-rules* to be described in Chapter 6). Although the action and development of each of these procedures could in principle be explained, at least *post hoc,* it is not obvious that any *set* of them will be systematically explicable. A psychologically useful short-cut, by definition, bypasses some computational processes – for which a systematic theory may be available. For example, experimental data supporting the idea of the phrasal lexicon suggest that syntactic analysis is sometimes bypassed by high-level lexical knowledge. That is, we apparently develop relatively direct computational rules which cause us to jump to a pre-stored interpretation on hearing a familiar phrase without going through any detailed step-by-step syntactic analysis. And idioms, by definition, are not best treated by a general syntactic analysis. So if we cannot know how someone interprets language unless we know about his or her scripts concerning restaurants, or unicorns, or . . . , there may be even less chance of understanding these matters scientifically than of understanding the movements of pebbles on a beach. Even though the general principles might be understood, it would not in practice be possible to explain (still less, to predict) why *this* pebble moved to *that* spot, or why *this* person interpreted a sentence in *that* particular way.

(There is an analogy here with vision. As we have seen, Marr not only picked what he admitted is the "easiest" psychological domain, but restricted himself to the most straightforward part of it: low-level vision. It is not obvious that his ideas on 3D-models can be generalized to cover all shapes. Moreover, high-level vision may involve efficient, but messy, computations that are not systematically related to the theory of optics.)

Johnson-Laird's ATNs test the input-words for the presence of certain syntactic features, and use the syntactic structure in constructing a semantic model or representation of the sentence's meaning. What sort of model is constructed and what the system does with it when it has been constructed depend on the meaning of the sentence. Thus an interrogative sentence will lead (among other things) to a search for the information asked for, whereas a declarative sentence will lead (indirectly) to a search only if this is necessary in order for the system to construct its semantic representation.

The flavour of this approach can be conveyed by considering Johnson-Laird's treatment of the semantics of active and passive verbs, which reflects our intuitive sense that these do – and yet do not – have the same meaning. His accounts of the sentences "Did Mary meet John at two o'clock?" and "Was John met by Mary at two o'clock?" shows them to have distinct processing implications. The active sentence instructs (*sic*) the hearer to search his or her memory for events in which Mary meets someone, to locate those in which she meets John, and to see if any of those happened at two o'clock. The passive sentence instructs the hearer to locate John's meetings first, then the sub-set in which he meets Mary, and finally the meeting (if any) which happened at two o'clock. Our intuition that active and passive forms have the same meaning is captured by the fact that, in cases where all the truth-conditions are met, the answer to both questions will be "Yes". Our intuition that they have different meanings is reflected in that different searches go on to comprehend them, and – where no such meeting is represented as having taken place – the answer ("No") is computed at different points.

This reference to the construction and searching of models involves the third theoretical problem identified above: accounting for our ability to compute truth and falsity, by showing "how to get the [infinite] possible worlds into the [finite] head". Because Johnson-Laird uses his account of truth-preserving mental models to explain not only language-understanding but also thinking and problem-solving in general, I shall postpone this discusssion until Chapter 6.

Ill-behaved sentences, well-conducted conversations

But what of the apparently non-logical aspects of natural language: If psycholinguistics is based on a logician's semantic theory, surely these aspects must remain unexplained? Let us ignore the facts that people often reason illogically (a topic discussed in the following chapter) and that word-meanings are notoriously difficult to formalize. Even so, we must admit that there are various puzzling phenomena relating to those very aspects of language which one might expect to be logically cut-and-dried.

For instance, some sentences appear not to have straightforward truth-conditions: "The present King of France is bald" and "When did you stop beating your wife?" Again, a declarative sentence may in practice be used as a question, or a question as a command: "I don't know the time" and "Can you open the window?" Third, sentences that are logically equivalent (in that their truth-conditions are identical) are not actually used as equivalents: Alice's reply to the Mad Hatter, "I believe I can guess that", is not interchangeable with "I am confident that I can divine the solution." And last, truth is not always sufficient reason to make a statement in real life: Why did Alice not say (what would have been true), "I don't know the answer to your question 'Why is a raven like a writing-desk?' but I believe I can guess that"?

Seemingly ill-behaved sentences like these raise a number of general issues about the nature of language and of the mental states and thought-processes involved in using it. These include: the use of definite descriptions to refer to individuals; the distinction between sentence-meaning and speaker's meaning; the nature of speech-acts; and the presuppositions and conventions which govern spoken (and, with suitable adaptations, written) communication. All these issues have been discussed in abstract (and sometimes in formal) terms by linguists, logicians, and philosophers, and some of the relevant theoretical insights have been adopted by Johnson-Laird and by other workers in the computer-modelling of language.

For example, in his attempt to base language on logic, Bertrand Russell [1905] analysed the meaning of the sentence "The present King of France is bald" in terms of a predicate-calculus expression which (by virtue of the existential quantifier) asserts that there exists one and only one person who is the present King of France. If there is in fact no such person, the sentence is therefore false. Half a century later, the claim was made instead that this sentence presupposes, without actually asserting, that there is a King of France [Strawson, 1950]. If there is no such person, then the sentence is neither true nor false (the question of its truth-value does not arise). This suggestion is attractive, since it allows for cases where Russell's analysis seems too rigid. But it cannot account for the fact that we would accuse an antique-dealer of lying if he said, "The present King of France once owned this table." Moreover, it has a distinctly paradoxical air, since in traditional logic a meaningful sentence must have a truth-value: either *true* or *false*.

The paradox disappears if Strawson's claim is interpreted procedurally rather than logically, in which case it may be literally true that the question of the sentence's truth-value does not arise. Thus in Johnson-Laird's procedural semantics, a definite description is interpreted as an instruction to search for some unique item which fits the description. Only if this search succeeds is the reference taken to have been established, and only then can the hearer add the extra information given by the sentence of which the definite description forms part. That is, the sentence as a whole instructs you: first locate your representation of the present King of France, and then label him as "bald". However, it is in general true that if you cannot locate such a representation, you may construct one there and then. This licence to construct – which explains Strawson's intuition that the sentence presupposes, without actually asserting, the existence of the King of France – is a consequence of the conversational postulate of truth-telling, discussed below.

Of course, this procedural account will only be convincing if one shares both Russell's and Strawson's contradictory intuitions. If one does not, then programming them will not make them any more acceptable. Similarly, if we do not understand how someone who says, "The headmistress gave a good speech yesterday" may be taken to have referred (successfully) to the woman who is in fact the deputy headmistress, then we cannot model that type of reference in a computer (except in unsatisfactorily *ad hoc* ways). Theoretical problems about reference, as about syntax or stereopsis, must be solved at the abstract "computational" level, the level of task-analysis, if they are to form part of a systematic psycholinguistics.

Such problems are typically discussed by philosophers, who thus have a potential for contributing to the theoretical base of psychology – especially if they adopt the "design stance" [Dennett, 1978] and try to relate their analyses to the requirements of language-users as computational systems. Philosophy is part of cognitive science not just because philosophers are interested in the mind (so are astrologers and spiritualists), but because their work addresses some of the radical theoretical questions which an adequate cognitive *science* must answer.

But this does not mean that psychologists must sit back and wait for the philosophers to do all the work, for the investigation of these matters is a dialectical process. Just as a depth-perception algorithm based on a faulty computational task-analysis can lead us to construct a better theory of stereopsis (by trying it out and finding where it fails), so the attempt to embody reference in procedural models may help to refine the basic theory of language. Indeed, if one adopts *cognitive science* as the appropriate label for one's intellectual endeavours, demarcation disputes about philosophical and psychological (and linguistic) questions should not arise. The task will rather be to identify the methods and techniques best suited to solving the problem at hand – no matter which single discipline was primarily responsible for developing those methods in the first place.

Seemingly ill-behaved sentences like "I don't know the time" and "Can you open the window?" remind us that the speaker's meaning and the sentence-meaning may not be the same thing, and that what a person intends to communicate must be distinguished from how he or she chooses to communicate it. How can this distinction be embodied in a procedural model of language? And is there any account of how hearers attribute communicative intentions to speakers which is sufficiently general to form part of the abstract computational base of psychology?

Some of these questions have been addressed by the philosophical theory of "speech acts" [Austin, 1962; Searle, 1969]. According to speech-act theory, every utterance is intended and interpreted as one of a limited class of communicative actions: asserting, asking, promising, warning, adjudicating, and the like. J. Austin, who pioneered work in this field, believed that there may be a few hundred distinct speech-acts, at most. However, he himself identified only a handful. Work on speech-acts was originally discursive, and founded on intuitive recognition of the different sorts of things one can do with words. But it has become increasingly systematic and formal in nature, recent treatments having identified axioms and general laws of an "illocutionary logic" [Gazdar, 1981a; Searle & Vanderveken, 1985].

A given speech-act is typically effected by a certain syntactic and/or lexical form, and many lexical forms (words) are normally used to perform a specific speech-act. Thus orders are expressed by imperative sentences, assertions by declaratives, and promises by way of the verb "to promise". Likewise, a warning may be expressed by "I'm warning you, don't do that again" and an expression of gratitude by "Thank you"; and "That's nice!" is normally used to express a mildly positive evaluation.

However, these linguistic regularities have many exceptions. The characteristic lexical items may be dispensed with, as in "Thin ice!" or "How kind!" Or they may even be used to express something contrary to their normal signification: given a different intonation-pattern, "That's nice!" is often used to express a strongly negative evaluation. Seemingly inappropriate syntactic forms may sometimes be employed, as when the interrogative sentence "Can you open the window?" is used, and recognized, not as a question but as a request or (polite) command. Indeed, seemingly inappropriate syntactic forms may even be used as the *standard* way of performing a certain speech-act: interrogatives are standardly used to express requests (this sort of example casts doubt on the orthodox view that different speech-acts are typically effected by distinct linguistic forms [Gazdar, 1981a]).

Any adequate psychological theory, or realistic computer model, of discourse must allow not only for the straightforward linguistic regularities associated with distinct speech-acts, but for the exceptions too. It is not enough for a program to parse an interrogative as a (syntactic) interrogative: it should be able, like us, to tell when it is meant as a question and when it is not.

Depending on the circumstances, "Can you open the window?" will be interpreted by a human hearer in one way or the other. Spoken by a physiotherapist to her wrist-injured patient, it may be interpreted as a question. It is more likely to be a request if the speaker is hot and believes that the hearer either knows or is willing to accept that he or she is hot; if the speaker is further away from the window than the hearer is, and knows that the hearer is aware of this fact; if there is any other reason why it would be difficult for the speaker to open the window; and if the hearer is a person of normal strength and intelligence, unencumbered by bonds or packages. These conditions, open-ended though they are, could be represented in a procedural model (one of the advantages of the ATN-formalism used by Johnson-Laird is that it enables pragmatic conditions like these to be added to an arc in the existing network). Rather different conditions, however, would have to be supplied for the sentence "Can you reach the marzipan?" Clearly, what is needed is a general account, one that captures what is going on here at a more abstract level.

Any such account must involve at least two features besides a classification of speech-acts, with their typical syntactic and lexical expressions. It needs to specify planning concepts, for without them no hearer could infer the speaker's intention and no speaker could rely on such inferences being made. And it must distinguish between the knowledge (or belief) possessed by the speaker and by the hearer – where the speaker's knowledge includes his model of the hearer's knowledge, and vice versa. It follows that no system can be computationally adequate to model the understanding of language which does not have sufficient complexity for these concepts to be represented and these distinctions made. And no theory of communicative language-use can be adequate if it is not based on first-level task analysis using these concepts (among others). Much as one cannot see the 3D-form of physical objects without being able to compute the distance and orientation of surfaces, so one cannot converse without being able to compute the beliefs and intentions of one's interlocutor, in distinction from one's own.

The importance of the speaker's model of the hearer's knowledge is recognized by philosophical work on "the logic of conversation" [Grice, 1975]. Effective conversation (and lecturing and writing too) demands a subtle adjustment of the speaker's utterances to the requirements of the hearer. For the hearer's sake, the speaker must be *truthful, brief, relevant, helpful,* and so on. (Because hearers assume – or postulate – that speakers observe these maxims, they are sometimes referred to as conversational postulates.) In general, utterances are interpreted on the presupposition that these conventions are being followed. If they are flouted, the hearer may assume that something different from the normal meaning of the words is intended.

It is crucial to realize that these are not "mere" conventions, like the rules that govern the use of *tu–vous* or different forms of address in Japanese. In general, utterances *could not* be successfully interpreted by finite, and time-limited, systems without such conventions being observed. They are conventions grounded in computational constraints, for they make effective communication possible. The laws of optics allow for many images to be formed, which would not be interpretable unless their range is constrained in some way (to exclude a world of fun-fair mirrors, for example). Analogously, the abstract rules of syntax and semantics allow for any well-formed utterance to be generated. But unless the utterances actually presented to language-users are constrained in certain ways, they will not be intelligible. Even talking Martians would need to exploit (and act in accordance with) these general constraints.

Truth-telling, for example, is essential if the speaker is to communicate a message (as opposed to merely being heard to assert it). If one had to check the truth of every assertion before accepting it, communication would be both impossible (because of time-constraints) and unnecessary (because the new information would have to be already inferable by the hearer). But a system of communication in which utterances were equally likely to be true or false would have no adaptive value, since the hearer could not effectively use any message at above chance level. Since natural language has evolved, it must be possible to rely, by and large, on the truth of what is said.

To put this point in terms of procedural semantics, only a general presupposition of truth-telling enables someone to know what to do on hearing an assertion. In Johnson-Laird's theory, for example, an assertion is interpreted as an instruction, or recommendation, to add the message-information to the hearer's pre-existing mental model. Sometimes this will involve adding one more description to a previously represented individual (as when one assimilates a novel item of gossip about an acquaintance). At other times, the message refers to an individual who has not yet been identified in the linguistic or perceptual context. If this is to inform the hearer of this individual, the hearer must be able confidently to construct a new item within his or her mental model of the discourse.

This explains the strangeness of the sentence "The present King of France is bald." A hearer who already knows that such an individual does not exist has reason to withstand the implicit instruction to add to his or her mental model. One who does not will normally construct a new item to represent the present King of France, then add the information that he is bald. This (together with our knowledge about intentions, both communicative and financial) is why we accuse the antique-dealer of lying who says, "The present King of France once owned this table." While such an account does not settle the strictly semantic question of whether the antique-dealer's sentence is *true* or *false,* it does help to explain the existence of contradictory intuitions (Russell's and Strawson's) about that question.

A total commitment to truthfulness, however, could be too much of a good thing. As our earlier discussion of semantic nets and text-processing recognized, every sentence has indefinitely many implications. Communication would be impossible if one tried to express not only the main message but all its implications too. Rather, one tells one's hearers only those things that they need to know in order to understand the message, and which they do not know already. This is why Alice did not answer the Mad Hatter by saying, "I don't know the answer to your question 'Why is a raven like a writing-desk?' but I think I can guess the solution." Brevity, then, is another conversational maxim that reflects a basic computational constraint on message-interpretation.

It is now widely recognized that, because of these sorts of constraint, the computational complexity of even the most banal conversation is very great. This is so even though, as argued above, everyday discourse involves many short-cut rules which remove the necessity for complex constructive processes and bottom-up inferences *at every step.* From the fact that "How are you?" may automatically, unthinkingly, elicit the response "Fine, thanks!" from someone who is both very ill and willing to talk about it, it does not follow that every interchange in the ensuing conversation is equally stereotyped. Recognition of the complexity of discourse has been helped by work in the computer-modelling of *conversation,* as distinct from the computer-modelling of *language* [Reichman, 1978; Joshi, Webber & Sag, 1981; Cohen, Perrault & Allen, 1982; Ringle & Bruce, 1982].

Someone might say that even the earliest language-using programs were computer models of conversation. For ELIZA was an interactive system that would respond to any input remark, and BASEBALL and STUDENT answered questions (about baseball-scores and algebraic problems respectively). Winograd's program not only answered questions but asked them too ("I'm not sure what you mean by 'on top of'. Do you mean: 1–directly on the surface, 2–Anywhere on top of?"). And early Schankian programs included question-answering systems, whose function was to illustrate the system's degree of understanding of a connected text by answering questions about it.

However, these models had no representation of a shared conversational goal, continually modified in the course of the conversation. They typically treated inputs as semantically isolated items (although some could resolve anaphora). They concentrated on conveying their own knowledge, without any concern for the knowledge-state of the hearer. And even those (Schankian) models of language-use which made inferences about intentions did not deal with specifically *communicative* intentions (where the goal is to get the hearer to recognize what it is that one wishes to communicate). In short, none of these systems focussed on the general computational constraints on communication.

These theoretical issues were first addressed in a computer system by a model of discourse that took as its domain a world containing two robots (John and Mary) with a bolted door between them [Power, 1979]. Only the robot on the bolt-side of the door could see whether the bolt was up or down. The conversational goal was to open the door. This involved not only problem-oriented planning concerned with how to get the door open (by moving the bolt), but *communicative* activities such as: attracting the other robot's attention; suggesting and then negotiating an agreed common goal (followed by a series of sub-goals); communicating or requesting information accessible to only one robot; confirming that this information has been duly noted; instructing another agent to do something which one cannot do oneself; and so forth. At various points in the conversation, a robot would have to find out what the other robot knew and compare that with its own knowledge. All these activities were modelled by processes that took account of each robot's (changing) knowledge and its (continually updated) model of the other's knowledge.

It is crucial to realize that communicative acts themselves have to be planned. Indeed, planning has a multiple relevance here. The speaker must plan how to express his or her meaning in such a way that the hearer can interpret it, and the hearer must be able to recognize the speaker's plan (the communicative intention) in order to interpret it. Indeed, the speaker's plan has to take account of the hearer's plan-recognizing abilities in the first place. The Gricean maxim of "helpfulness", for example, is largely a matter of providing cues by which the hearer will be led to recognize the speaker's intention for what it is. (It is also a matter of allowing for questions based on wrong assumptions, such as "Is the present King of France bald?", a co-operative activity which has featured in computer models [Kaplan 1981].)

The complexity of the plan-generating and plan-recognizing processes required are even greater when the speech-act employs some non-standard expression. Let us take our previous imaginary example: Alice's saying, "I don't know the answer to your question 'Why is a raven like a writing-desk?' but I think I can guess the solution." The Mad Hatter would have recognized this sentence as intentionally uttered, and also as anomalous (because it flouts the brevity-constraint). He could infer that, since it was uttered intentionally, there must be some reason for the anomaly. One possible reason is that Alice is trying to be funny. Another is that there is some other person now present who did not hear the original riddle, in which case this sentence would be appropriate. Accordingly, the Mad Hatter might glance sharply at Alice to see whether she was laughing, and then look over his shoulder to see whether any new arrival (the White Rabbit, perhaps) is standing in the doorway.

Recent computer models of conversation, accordingly, take advantage of the large body of work in the computer-modelling of planning, as well as incorporating theoretical ideas about speech-acts, conversational postulates, and focus [Allen & Perrault, 1980; Grosz, 1981; Cohen, Perrault & Allen, 1982]. General planning notions such as *goal, sub-goal, precondition, enablement, effect,* and *means* are exploited in understanding each utterance. These models involve multi-level representations of the plans of the conversationalists, and specify ways in which the two sets of plans can be mutually adjusted (in the light of ongoing perceptions and interpretations) so that communication is achieved. In general, the hearer uses its current model of the probable beliefs and intentions of the speaker in order to distinguish the literal meaning of the sentence from the speaker's meaning in uttering it – which may of course be very different.

For the same reasons that were mentioned above with respect to the phrasal lexicon (and in Chapter 3 with respect to vision), a computer model which uses general planning notions to interpret *each* utterance from scratch is implausible as a theory of conversational *performance*. Given time- and access-constraints, the need for computational efficiency in performance will favour the development of many pre-compiled plans, such as those exploited by practised interviewers or interviewees. Even so, conversation will normally involve some planning: one can practise interview-technique, but few interviews go entirely according to one's pre-stored plans. Moreover, the role of pre-stored plans can be fully understood only by way of a theory of conversational *competence,* in which planning is identified as an essential process without which conversation would not be possible.

Further developments in the abstract theory of planning (from which all of Dyer's TAUs, for example, could be generated) should be relevant to the modelling, and the psychological understanding, of conversation. It is no accident that chimpanzees, whose capacity for mechanical bolt-and-door planning is very limited, cannot converse. (They can communicate a limited class of messages in other ways, to be sure; and a few famous individuals can even do so by using learnt symbols whose semantics is arbitrary rather than natural.) It is perhaps conceivable, though not evolutionarily plausible, that a creature's planning powers might be used within its linguistic activities alone. But it is not conceivable that a creature wholly lacking in complex planning abilities should be able to converse with its fellows.

Psychologists' theories about, and experiments on, conversation have gradually moved towards an explicit recognition of these points. Recent psychological studies of indirect speech-acts [H. H. Clark, 1979; Gibbs, 1981] and demonstrative reference [Clark, Schreuder & Buttrick, 1983] have added to the pragmatic insights of linguists, philosophers, and computer modellers. One elegant experiment, for example, showed that utterances may be collaboratively designed by two conversationalists, so as first to establish a mutually intelligible convention for talking about the task-domain before finally achieving the task [H. H. Clark *et al.,* 1983]. Two subjects were seated on either side of an opaque (but not soundproof) screen, and each was given an identical set of somewhat similar nonsense-diagrams and a square matrix-card. They were then asked to place their diagrams on their cards so that they ended up with the same array. This conversational goal could not be achieved unless the speakers could negotiate a mutually intelligible description for each diagram (for example, one arrangement of overlapping triangles came to be referred to as "the ice-skater" and another as "the bird"). Over a series of six trials, the subjects spontaneously initiated, refashioned, and evaluated their proposals for the various diagram-descriptions. During this interactive process, each subject took particular account of the addressee's knowledge, and distinguished knowledge-items that were shared from those that were idiosyncratic. These human subjects were considerably more subtle than the conversing robots John and Mary, but they were engaged in an essentially comparable enterprise.

Computer models of speech

As the reference to non-soundproof screens reminds us, natural language has evolved as spoken utterances: speakers actually speak and hearers literally hear. Psycholinguistics, then, must deal with the auditory signal as such and with its production and interpretation as spoken words.

Experimental studies of speech are increasingly being complemented by the computer-modelling of speech-recognition, -understanding, and -generation [Hill, 1980; Isard, 1986]. It has become increasingly clear that, as in vision, there is a highly complex and many-levelled mapping between the purely physical features of the sensory signal and its interpretation.

The purely physical features of the sound-signal are the auditory equivalent of the wholly uninterpreted visual image, or light-array – namely, the *wave-forms* reaching the ear. Sound-waves can be digitally represented, giving what one might call auditory pixels, in terms of successively measured amplitudes (10,000 measures per second is a typical sampling-rate for speech-research). Spoken wave-forms could in principle be described in this way by a physicist ignorant of the existence of human beings, never mind human speech.

The next level of description concerns the *acoustic–phonetic* signal. This level includes a number of different representations. Some of these are relatively close to the physical level, involving (for example) statistical averaging of the digitized first-level representation. Others rely on specific knowledge of human anatomy. Much as intensity-gradients and line-orientations can be represented only after interpretation based on specific physical constraints on surfaces in general, so the various speech-sounds of natural languages (each of which employs only a subset of all speech-sounds) are classified and identified in terms of physical constraints grounded in the anatomical properties of the vocal tract. The systematic acoustic differences between vowels and consonants, for example, or between plosives and fricatives, depend on varying movements of the mouth, tongue, and lips. This level of representation allows two significantly different wave-forms (whispered or shouted, soprano or bass) to be recognized as the same vowel. It could in principle be used by an anatomically informed physicist who thought that human beings use their vocal apparatus to *make sounds* (not to *speak*).

Next to phonetics, phonemics. Phonemes are those speech-sounds which, in a given linguistic community, code significant differences between linguistic units (morphemes or words). Much as edges have no dependable mapping onto either the light-input or light-intensity gradients, so there is no one-to-one correspondence between phonemes and physically distinguishable features of the acoustic input, whether the latter are described at the level of wave-forms or of phonetics. This is not a question of a slightly fuzzy match: the variation in the way in which a given vowel is spoken by a single speaker is greater than the mean variation between different vowels. Accordingly, computer models of speech-understanding cannot simply read off the phonemes from the phonetics. The phonemic level of description, which comprises the most basic *linguistic* units, can be employed only by someone who knows that the vocal sounds produced by human beings are meaningful words (and morphemes).

Just what people mean by their spoken words is something else again. In discussing some of the many syntactic, semantic, and textual features that contribute to language-understanding, we have thus far concentrated on written text. But such features, involving several distinct levels of description, are no less crucial when the language is spoken. Consequently, a comprehensive speech-understanding program would embody representations of these higher-level matters as well as of the properties of the sound-signal.

If speech is to be understood, it must first be spoken. Just as a theory (or computer model) of language-use should explain not only the understanding of language but also its generation, so a theory of speech should explain the competence of both listener and speaker.

It is more difficult to describe speech-production than image-formation, because the speech-signal, unlike the mind-independent 2D-image, is generated by complex psychological processing in the first place. This processing determines not only the individual words and their order (including their specific syntactic form, as in A. Davey's [1978] model described in the preceding chapter) but their pronunciation and intonation too. For example, we saw that the pronunciation of the words "used to" can be contracted to "useta" only in certain syntactic contexts, and that the intonation given to the phrase "That's nice!" depends on which of its two opposite meanings is intended. On the hearer's side, intonation often helps one to interpret a sentence correctly: Chomsky's well-known example "They are eating apples" is syntactically ambiguous only if it is written, not spoken.

In general, then, spoken words are both generated and interpreted under the influence of linguistic processes defined on many distinct levels: acoustic, phonetic, phonemic, lexical, syntactic, semantic, and pragmatic or communicative. It follows that psychologically significant computer models of speech-understanding and speech-generation should take all these levels into account. (Purely commercial systems, of course, need not: unrealistic algorithms can already achieve 99 per cent accuracy in recognizing a hundred carefully spoken single words.)

One speech-understanding model which embodies multi-level processing, to some degree, is the HEARSAY system [Erman & Lesser, 1980; Erman, London & Fickas, 1981]. HEARSAY plays chess with human opponents who describe their individual moves verbally (as one might to a blind player). The program uses its knowledge of phonetics, vocabulary, syntax, semantics, and chess-pragmatics to understand sentences like "Bishop to Queen-4". It rarely confuses this utterance with the physically and phonetically similar "Bishop to King-4", because its interpretation uses knowledge of chess as well as of language. That is, HEARSAY uses the fact that a move which is both legal and sensible if the Queen is in question may be illegal or stupid if the King is named instead.

The linguistic ambitions of this speech-understanding program are deliberately limited in many ways. Its vocabulary and world-knowledge are restricted to the game of chess. Unlike the noughts-and-crosses program described in Chapter 4, it has no representation of, and therefore no use for, the fact that syntax can be subtly modulated by the strategy of the game. And unlike conversational programs, it does not distinguish a range of different speech-acts, still less worry about whether an interrogative is really meant as an interrogative. Even so, it misunderstands a significant proportion of its opponent's utterances. And it responds satisfactorily only to the handful of human voices that it knows, finding other people about as intelligible as they find Donald Duck. As with vision, then, the attempt to construct a machine capable of performing a basic human task has helped to show just how complex the human mental processor must be.

A point of general psychological interest is that HEARSAY uses many different knowledge-processes co-operatively, in parallel. It does not (like Winograd's program) run through a sequence of interpretative steps and cross-validations: first hearing the input-signal as "Bishop to Queen-4", then checking this judgment to see whether it is plausible, and then backtracking if it is not. Rather, it carries out all the relevant tests simultaneously. HEARSAY's independent knowledge-processes communicate indirectly, by writing and modifying hypotheses on a public "blackboard", or communal working memory. The program is close in spirit to the *production-system* approach (discussed in the next chapter), but has a more dynamic form of conflict-resolution. Instead of rule-priorities' being pre-decided once and for all, they are assessed on the fly, with respect to the specific context, by knowledge-processes defined at the various linguistic levels. This allows HEARSAY's attention to shift if a promising hypothesis is activated (an idea which led to the computer-modelling of *opportunistic planning* [Hayes-Roth & Hayes-Roth, 1979]).

HEARSAY is parallel only in spirit, not in basic implementation. Because it is implemented on a von Neumann machine, the processing is actually sequential. But the various knowledge-processes are *logically* independent: the action of any one does not have to wait on the results achieved by any other. Consequently, the various tests might just as well be, and in a "non-von" machine they could in fact be, performed *simultaneously*.

The HEARSAY program was one of the earliest (simulated) parallel-processing models of any complexity. It differs from G. E. Hinton's [1981a] parallel system (discussed in Chapter 3) on a number of counts, of which the most significant is the way in which knowledge is represented. HEARSAY's knowledge is organized as various *sets* of rules, which act as distinct computational units. Each of HEARSAY's knowledge-processes is thus a mini-program, functioning with some degree of "intelligence". The units in Hinton's model, by contrast, are very stupid: each of them can only vary the strength with which it asserts its (unalterable) opinion. (Admittedly, the individual production rules in HEARSAY cannot vary the enthusiasm with which they do their one and only task; but this task often involves testing for a highly complex condition-set.) As a corollary of this difference in their computational power, there are only some scores of individual units in HEARSAY, whereas connectionist (PDP) models in general are conceptualized as involving many thousands (or even millions) of units.

The difference in the topic, or content, addressed by the two systems is less important. Hinton's work on shape-perception concerned 2D-to-3D visual mapping, but other types of knowledge (other mappings) could in principle be provided by connectionist models such as those he outlined. Hinton himself has applied his ideas to language and memory, and recently (in a very interesting paper) to motor-control [Hinton, 1981b; 1984]. Indeed, his ideas have been influenced by early parallelist models not only of 3D-vision but also of word-recognition, semantic nets, and associative memory.

These models are largely due to psychologists, and some take account of extremely detailed experimental data [Norman & Rumelhart 1970; Collins & Quillian, 1972; McClelland & Rumelhart, 1981; Rumelhart & Mc-Clelland, 1986a]. One highly developed example is J. R. Anderson's ACT* system ("ACT" stands for Adaptive Control of Thought). This has evolved over the years, passing from ATNs to production-systems in the process [Anderson, 1983]. In its current form it is a synthesis of the author's work on psycholinguistics, learning, and cognitive psychology.

"Synthesis" here does not mean the orderly integration of distinct psychological modules, or theoretically independent capacities. Anderson's approach is radically different from that of Marr, Chomsky, and Fodor: he explicitly rejects the modularity thesis [Chomsky, 1980; Fodor, 1983], except with respect to peripheral sensory processing. He believes instead that it is possible to speak of *cognitive architecture* in general. His theory attempts to describe the basic principles of operation built into the cognitive system (where language is distributed throughout the cognitive system rather than being a procedurally distinct sub-system), focussing on the control of cognition rather than its task-specific content. The assumption that some general cognitive architecture is in principle discoverable will be discussed in the following chapter, in relation to the work of A. Newell and H. A. Simon.

The discussion of this and the preceding chapter suggests that there is some hope of achieving a psycholinguistics based on a theoretically precise analysis of what people are doing when they speak to each other. Hope is more apt than confidence here, to be sure. The physical aspects of the speech-signal are relatively well understood; candidate-theories of syntax exist; and embryonic theories of semantics and speech-acts arguably exist also.

But various aspects of language may be essentially unsuited to a computational-level, processing-independent task-analysis – as high-level vision may be too. Quite apart from unprincipled phenomena serving computational efficiency (such as the phrasal lexicon), we have seen that language-understanding sometimes requires commonsense reasoning – about antique-dealers or closed windows, for instance. And it often leads to such reasoning, whether at conscious or unconscious levels. We must now ask if it is plausible even to *hope* for a principled psychological theory of reasoning, or problem-solving, in general.

6　Reasoning and rationality

Racking one's brains over a problem and solving a problem "effortlessly" are experiences familiar to us all. The problem may be a trivial puzzle, an intellectual difficulty in science or the humanities, or a practical perplexity in one's daily life. Many psychologists have hoped for a theory covering all these diverse cases. But others regard the hope of a general theory of problem-solving as in principle illusory.

Sometimes the suitable problem-solving actions – and even the solution or end-point itself – are clear from the start, the problem being to reach the latter by way of the former. More often, the problem (*problem*, not *puzzle*) requires what the psychologist F. C. Bartlett [1958] called adventurous thinking, wherein the potentially relevant ideas are not all obvious beforehand, and the solution may not be easily recognized as such even after it has been formulated. Adventurous thinking involves some degree of creativity, but many relatively unrestricted problem-solving methods are not called creative, because they are so commonplace. Instead, they are attributed to common sense.

Commonsense reasoning is richer and more subtle than is often realized. Not surprisingly, then, the computer-modelling of everyday thinking is less well developed than the simulation of relatively formal problems, or puzzles. Even here, however, there is disagreement over the extent to which *informal* methods are used in the solution of logical or mathematical problems. (In this chapter, problem-solving skills are treated as static, or given; the question of how such skills improve with learning is addressed in Chapter 7.)

From GPS to production-systems

Most of the huge body of work on computer problem-solving falls within artificial intelligence rather than computational psychology. To be sure, the distinction between these two approaches (as previous chapters have shown) is not clear-cut. Like other advances in AI-technology, problem-solving programs exploit psychological intuitions of a very general kind. And some of the central ideas in the current technological research are drawn from the psychologically motivated models to be described in this chapter. But by and large, work on the automation of problem-solving has been done with little or no regard for *detailed* psychological verisimilitude.

151

The glaring exception is due to two pioneers of artificial intelligence: A. Newell and H. A. Simon. Their various computer models of problem-solving were intended from the start as psychological simulations, and have been a seminal influence not only on AI-technology but on psychology too. Their emphasis on the theoretical importance of abstract *task-analysis* predated D. Marr's concept of the *computational level* by two decades. A number of prominent psychologists (such as J. R. Anderson) have developed computational models of the higher mental processes which owe much to their example. And Z. W. Pylyshyn's methodological stress on the mind's *functional architecture* (discussed in Chapter 2, above) also derives from their theoretical approach.

However, Newell and Simon have fierce critics even within the computationalist camp. These critics do not merely complain about detailed flaws or mistaken hypotheses. Some object that Newell and Simon have been intellectually seduced by the digital computer, positing psychological properties that are possessed by the computational processes in von Neumann machines but not by minds implemented in connectionist hardware. Other critics dismiss Newell and Simon's whole approach as fundamentally irrelevant to psychology, saying that they have not identified the appropriate questions to ask. Still others doubt the possibility of our ever arriving at a psychological theory of problem-solving in general, whether Newell and Simon's or anyone else's. These disputes rest on radically different concepts of what a computational psychology should, and can, be like.

One of the main reasons for Newell and Simon's influence on psychology is that their computer models of problem-solving have led to, and incorporated the results of, a wide range of highly detailed psychological experiments. As long ago as the 1950s, they compared their early problem-solving programs with the experimental results of the Gestalt psychologist M. Wertheimer. Since then, they have increasingly combined a programming methodology with the observation and simulation of individual human subjects. Their later models of problem-solving [Newell & Simon, 1972] and motor-skills [Card, Moran & Newell, 1983] achieve a remarkably detailed match between program-performance and behaviour (including eye- and finger movements, "ums" and "ahs", and introspective reports). Likewise, recent studies done by them and their students of learning and discovery in science (some of which are discussed in Chapter 7) rest on the painstaking collection of experimental and historical evidence [Larkin *et al.*, 1980; Langley *et al.*, 1987].

Newell and Simon's [1961] pioneering General Problem Solver, or GPS (described in more detail in Boden, 1987 [chap. 12]), was a hierarchically structured program that employed *means–end analysis* to structure the *problem-space*, and *heuristics* to guide its *search* of the problem-space in promising directions.

The *problem-space* is defined in terms of the solver's representation of the problem, and it comprises the set of all problem-states that could possibly be reached by the available operators. An *operator* is a way of getting from (or transforming) one problem-state to another. Even a small set of operators can generate a problem-space too large to search exhaustively. So GPS used *means–end analysis* to limit the effective size of the problem-space. This strategy converts the overall problem into a series of goals, sub-goals, and sub-sub-goals . . . on distinct hierarchical levels, all related as *means* to the *end* of achieving the overall goal: solving the problem. (The goals and sub-goals were embodied in a push-down goal-stack like those described in Chapter 4, above.) Rules of thumb, or *heuristics,* were used to guide the search in directions likely but not guaranteed to lead to success.

On whichever level it was working at the moment, the program's aim was to reduce the difference between the current state and the goal-state. The set of operators on which it relied to do this was supplied by the human user, depending on the particular application area. In logic-problem applications, for instance, it was supplied with a set of operators for transforming symbolic expressions in specific ways (substitution, deletion, and the like). It decided which operator to apply next by referring to its *decision-table.* The decision-table specified the preconditions and the results of each operator, and so showed which operators were applicable and likely to be helpful in which situations.

As a simulation of human thinking, GPS was very limited. It could solve only problems having a simple logical structure. It could tackle the small-scale problems only: complex problems of the same general type were unsolvable, partly because of the demands made on its memory and goal-stack. The problem-representations and task-knowledge used by the program were all abstract and internally stored. There was no external or physical task-environment, changes in which might act to jog the problem-solver's memory. (Still less was there any opportunity for serendipity.) Partly for the same reason, GPS was unlike human problem-solvers in being rigidly single-minded and non-distractible. And it made no attempt to model real time.

The most radical failing of the GPS approach was the assumption, implicit in the term "*general* problem-solver", that all problems can be represented by a state-space, and that all solutions consist of search in a state-space. This assumption, which also characterizes Newell and Simon's later work, is not acceptable. For instance, many problems require a representation allowing for the exploration of analogies. Others involve perception, as in the use of diagrammatic representations and three-dimensional models, or of spatially distinct columns of symbols (like those used in the arithmetical problems discussed below). Indeed, the definition of the state-space itself may depend on prior semantic and/or perceptual processes of some complexity. In general, *operators* must be identified before they can be applied; likewise, the *matches* that can be recognized by the rule-based programs described below depend on the rules specifying what range of patterns can be matched. The psychological processes of reasoning and perception by which useful operators are identified, and relevant patterns specified, are taken for granted by state-space or rule-based theories of problem-solving. But they may be much richer than the processes actually described by the theorists concerned.

Nevertheless, our still-incomplete understanding of the origin and importance of different types of problem-representation owes much to the questions raised by GPS and by Newell and Simon's more recent work. Despite its many weaknesses, GPS was psychologically important in alerting psychologists to the potential of computer simulation in general. (It also led to significant developments in technological artificial intelligence.) Moreover, it introduced some useful theoretical ideas for describing the psychology of a significant sub-class of problem-solving, such as: the *search* through a *problem-space;* the role of current *goals* (*sub-goals*) in *guiding* search and selecting the *operator* (or computational *rule*); and the use of information about the *preconditions* and the *results* of different operators in the *control* of processing.

These early theoretical ideas about the abstract computational structure of problem-solving are still recognizable in Newell and Simon's later, and even more influential, models. In their current models, all but the last of the weaknesses listed above have been overcome, as we shall see. They still view problem-solving as search through a state-space, so their approach is limited to problems which can reasonably be so regarded. Subject to this qualification, they can now tackle problems with a more complex logical structure, in a more human way.

Newell and Simon's recent computer models have the form of *production-systems*. Production-systems are a class of computational system first outlined in the early 1940s by the logician E. Post. In general, a production-system is a set of logically independent condition–action rules, or "productions". And a production is, in essence, an *if–then* pair: *if* the condition is satisfied, *then* the action is executed.

(There is an obvious theoretical similarity to stimulus–response associations: indeed, Newell and Simon see productions as expressing "the kernel of truth that exists in the S–R position" [1972, p. 804]. But whereas the behaviourists considered only associations between observable items, Newell and Simon – like all computational psychologists – focus primarily on internal information-processes, whose input and output are not directly observable.)

On this very general definition of production-systems (as sets of *if–then* pairs), they can be seen as a universal programming language. As such, they are no more relevant to psychology than to any other domain. The *conditions* and *actions* could be anything at all, and could be matched, generated, and effected in any way whatever.

A production-system specifically intended as a psychological model must be *constrained* in certain ways – ideally, in just those ways in which the human mind is constrained. The potential computational power of the system will thereby be reduced. This would not please the technologist (whose use of production-systems need not be bound by such constraints), but from the psychologist's point of view it is an advantage. For it is a familiar observation in the philosophy of science that the more phenomena are excluded by a scientific theory, the stronger it is [Popper, 1963]. Accordingly, Newell and Simon deliberately impose a number of stringent processing constraints, and seek to match them with experimental observations (their own and other people's) of human behaviour.

One can think of these purposely imposed theoretical constraints as of two types. First, there are general constraints on the permissible complexity of individual conditions or actions. Second, there are background architectural constraints on the way in which these are generated, matched, and effected.

This distinction is somewhat artificial, however, since the two types are of course intimately related. The form of *individual* conditions must be affected by architectural constraints on how *all* conditions are tested. Consequently, if we first discuss constraints on the nature of individual rules, we shall find (when we are done) that most of the background architectural principles suggested by Newell and Simon will already have been implied. (Analogously, if in Chapter 2 we had managed to identify inherent features of individual images, such as the quasi-spatial properties posited by S. M. Kosslyn, these features would have provided crucial information about the underlying functional architecture.)

To understand what the individual productions are like, we must consider their *content*, their *form*, and the way in which they are *processed or executed*.

As regards their specific *content*, it is clear that they must reflect the possible contents of the human mind. There can be no conditions requiring ultra-violet perception, and no actions of felling trees with one's teeth (acceptable in models of bees and beavers, respectively). What are the relevant contents?

Hundreds of individual productions have been specified by Newell and Simon, based in their experimental studies of chess, logic, and cryptarithmetic. Their content reflects the abstract constraints on the tasks concerned which apply to all subjects. For example, everyone is constrained by the fact that $2 + 5 = 7$. More interestingly (because it affects the organization of the problem-space), everyone doing a pencil-and-paper addition sum is constrained by the fact that adding a 9 to a 7 will

```
  DONALD        D ◄──────── 5
+ GERALD
  ROBERT
```

Fig. 6.1. A cryptarithmetic problem. (From A. Newell & H. A. Simon [1972], *Human Problem Solving*. Englewood Cliffs, N.J.: Prentice-Hall. P. 143.)

require carrying – which influences the computations in the neighbouring left-hand column.

The productions are also intended to capture the details of people's actual problem-solving behaviour, which varies across individuals. Because different people organize the problem-space differently, individuals solving the same problem are assigned distinct production-systems. Even so, a given production-system can generate superficially varying problem-solving behaviours: if someone happens to notice something relevant, his or her subsequent behaviour will differ from what it would have been if at that moment he or she had noticed something else or nothing at all.

For instance, consider Bartlett's coded arithmetical problem "DONALD + GERALD = ROBERT (D = 5)", presented to Newell and Simon's subjects as shown in Figure 6.1. The task is to assign digits (values) to letters (variables) such that each column in the numerical version of Figure 6.1, obtained by substitution of all letters, is arithmetically correct.

Clearly, from time to time one will need to make definite assignments – *this* digit to *that* letter. One will need also to make lists (disjunctive sets) of possible assignments, which will be useful in checking hypothetical assignments for contradiction. For example, one might infer that a letter must have a value larger than 5 without yet knowing whether it is 6, 7, 8, or 9. And these possibilities will have to take account of inferred numerical equalities and inequalities, and allow for any carrying operations that might be needed.

This cryptarithmetic problem can be intelligently tackled in a number of ways, each requiring a distinct production-system. Newell and Simon describe the behaviour of one of their experimental subjects by the fourteen productions formally expressed in Figure 6.2 (English versions of some of them are given below).

However, Newell and Simon's aim is not to collect individual productions: fourteen more is not fourteen better. Rather, it is to discover the general principles explaining how the mind's activity is controlled from moment to moment. The task-content has to be specified in great detail, because it affects what happens in problem-solving. But control, not content, is the theoretical focus.

What is of theoretical interest about the rules of Figure 6.2, for example, is how they determine *what the problem-solver will do next*. It is intuitively obvious that the first aspect receiving attention should be the rightmost

P1: <assignment-expression> new →
    FC(variable of expression) (⇒ column); PC[column]
P2: get <variable> | get <variable> = <general-digit> →
    FC(variable) (⇒ column); PC[columns for variable]
P3: get <letter.1> → FA(letter.1) (⇒ column);
    AV(letter.2 of column); PC[column for letter.1]
P4: get <variable> and (<constraint-expression> new) with variable →
    GN(variable) (⇒ digit-set); size (digit-set) = small →
    AV(variable)
P5: check <column-set> → GNC(column-set) (⇒ column); PC[column]
P6: <expression> unknown → (get expression)
P7: <expression> □ → (get variable of expression)
P8: check <expression> new → (get expression)
P9: get <letter-set> → FL(letter-set) (⇒ letter); (get letter)
P10: <expression> note → (check expression)
P11: <letter> = <digit> new | GN(<letter>) (⇒ <digit>) →
    TD(letter, digit)
P12: <expression.1> □ → FA(expression.1) (⇒ expression.2);
    (expression.2 □)
P13: <operator> ⇒ (<expression> unclear) →
    (get variable of expression); repeat operator (variable)
P14: check <expression> → FP(expression) (⇒ production);
    (get expression); repeat production on expression

Fig. 6.2. Productions for cryptarithmetic. (From A. Newell & H. A. Simon [1972], *Human Problem Solving*. Englewood Cliffs, N.J.: Prentice-Hall. P. 192.)

column. (To say that something is intuitively obvious is to say that we know it to be true, but do not know *how* we know: it is *not* to say that we arrive at this knowledge by some special, quasi-magical power of intuition.) It is equally obvious that the first new assignment will be "T = 0", which will involve a carry affecting the neighbouring column. But precisely how is this decided? And what, if anything, should be done *now* about the carry? As the person works through the problem, countless decisions have to be made as to which letter and/or column should be attended to next.

Or, rather, decisions are made which Newell and Simon claim *can* be counted. What happens next, in each of these numerous cases, depends on which of the fourteen productions is triggered (by having its condition satisfied).

It would be unnecessarily tedious to work through their model in detail here (a simpler production-system [Young, 1976] is presented in Chapter 7, below). The content, and interactions, of their production-rules can for present purposes be indicated by the English translations and explanatory comments they give for four of the rules in Figure 6.2 [Newell & Simon, 1972, pp. 193–195]:

P1:   If a new expression determining an assignment (either = or ←) has been produced, then find a column that contains the variable involved in the exxpression, and process that column, PC [column].

    Comment: If no column is produced by FC [the operator that finds a column], then of course PC [the operator that processes a column] is not evoked; that is, the sequential action is conditional on appropriate outputs' being produced by prior actions. This production represents the subject's ability to take new information and apply it elsewhere to get yet more new information. Its evocation depends only upon some new information's being available. Successful execution of the production removes the *new* tag from the recognized *assignment-expression;* thus the production will not be repeated. [Note that *P1* applies to variables – i.e., to letters or carries. Some rules apply only to letters, such as *P9*, below. Note also that the subject can distinguish *equality* (=) from *assignment* (←), even though P1 responds to each in exactly the same way. Inferring that a letter must (given certain assumptions) be *equal* to a particular digit is quite different from *assigning* it (whether provisionally or not) to a particular digit.]

P4:   If the goal has been set to evaluate a variable that is constrained in its set of possible values – i.e., occurs in a constraint-expression – generate its admissible values. If there are only a few values satisfying it, assign a value, AV(variable); otherwise do nothing.

    Comment: Again, as with *P1,* the tag, new, is stripped from the constraint-expression by *P4.*

P9:   If the goal is to evaluate a set of letters, find one of them (by means of [the production FIND-LETTER]) and set up the goal of evaluating it.

    Comment: This production simply selects a member from a set. Its role is essentially to find something to work on when all else fails, since the initial problem is stated as: get all-letters.

P12:   If it is determined that expression.1 is not possible, then find expression.2, which was used in deriving expression.1, and declare it not possible also [this is the meaning of the square symbol in the right-hand side of *P12* in Figure 6.2].

    Comment: This production provides back-tracking on a succession of implications when a contradiction is discovered. [Simple backtracking, such as this, merely returns the problem-solver to the immediately preceding choice-point; some computer models allow for dependency-directed backtracking, in which the previous choice-point to which the problem-solver is returned depends on the specific nature of the contradiction that has been found.]

Such examples show that the *current goal* is crucial in constraining what happens next. These four rules and their ten fellows, like all productions, are logically independent: they can be stated separately, and can be inserted or deleted as single items. But taken together as a system, they implicitly define the (goal–sub-goal) structure of the problem-space and locate the various operators within it. Significantly, the *conditions* of seven rules require that a specific goal has already been set up, and the *actions* of seven rules establish a new goal; in *P9,* above, the condition seeks an existing goal and the action sets up a new one.

But what is it to set up a goal? In GPS, this was done by pushing or popping to a different level in the hierarchical goal-stack. In a production-system, a goal is set up by adding a new item to short-term memory, or STM. To understand this, we must now consider the *general form* of Newell–Simon productions and the way in which they are *processed* (executed, or interpreted) by the system.

Both these aspects are highly constrained, in ways supposed by Newell and Simon to be equivalent to processing constraints inherent in the functional architecture of the human mind. Their theoretical psychology is parsimonious to a high degree, for there are severe – and uniform – constraints on the form and processing of the rules. (This is not true of all production-systems: for instance, Anderson describes his psychological model as "baroque" in comparison with the purer Newell–Simon version. Many technological applications, too, go against the spirit of the pure production-system approach [Davis & King, 1977].)

The elementary information-processes defined by Newell and Simon are extremely simple symbol-manipulations, which can be combined in strictly limited ways to give productions such as those listed in Figure 6.2. In general, a *condition* is specified as a pattern, or (small) set of patterns, to be matched against those currently in the system's STM. The type of match allowed is very simple, being defined in terms of syntactic identities and straightforward variable-substitution. There is no sub-set of rules, no mini-program, which could be called to work out whether a condition matches STM in a more complex fashion than this. (Nor is there any allowance for powerful perceptual mechanisms capable of effecting matches of a richer and more subtle kind.)

The allowable *actions* are highly constrained too: an action effects a motor-movement, and/or writes a new pattern into STM, and/or reads a specific pattern in the system's long-term memory (LTM). Moreover, if a condition is matched, its action cannot be postponed: the system cannot go away from STM and think (for example, by calling a mini-program to explore the implications of the action).

The constraints on *what can count* as a match between patterns are theoretically significant. That is to say, Newell and Simon believe that purely syntactic matching suffices to control processing in the human mind. It is this belief (shared with Pylyshyn) which leads J. A. Fodor to characterize their theory as "methodological solipsism", and J. R. Searle to charge them with psychological irrelevance (both discussed in Chapter 8, below).

But the way in which their programmed pattern-matcher actually works is – to them – theoretically unimportant, since they are not primarily interested in the corresponding mental process. They allow that (syntactic) pattern-matching in the human mind may involve computational mechanisms very different from those used in their models – such as massively parallel processing, like that described in Chapter 3. But they do not ask what these might be. They have nothing to say (or to deny) about the microstructure of pattern-matching in the mind: their theory treats it as a given, as something that just happens.

It follows that criticisms of their work that are grounded in "alternative" theories about pattern-matching are not strictly relevant, unless they offer a different criterion of *what should count* as a match. It was implied above, for example, that an adequate theory of perception might account for the recognition of complex structures and analogies that could underlie matches of a kind much richer than that allowed by Newell and Simon. And in later sections we shall consider the connectionist argument that the nature even of formal problem-solving relies on specific properties of pattern-matching which Newell and Simon ignore.

The role of STM is crucial, for behaviour (including internal information-processing) can be *directly* influenced only by items currently in STM. In other words, moment-by-moment control is mediated by changes in the content of STM. Citing the varied experimental evidence for G. A. Miller's [1956] "magical number seven, plus or minus two", Newell and Simon argue that STM (attentional) capacity is limited to seven items. But, as in the case of the three-place parsing buffer described in Chapter 4, an individual item can have a complex inner structure.

Perception influences behaviour *indirectly*, by writing new items into STM. Newell and Simon see perception of the task-environment as crucial in controlling problem-solving (although, as already remarked, they do not ask how perception works but take its functioning for granted). The task-environment involves both internal (mental) and external structures. Paper and pencil, for example, act as externalized memories (EM) holding a changing collection of patterns that can be brought into STM to be matched against the conditional side of productions. Much of Newell and Simon's experimental work is directed at showing the importance of detailed aspects of the physical task-environment. Like the behaviourists before them, they stress that what may look like purely spontaneous or autonomous behaviour often turns out to be closely controlled by environmental factors.

Important as pencil and paper are in cryptarithmetic problem-solving, such externalized memories are not enough: one also needs some idea of how to do arithmetic. More generally, one needs some background-knowledge about the problem-spaces and search-strategies relevant to different tasks. This knowledge is stored in LTM, to be selectively retrieved and brought into STM at appropriate moments during the problem-solving process.

Many individual productions, then, are stored in LTM. LTM is represented by Newell and Simon as a large collection of independent rules, with no inner structure or activity. Many psychologists see this passive account of memory as inadequate, even if they themselves have been strongly influenced by Newell and Simon. For instance, Anderson [1983] models LTM by a semantic net allowing for spontaneous activity, even though he allows *control* to be handled by a production-system. But Newell and Simon's theoretical interest is less in how an item is stored or found than in why it was sought in the first place and what the system does with it when it has found it.

As we shall see when discussing their architectural principles, Newell and Simon answer these questions on the assumption that thought is serial. That is, only one production can fire (only one action can be executed) at a time: the one, and only one, whose condition is currently satisfied by the contents of STM.

This single-channel account of attention demands some mechanism of conflict-resolution. For the contents of STM will often satisfy the conditions of more than one production. This is bound to happen, unless the logical (syntactic) form of conditions is restricted in a psychologically unrealistic way.

For instance, *conjunctive* conditions are needed to state productions of the type "If your current goal is so-and-so, and you see such-and-such, then do thus-and-so." But any pattern which satisfies a condition demanding p *and* q must also match conditions seeking p alone or q alone (and the disjunctive p *or* q as well).

It seems intuitively plausible that a successful match of a conjunction should take precedence over a match of only one conjunct. This is often sensible, because the former, more discriminating, condition is necessarily harder to achieve. Newell and Simon generalize this intuition, potential conflicts being resolved by selecting the "stronger", more restrictive condition. As in this example, the selection is in general made on *syntactic* grounds, although *recency* is allowed some influence too.

(This syntactic method of conflict-resolution is sensible only to the extent that no rules exist which might give precedence to premature tactical actions rather than strategic planning. In the case of closed problems like logical or arithmetical puzzles, the rule-set can be carefully crafted so that no such rules are included. In real life, they cannot. Admittedly, explicit conjunction-rules are sometimes provided; for example, airline-passengers are warned that, in the event of depressurization, adults travelling with children should not immediately satisfy the children's need for oxygen-masks, but should fit their own masks first. In general, however, we must be able to plan a strategy while ignoring details – details that would normally trigger particular actions but that in the actual situation are irrelevant. But irrelevance is a matter of semantic content; it cannot be evaluated in terms of syntactic form.)

So much for the nature of individual production-rules. What of the general architectural constraints imposed on Newell and Simon's computer models? These are crucial. For Newell and Simon's core theoretical claim is that there is some universal *functional architecture* common to every human mind. This must be identified if we are to achieve computer models providing principled psychological explanations as opposed to mere computer mimicry of performance. Likewise, experimental psychology should rest on some integrative theory. Much psychological argument and experimentation is a waste of time, being based on a ragbag of empirical findings most of which are boring in the extreme: as Newell put it in an influential paper, "You Can't Play Twenty Questions with Nature and Win" [Newell, 1973]. The attraction of the notion of functional architecture, for Newell and Simon, is that it promises to provide the remedy: an integrative theory of the mind.

The concept of functional architecture (as we noted in Chapter 2) is drawn from computer science. It is defined in computational, not hardware, terms. It comprises the set of basic information-processing operations that can be carried out by the system concerned. These basic operations define what computer scientists call the *virtual* machine: the machine which the programmer can *think* is being used.

It is often helpful to use these terms so as to identify *several* types of functional architecture, *several* virtual machines, within one and the same system [Sloman, 1983]. For example, one might say that each of the levels of visual representation posited by Marr provides the functional architecture for the level above, that each acts as a different virtual machine. Likewise, we may speak of several virtual machines (several different architectures) when considering an AI-program written in a high-level programming language: thus PLANNER procedures are made up of LISP instructions, which are interpreted in some lower-level assembly-language–which in turn rests on the machine-code. Even the everyday use of "architecture" allows of multi-levelled reference: it is often useful to talk about the architecture of a building not just in terms of bricks and mortar and rafters, but of storeys, parapets, and porticos.

However, these two concepts are used by Newell and Simon (and Pylyshyn) in a more restricted way, which does not permit identification of virtual machines at more than one level. In their usage, "functional architecture" and "virtual machine" refer solely to information-processes that can be explained (not in terms of any other information-processes but) only by direct reference to the hardware.

Specification of a virtual machine, whether understood in the more or the less restrictive way, leaves open the details of its lower-level make-up. In computer science, what the programmer regards as a *basic* operation of the virtual machine may, in its actual implementation, be either absolutely elementary or composed of smaller-scale operations. In the first case, it is represented by a single instruction at the level of the computer's machine-code; in the second, by a higher-level instruction that is automatically translated into a set of machine-code instructions (which set may be fixed or, by way of a flexible interpreter, context-sensitive to some degree). Provided that the operation's input–output relations are the same in either case, however, it clearly does not matter to the programmer which of these is actually true. Being primarily interested in what the operation does, one can ignore the details of how it does it if these do not affect its behaviour in varying circumstances. (Admittedly, the time an operation takes, all things being equal, will depend on whether it is simple or composed. This is a prime reason for building faster computers, in which previously composite operations are hardwired as single instructions. But in using *this* or *that* computer, one must accept its temporal properties as given.) Likewise, as Newell and Simon themselves point out, knowing what the mind's (basic-level) virtual machine is tells us nothing about its implementation in the *physical* machine – the brain.

In Newell and Simon's usage, then, the "functional architecture" describes the basic *virtual* machine on which our psychological processing is done. Knowing what this is guarantees nothing about the way it is implemented in the brain. An "elementary" information-process may, in fact, require complex neural activity (to pattern-match its condition and/or to effect its action). This is a special case of the general point already noted in Chapter 3, that psychological or computational explanations are logically independent of neurophysiology. In particular, one must avoid taking "architecture" as a pun. There may be some physical structures in the brain which a neuro-anatomist might describe as the brain's architecture (for instance, the columns of functionally related cells in the visual cortex). But this is irrelevant to the sense in which the term is used here. Newell and Simon are interested in the (virtual) architecture of the mind, not the brain.

It is because this is their primary interest that they are content to focus on a narrow range of problem-domains. The functional architecture (by definition) controls all the so-called higher mental processes. That is, it controls all of what Pylyshyn would call the cognitively penetrable phenomena. Architectural principles apply to all tasks, irrespective of task-content, because they are themselves content-free. They are not representations (which by definition have semantic content). Rather, they are the basic information-processing mechanisms for storing, retrieving, and comparing symbols and for controlling which symbols should receive attention at any given time.

Newell and Simon summarize their theory in terms of eight empirical hypotheses about the architecture of the human information-processing system. (As explained above, these are at the level of bricks and mortar and rafters, not windows or parapets.) As outlined in the following section, some of these are rejected by other computational psychologists – who would nevertheless agree, on general methodological grounds such as those outlined above, the mental architecture is in principle important. Ignoring such disagreements for the present, let us see what Newell and Simon [1972, pp. 808–809] consider to be the eight main architectural features of the human mind. In their own words, these hypotheses are:

1. It [the human mind] is a serial system consisting of an active processor, input (sensory) and output (motor) systems, an internal LTM and STM and an EM.
2. Its LTM has unlimited capacity and is organized associatively, its contents being symbols and structures of symbols. Any stimulus configuration that becomes a recognizable configuration (chunk) is designated in LTM by a symbol. Writing a new symbol structure that contains K familiar symbols takes about 5K to 10K seconds of processing time. Accessing and reading a symbol out of LTM takes a few hundred milliseconds.
3. Its STM holds about five to seven symbols, but only about two can be retained for one task while another unrelated task is performed. All the symbols in STM are available to the processes (i.e., there is no accessing or search of STM).
4. Its STM and LTM are homogeneous, in that sensory patterns in all sensory modalities, processes, and motor patterns are symbolized and handled identically in STM and LTM.
5. Its elementary processes take times of the order of fifty milliseconds, but the overall rate of processing is fundamentally limited by read rates from LTM and EM.
6. EM (the immediately available visual field) has access times of the order of a hundred milliseconds (the saccade) and read times to STM of the order of fifty milliseconds. Write times are of the order of a second per symbol for overlearned external symbols.
7. Its program is structured as a production system, the conditions for evocation of a production being the presence of appropriate symbols in the STM augmented by the foveal EM.
8. It possesses a class of symbol structures, the goal structures, that are used to organize problem solving.

Many of these eight hypotheses about content-neutral processing principles have already been mentioned, for there must be a close relation between general architecture and the form and execution of individual rules. Newell and Simon's claims about the ubiquity of productions, the limited capacity of STM, the seriality of thought, the passiveness of LTM, and the importance of goal-symbols have been explicitly remarked. The large size of LTM and the homogeneity of information-processes have been implied. My previous discussion suggests that a relatively simple computational mechanism could suffice to interpret these rules – for matching (according to Newell and Simon's theory) is syntactic and simple, and actions are executed immediately.

What have not been mentioned in this chapter are time-factors, which enter into no fewer than three of the eight architectural features just listed (and which are extensively addressed by some of Newell and Simon's detailed experimentation). Temporal constraints are seen by Newell and Simon as theoretically important because they are believed to affect not only *when* things happen but *what* things can happen. Whatever the accuracy of their numerical measures (in items 2, 5, and 6), temporal constraints are surely important. We noted in earlier chapters, for instance, that certain computations–such as the purely bottom-up construction of a 3D object-model or sentence-representation–may take too long to be relied on *in general.*

Critiques of Newell and Simon

If the psychological importance of a program rests on its degree of match to empirical observations, Newell and Simon's models are impressive indeed. One can readily understand why they have so many admirers. But they have stern critics, too.

Some criticisms are not specifically relevant to issues about *computational* theorizing, but posit inconsistencies within Newell and Simon's theory. For example, they have been charged with belying their stress on mental architecture when they say their theory "places the constraints upon the possible forms of behaviour in the environment rather than attributing these constraints directly to psychological mechanisms" [1972, p. 866; cf. Bainbridge, 1973]. This criticism is not decisive. For the quoted remark occurs within Newell and Simon's discussion of individual differences, as an explanation of why psychological *laws* capturing the detailed content of people's behaviour are so elusive. Because our life-environment, as opposed to closed task-environments, is largely independent of our current goals, distractibility and behavioural *interrupts* (which production-systems can model very readily) are highly adaptive forms of behaviour. The role of background-architecture may drop out of sight when the environment offers a stream of surprises, but the architecture is mediating control nonetheless. (This reason for pessimism regarding the formulation of general laws of problem-solving should be distinguished from the cognitive-penetrability reason mentioned later.)

What is more significant for our purposes, some objections to Newell and Simon's work rest on differences about the value of their–or even of *any*–computer-modelling methodology.

Among their most vociferous critics are some people who disagree with the computational approach in general. Such people are unimpressed by empirical matches and ignore experimental specifics. They reject Newell and Simon's basic premise: that the human mind is, literally, an information-processing system in their sense. They may (like Searle) praise Newell and Simon's honesty in putting their theoretical cards so clearly on the table, comparing them favourably with psychologists whose computational claims are intended only metaphorically. But they repudiate these computer models along with all the others. This philosophical critique of Newell and Simon's work, which if correct would discredit other work in computational psychology too, will be discussed in Chapter 8.

Some critics, however, are themselves psychologists committed to computational theorizing. Even so, they question the general assumptions and methodology of the Newell–Simon paradigm, rejecting one or more of the eight architectural hypotheses listed above. For instance, item 4 on the list is rejected by people who claim that vision involves either a special medium, or a special manner, of representation – a group that includes theorists as different as S. M. Kosslyn and Marr (see Chapters 2 and 3, respectively).

Again, many computational psychologists believe thought to be an essentially *parallel* activity. D. A. Allport [1980], for instance, charges that Newell and Simon's theoretical commitment to seriality (the first item of their eightfold list) has no independent psychological motivation, but is a hangover from the architecture of von Neumann computers. (He makes the same objection with respect to the limited capacity of the Newell–Simon STM, the passiveness of their LTM, and their assumption of general-purpose rather than dedicated machinery.)

Even some of those psychologists specifically inspired by Newell and Simon to use production-systems in modelling the mind have assumed a non-sequential architecture. For example, Anderson's [1983] ACT* system – which he describes as a "baroque" variation of the "neoclassical" architecture defined by Newell and Simon – is partly probabilistic rather than fully deterministic, and parallel rather than sequential: in ACT*, several rules can fire at once (although higher-level, goal-directed, cognition is modelled sequentially). In addition, the method of conflict resolution involves reference to ACT*'s current goal, a fact which Anderson regards as a "major departure" from syntactic data-driven methods of directing the flow of control. And the system's long-term memory is represented as a semantic network involving spreading activation, rather than a set of fixed rules modifiable only by activity in the focal short-term memory. Anderson's partial abandonment of seriality was due to the fact that he was deeply influenced not only by Newell and Simon but also by connectionist ideas [Rumelhart & Norman, 1975; 1982; McClelland & Rumelhart, 1981].

For their part, Newell and Simon argue that seriality is not only theoretically elegant (because highly constrained), but also experimentally justified. Studies of binaural hearing, for instance (in which different messages are input to the two ears), suggest that what at first looks like parallel activity is actually achieved by rapid time-sharing: the two ears take turns to process their information. This finding requires that the experimenter's time-scale be made small enough to discern the switching involved. Likewise, precise temporal measures of (psychological and neurological) latencies counter the common view that thinking happens so fast that it cannot be a step-by-step process. Suppose that the time needed for one information-processing operation were only 10 milliseconds, instead of the 50 favoured by Newell and Simon (the rate of neural firing sets a lower limit to the unit-time). In that case, 200 milliseconds would suffice for a sequence of 20 binary choices, which in principle could discriminate up to a million different patterns: but one cannot recognize even one's mother in only 200 milliseconds [Simon, personal communication]. And conscious thinking, of course, is eminently serial in nature.

Arguably, the serial–parallel argument *when put in the terms assumed by the preceding paragraph* does not address the theoretically crucial issue: the extent to which distinct psychological processes are – and/or (for reasons of computational efficiency) must be – potentially functionally independent. For seriality and parallelism could, in a sense, be combined. There may be *logically* independent and potentially asynchronous processes, which are *actually implemented* in the human brain by time-sharing in one processor, as opposed to being implemented on several or even indefinitely many processors. In this sense, Newell and Simon themselves model parallelism: all their rules are *in effect* tested at once, in that they all have simultaneous access to STM (the computational blackboard is visible to all the productions). Moreover, although Newell and Simon insist that the higher mental processes involve serial processing, they allow that perceptual pattern-matching may be effected in parallel. (They could allow, too, that *some* pattern-matching processes are modular: however, they believe – *contra* modularity-theorists – that language and imagery are generated by the same underlying system, or mental architecture, as problem-solving is.)

Even if one questions Newell and Simon's whole-hearted commitment to seriality, there is persuasive evidence of seriality in some types of thinking. This poses a challenge to connectionist theories (as noted in Chapter 3). It is not clear that processes of relaxation using multiple constraints, powerful though they may be for pattern-matching, are well suited to modelling conscious planning or cryptarithmetic – or even mere arithmetic, for that matter.

The theoretical challenge for connectionism is thus to show that "we succeed in solving logical problems not so much through the use of logic, but by making the problems we wish to solve conform to problems we are good at solving" [Rumelhart *et al.*, 1986, p. 44]. (We shall see below that an essentially similar challenge has been taken up, by P. N. Johnson-Laird [1983], independently of arguments about implementation-issues.) In effect, then, proponents of parallel distributed processing must show how it is possible for a PDP-architecture, originally evolved for speed and efficiency in perceptuomotor tasks, to simulate a von Neumann machine.

How this might be done is still obscure. A recent suggestion is that the pattern-matching functions of cerebral hardware are employed for serial thought by utilizing *multi-level* networks that exploit our natural ability to perceive and manipulate the external environment [Rumelhart *et al.*, 1986]. Broadly, the idea is that patterns in the environment can be internalized, and then successively function so that (by the usual processes of relaxation) the pattern in a network on one level affects the next equilibrium-state (the next pattern) in some network at another level, which in turn partially constrains the following equilibration of the first network.

The authors outline ways in which successive pattern-matching might be exploited to do elementary arithmetic, of the kind which we can do only if the sum is set out in a spatial array. And they describe a simple computer model which uses two mutually influential relaxation-networks to produce the sequential moves of a game of noughts and crosses (tick-tack-toe). The relaxation-constraints of both networks embody the rules and strategy of noughts and crosses, but one network represents player's move while the other represents opponent's move. The opponent's moves might be represented only by a *perceptual* network, one reflecting actual events (the opponent's moves) in the outside world; in that case, the player could play the game by repeatedly settling into some equilibrium-state in response to the opponent's moves but would be unable to think about it, or plan ahead. But if these perceptual patterns can be internalized, they can then be used *in the mind* to drive the equilibration of successive patterns representing the player's own carefully thought-out moves.

As its authors frankly admit, this suggested connectionist paradigm for serial reasoning is highly speculative. Nor is it entirely opposed to Newell and Simon's work. It echoes their stress on the importance of the external environment (and manipulations thereof) in controlling what happens next, and even acknowledges that many of the problem-solving strategies and rules defined by them may indeed be significant at some level. Connectionists can allow that "people do seem to have at least two modes of operation, one rapid, efficient, subconscious, the other slow, serial, and conscious" [Norman, 1986, p. 542], and that production-rules may well be appropriate for modelling the second type of thinking. Indeed, connectionist implementations of production-systems are being developed precisely to deal with logical processes such as variable-binding (in which a variable x in a general rule-schema is temporarily bound to, or substituted by, a particular individual – such as 5, or Lucy) [Touretsky & Hinton, 1985]. But many of the lower-level problem-solving processes described by Newell and Simon in terms of production-rules would be attributed by connectionists to processes of pattern-matching by relaxation in neural networks.

The connectionist suggestion considered above is relevant to Marr's radical criticism of Newell and Simon's work. Marr complained that they fail to recognize the importance of task-definition. This failure (he said) nullifies their constant appeals to experimental evidence, because the goal of empirical matching is "mimicry rather than true understanding". Despite their empirical verisimilitude, Newell and Simon's programs do not model "what is really going on". As Marr puts it, "Studying our performance in close relation to production systems seems to me a waste of time, because it amounts to studying a mechanism, not a problem" [1982, p. 348]. Computer models (and psychological theories) are theoretically interesting only insofar as they take seriously the abstract constraints necessarily involved in a given information-processing task – which, according to Marr, Newell and Simon did not do.

Is this criticism fair? At first sight, it is not. Not only did Newell and Simon repeatedly emphasize the importance of the "task environment", but they first recommended careful task-analysis long before Marr did (and applied this idea to AI-research [Newell, 1982]). They saw prior analysis of the abstract constraints implicit in the task-environment as essential (hence their emphasis on the "problem-space"). Understanding *what* has to be done in solving a problem is necessary for understanding *how* it could be done. And they stressed that computer-modelling must rest on prior theoretical analysis, if it is not to degenerate into mere tinkering.

One can hardly deny their point. We have already seen that fruitful work in vision and parsing relies on abstract theories of projective geometry and grammar, in terms of which the underlying task can be defined. If necessary, these must be specifically developed, as in the "geometrical progression" culminating in the work of A. K. Mackworth and S. W. Draper. Similarly, reliable computer-modelling (and psychological understanding) of musical perception requires a grasp of the abstract theory of harmony; this too has recently been further developed in the context of computational work [Longuet-Higgins & Steedman, 1971; Longuet-Higgins, 1979; 1987]. All of this fits well not only with Marr's approach, but also with Newell and Simon's. Why, then, should Marr demur?

To understand why Marr was so dismissive, one must remember that the *identification* of the basic task of some psychological domain is logically prior to its *analysis*. Marr did not query Newell and Simon's emphasis on task-analysis, nor even their analyses of their chosen tasks. Rather, he attacked their choice of tasks to be analysed.

Modularity-theorists in general, of whom Marr is one, are most interested in the sorts of tasks which we all perform very well. It appears to be an empirical fact that these tasks are to a high degree psychologically encapsulated, in that they cannot (or can only very rarely) be controlled by psychological processes outside the module concerned. To the extent that this is so, it follows that they are (in the terminology introduced in Chapter 2) cognitively impenetrable: they cannot be affected by the person's goals and beliefs. *A fortiori*, they are not open to conscious control: they are usually not even accessible to consciousness.

Low-level vision, parsing, and basic aspects of musical perception are examples of such tasks. But mental arithmetic is not. We do it largely by means of conscious operations, reported in the subjects' verbal protocols. Admittedly, with repeated practice of arithmetic, some of these may be replaced by reflexes (or pattern-matching) operating subconsciously. Admittedly also (as we saw in Chapter 2), introspective reports cannot necessarily be taken at their face value. But Newell and Simon's detailed models suggest that many of their subjects' claims about what they are doing may indeed be based in psychological reality. Mental arithmetic is cognitively penetrable to a high degree. Indeed, we have seen that the setting and following of specific *goals* is crucial in deciding what is to be done next. And most of us perform it badly – so badly that we reward success with special admiration.

Marr comments: "I have no doubt that when we do mental arithmetic we are doing something well, but it is not arithmetic" [1982, p. 348]. Moreover, he believes that "we are very far from understanding even one component of what that something is". (The discussion of connectionism earlier in this section suggests that the answer may concern pattern-matching processes in multi-level networks.) If Marr is right, it would not be only Newell and Simon who are wasting their time: similar strictures would apply to recent computational work offering a systematic account of children's successes and errors in subtraction [Brown & Burton, 1978; Burton, 1982]. In short, according to Marr, *all* psychological research on arithmetical (and other types of) problem-solving is a theoretically useless activity. It will remain so until we can identify the basic task(s) and the relevant information-processing constraints. Until then, we had better concentrate on what Marr would term simpler (though by no means simple) problems – such as low-level vision, parsing, the perception of music, and (possibly) semantics.

Can there be a theory of problem-solving?

One might argue that Marr's view is too stern. One might say that, much as work in scene-analysis gradually achieved a better analysis of the visual task-environment, so Newell and Simon's work could eventually help lead towards a better understanding of problem-solving (where problem-solving includes not only logically closed puzzles such as cryptarithmetic but scientific and everyday problems too).

Such a reply, of course, assumes that there *can be* a principled theory of problem-solving, as opposed to an unsystematic collection of problem-solving procedures and suggestive anecdotes. This assumption itself has been firmly rejected by some devotees of modularity [Fodor, 1983]. They point out that problem-solving (like other higher mental processes) is not computationally encapsulated, but involves *cognitively penetrable* phenomena. As we saw in the discussion of Pylyshyn's work in Chapter 2, this means that problem-solving can be influenced by desires and beliefs – *any* desires and beliefs that the problem-solver takes to be somehow relevant to the problem.

To explain cognitively penetrable phenomena in general, we adopt what

Dennett [1971] calls the intentional stance. That is, we assume that the computational relations between representations are *rational* ones, that they are intelligible in terms of goals and beliefs. The behaviour of an intentional system (by definition) is best interpreted on the assumption that, by and large, it will do whatever it judges to be the best thing to do, given its goals and beliefs.

Admittedly, experimental studies of the everyday estimation of probabilities, and of social-psychological thinking (which show that people often flout abstract principles of reasoning), are commonly taken to prove that we are *irrational* [Tversky & Kahnemann, 1974; Nisbett & Ross, 1980; L. J. Cohen, 1981]. Studies described at length below suggest that we very rarely use the laws of logic in reasoning, even when faced with problems couched in the form of syllogisms [Johnson-Laird, 1983]. And Freud's account of the dream-work, and of primary-process thinking in general, seems to show the irrationality of the unconscious.

But these apparent counterexamples are not decisive. We call such thinking irrational to distinguish it from more logical or realistic thinking. It is, nevertheless, rational as opposed to non-rational. Roulette-players who commit the Monte Carlo fallacy, who believe (wrongly) that a preceding run of blacks increases the probability of the next throw's being red, are unlikely to win a fortune. But they are acting rationally, in the sense that their behaviour is determined by the semantic content of their beliefs and desires. Even Freud's most baroque dream-interpretations are intelligible (whether they are also true, or even illuminating, is irrelevant here), and intelligibility is a fundamental property of rational as opposed to non-rational structures. We can understand, for instance, that the crumpled giraffe in Little Hans' dream could have been a symbol for his mother; there are specifiable semantic analogies (including those suggested by Freud himself) between the concepts of "giraffe" and "mother" which could have mediated a relatively direct association between them in Hans' mind. Indeed, if we allow for relatively indirect associations based on shared semantic properties and experiential coincidences, then what someone may understand to be relevant to a certain topic is unlimited. It is impossible to set general bounds on rational thinking so as absolutely to rule out specific semantic content.

Accordingly, modularity-theorists argue that problem-solving is potentially open to far too many influences to be theoretically manageable. If they are right, there can be no principled theory of problem-solving in general, and no truly *cognitive* science (as opposed to *modular* sciences of perception, parsing, and the like). – But are they right?

We have just noted that, because of the semantic richness and interpretative power of the human mind, the influences on thinking are indefinitely various. Cryptarithmetic and chess are special cases. In closed problems like these, the class of (what are generally agreed to be) potentially relevant cognitive factors is relatively small and well defined. The qualification in parentheses is needed because, even here, success in problem-solving could occasionally be aided by a seemingly irrelevant thought. For example, someone doing mental arithmetic might succeed partly as a result of remembering joining in a formation-dance wherein he or she was told to "add yourself to the head of the next column on the left". But where commonsense or adventurous thinking is concerned, there is in principle no theoretical limit to the semantic contents or representations that could intelligibly be (believed to be) relevant: problems that are not closed problems can lead people to think all manner of thoughts. Logicians can (perhaps) ignore this fact, but psychologists certainly cannot [Boden, 1980].

Hence, there cannot in principle be a psychological theory of problem-solving capable of generating – still less, predicting – all the details of every instance of human problem-solving behaviour. Newell and Simon's carefully tailored production-systems can perhaps do this for a few individual subjects, solving a tiny class of closed problems. But any theorist who tried to specify all the indefinitely many thoughts that might possibly arise, or even all those which had in fact arisen, during adventurous thinking would be doomed to failure. To this extent, scepticism about the power of psychological theories of the higher mental processes is justified.

It does not follow, however, that there can be no scientific study of thinking. Those (such as some modularity-theorists) who say that there can be no scientific account of cognitively penetrable phenomena have too limited a view of what counts as a scientific explanation.

Many scientific explanations rest on *laws* linking dependent and independent variables, which (together with knowledge of initial conditions) allow for detailed *predictions* of individual events. Such laws are found in abundance in physics and chemistry (and are sought by operationalist psychologists). They are found, too, in genetics and molecular biology – but not in Darwin's evolutionary theory, which predicts nothing (except in very general terms). Yet the theory of evolution is a scientific theory. For it explains how the many species of living things, and the fossil record, could have evolved by natural selection (given individual variation and some mechanism of heredity). Also, it provides a way of classifying species and explaining their degrees of relationship in terms of anatomical similarities and differences. Before Darwin, many people had been persuaded of the fact of evolution, but how it *could* have happened was still a mystery. Thus Darwin's theory was acclaimed because it satisfied an important – perhaps the most basic – aim of science: understanding how something is *possible* [Sloman, 1978].

The difference between understanding how something of a certain type is possible and predicting the occurrence of individual phenomena in detail underlies Noam Chomsky's distinction between *competence* and *performance*. A competence-theory specifies abstract generative rules, which distinguish those logically possible forms that are impossible according to the theory from those which are possible (not all of which need actually occur). Ideally, if the competence-theory suffices to explain the phenomena concerned, only the latter forms are ever encountered; but if performance can be influenced also by factors not included within the theory, anomalous forms will occur (speakers do utter ungrammatical word-strings). Likewise, a theory that is generative (not only in the mathematical sense but also) in the sense that it describes a *temporal process* will fail to cover processes which arise in different ways (a phrasal lexicon may enable short-cut computations bypassing the need for detailed parsing). A competence-theory exhibits structural similarities among various phenomena and can explain the potential for various types of anomalous forms (such as syntactically ambiguous sentences).

In all these ways, a generative theory of mental competence offers a *scientific* account of psychological phenomena. Certainly, generative power is not the same as predictive power. To the extent that the influences on a specific case of thinking cannot be completely predicted (or even confidently itemized *post hoc*), psychology is unlike those parts of the natural sciences which allow for detailed prediction. But theoretical psychology can satisfy the scientific aim of helping us understand how mental processes are *possible*. (Indeed, it is a main attraction of computer models that they seem to show that mental processes are possible in a basically mechanistic system [Boden, 1972]. The abstract proof that any effective procedure can be computed by a Turing machine is psychologically significant for a similar reason.) In the case of problem-solving in particular, one would ask of a psychological science that it provide a generative theory of types of problems and problem-solving strategies (though not necessarily any *laws* about which strategy will be used when).

To illuminate how human thought can possibly happen, and what sorts of thought can happen, psychologists may reasonably hope to provide three types of information.

First, they can collect detailed behavioural protocols in particular cases, including the subjects' verbal accounts of what they are doing and why. These can be used *post hoc* in explaining those specific examples of thinking: in showing how they were possible.

Newell and Simon's studies of individual episodes of problem-solving provide many such examples. Clinical and idiographic psychological casework, focussed on a particular individual person, does so too [G. W. Allport, 1942]. Occasionally, such casework is expressed as a computer model embodying highly idiosyncratic goals and beliefs [Colby & Gilbert, 1964; Colby, 1981; Boden, 1987, chaps. 2 and 3]. As remarked above, the actual content of individual rules, concepts, schemata, or beliefs will be of little or no general theoretical interest (especially for non-closed problems). What is more interesting is their potential for surprising interactions. The production-system approach is strong here. It shows clearly, for instance, that the addition or deletion of a single rule can sometimes achieve a holistic restructuring of behaviour. (Newell and Simon's work shows many instances of this, and a similar example will be discussed in Chapter 7.)

Second, psychologists can garner empirical evidence about which cognitively penetrable phenomena are *relatively* predictable. This involves seeking the semantic links and sometimes "irrational" heuristics that people actually tend to use in certain classes of problem-situation.

Some such regularities, of an abstract and presumably relatively culture-free type, have been identified by psychological studies of cognitive *strategies* in concept-attainment: for example, people find it very difficult to accept disjunctive information [Bruner, Goodnow & Austin, 1956]. Social psychologists of varying philosophical persuasions (from behaviourists to phenomenologists) have identified a multitude of others, though many of these are restricted to specific sub-cultures at specific historical periods [Gergen, 1973]. Even social psychology can come up with some surprises about the goals and beliefs affecting our behaviour if it relies not merely on intuition but on empirical study. For instance, it turns out that the explanation of the Kitty Genovese phenomenon (where not one of many onlookers does anything to help someone in distress) depends less on inner-city alienation or cowardice than on each onlooker's belief that one of the others will help; if an onlooker believes that there is no one else available, he or she is much more likely to act [Latané & Darley, 1970].

Within computer-modelling, the Schankian scripts, MOPS, TOPS, and TAUS described in Chapter 5 are examples of attempts to codify such matters, albeit based more on intuition than on systematic empirical study. Also relevant are R. P. Abelson's computer models of political belief, and his structured representation (based on concepts of *role* and *plan*) of various interpersonal themes used in the interpretation of social life [Abelson, 1973; Boden, 1987, chap. 4]. Current AI-work on *naive physics* investigates the concepts and beliefs involved in our everyday commerce with the material world (although it is an open question to what degree these largely tacit processes are cognitively penetrable) [Hayes, 1979; 1985]. And Newell and Simon themselves have suggested many examples of rules (reflecting, for example, arithmetical constraints or elementary chess-strategies) that are widely shared among subjects. (Some of these studies are germane to learning: as we shall see in the next chapter, a student of Newell and Simon has found significant differences in the representations of physics-problems used by novices and experts [Larkin, 1979; Larkin *et al.*, 1980].)

The third thing psychologists might do to show how thought is possible is to provide a very general account of computation, representations, and cognitive penetrability. This account would include theories about the mind's functional architecture and/or modular sub-systems, and about the types of information-processing that it allows (to be combined with abstract task-analysis of the various information-processing tasks specific to distinct psychological domains). It should also include ideas about the structure of long-term memory, and about various very high-level computational processes of a generally useful kind.

Some work in AI (not all of which is psychological in emphasis) addresses these latter issues. Research on planning (from GPS onward) is one source of relevant ideas. Most of it focusses on closed problems, including mathematical reasoning [Bundy, 1983; Boden, 1987, chap. 12], but some relates to semantic data-bases (models of belief-systems) built of schemata and related conceptual structures [Dyer, 1983; Wilensky, 1983]. A few computer models of metaphor and analogical thinking have been attempted (including a psychologically motivated aspect of Anderson's ACT* model) [Carbonell, 1982a, 1982b; Anderson, 1983; Boden, 1987, chap. 11; Ortony, 1979]. And some current AI-work aims to provide computers with something like common sense: this includes research on "non-monotonic" reasoning (in which a statement reasonably judged to be true, by default-reasoning allowing the system to jump to a sensible conclusion, can later turn out to be false) and on "truth-maintenance" (in which continual revisions preserve consistency in the knowledge-base) [Doyle, 1979; McDermott & Doyle, 1980, 1980; Davis, 1980; McCarthy, 1980; 1986]. As yet, however, these efforts to humanize AI-programs by providing them with commonsense reasoning have met with little success. According to the theorist discussed in the next section, this failure is inevitable so long as people try to model reasoning by using purely *formal* methods.

Mental models versus logical rules

One general process often attributed to the human mind is logical, deductive, reasoning. Many psychologists assume that we (often) make inferences by means of logical principles, not only in abstract problem-solving but in many everyday problems too. Piaget, for instance, held that, having achieved formal operations in adolescence, adults typically employ abstract hypothetico-deductive reasoning where it is appropriate; when they do not, he said, they are regressing to a previous developmental stage. In short, he claimed not merely that adults can somehow recognize and deploy deductive relationships (which could hardly be denied), but that they use specifically formal-deductive reasoning to do so.

There is extensive evidence, however, suggesting that we do not normally rely on logical deduction – not even when we are solving problems of apparently logical types. People (including logicians) not only make mistakes in probabilistic and everyday thinking [Tversky & Kahnemann, 1974; Nisbett & Ross, 1980; Cohen, 1981], but often do not use logic where one might expect them to do so. For example, the success-rate on problems of identical logical form can vary between 19 percent and 98 percent, given abstract or commonsensical subject-matter respectively; even professional logicians are affected by the specific content of the problem-schema [Wason, 1977]. And when solving problems expressed as syllogisms – for which logical inference may seem the obviously most appropriate strategy – people make a multitude of errors, and normally draw only *some* (if any) of the valid inferences that logic would allow [Johnson-Laird, 1981; 1983].

If our problem-solving does not involve the use of deductive logic, how is it done? An alternative hypothesis is that people reason by using *mental models* – where these comprise only a sub-set of all mental representations: namely, those having some significant structural similarity with what they represent.

In the 1940s, K. J. W. Craik [1943] suggested that a cerebral model can embody veridical thinking because it "has a similar [physical] relation-structure to that of the process it imitates" [p. 51]. This idea, often generalized to include similarities of *symbolic* structure too, has since been recommended by various computational theorists, including proponents of analogical representations of one kind or another (see Chapter 2, above). The most ambitious and systematic example is the recent work of the psychologist Johnson-Laird [1983]. His nine theoretical constraints on what can count as a mental model include not only the condition that their construction and interpretation be *computable,* but also the principle that "the structures of mental models are identical to the structures of the states of affairs, whether perceived or conceived, that the models represent" [p. 419].

Johnson-Laird's concept of mental models was mentioned in Chapter 5, in the discussion of his procedural semantics. We saw there that his explanation of language-understanding posits not only propositional representations (whose form closely reflects the structure of the verbal input), but also mental models (which reflect the structure of the world-state being talked about). He shows how these may be used in interpreting a wide range of grammatical constructions and functor words, and in understanding a story or discourse whose thematic structure is reflected by (for example) the pronouns used. And his "psycholexicology" (discussed also in Chapter 7, below) betrays a commitment to innate semantic primitives, which appears also as one of the nine constraints on mental models: that they be constructed out of a *finite* set of innate conceptual primitives and operators, giving rise to a corresponding set of semantic fields.

Although Johnson-Laird took logic seriously in his procedural semantics (accepting the need to account for English words with near-equivalents in formal logic such as the quantifiers and connectives "all", "some", "most", "and", "or"), it was not the core of his theory. We saw, for instance, that in discussing definite descriptions (as in "The present King of France is bald") he rejected the two formal analyses previously suggested by logicians, and did not offer a third. Instead, he specified ways of building and using mental models in interpreting the sentence and assessing its truth-value.

In his account of problem-solving, likewise, Johnson-Laird takes logic seriously but does not explain reasoning in terms of logical rules. His central claim is that people solving problems (even problems that are amenable to the methods of logic) typically do not use logic, although occasionally some individuals do. Rather, they reason by constructing and transforming a class of representations of a more natural kind than lists of logical rules. He argues that mental models can support valid reasoning (although some lead to error), and that computational efficiency favours them over formal rules of inference. In short, whereas formal logic is a culture-specific cognitive resource (which even professors of logic often ignore), the ability to construct and reason with mental models is a general feature of the human mind.

The idea that, even when we *succeed* in solving "logical" problems such as syllogisms, we need not be using formal rules of inference did not originate with Johnson-Laird. Some psychologists had already claimed that their experimental subjects relied on alternative representations – such as Euler circles or Venn diagrams (and they seemed able to explain some, though not all, of the common errors made by experimental subjects). But he objects that, with respect to how these non-logical representations could be used, previous psychologists had posited information-processing of such a complicated kind that it can be plausibly attributed only, if at all, to a tiny minority of subjects. Using Euler circles, for instance, a single premise may need several different representations to cover all possibilities: thus "All of the artists are beekeepers" needs the two circles shown in Figure 6.3a, while "Some [i.e., at least some, and perhaps all] A are B" requires the four representations shown in Figure 6.3b; a syllogism with two premises may involve consideration of well over a dozen pairs of Euler circles.

Johnson-Laird relates his own account of our natural reasoning competence to an abstract semantic theory: possible-worlds semantics. This holds that the truth-conditions of a sentence are determined by the set of all possible worlds that can be taken as models of that sentence. Accordingly, he aims to show how valid reasoning is enabled by the construction and manipulation of *mental models* – as he puts it, by "getting the [infinite] possible worlds into the [finite] head". His nine constraints on mental models are grounded in semantic–ontological assumptions (such as a commitment to a finite set of semantic primitives). Many computable representations are not mental models in his sense, because their semantics are not specified as required by the other eight constraints: frames, scripts, schemata, and their many computational cousins (discussed in Chapter 5), for example, are not. His theory of problem-solving defines effective proce-

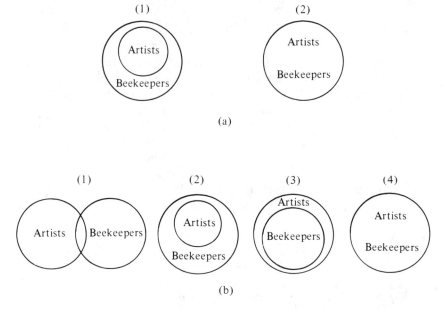

Fig. 6.3. (From P. N. Johnson-Laird [1983], *Mental Models: Towards a Cognitive Science of Language, Inference, and Consciousness.* Cambridge: Cambridge University Press. P. 78.)

dures for seeking counterexamples (which can exist only in some as-yet-unconsidered possible world) and for revising the current model as appropriate. Varying degrees of difficulty are explained in terms of the number and complexity of models needed to define the potentially relevant search-space (he claims that, of the sixty-four types of syllogism, those which are exceptionally difficult require the construction and integration of three distinct models). And systematic errors (failures to allow for all possible worlds) are attributed to specific inadequacies in mental models or the procedures for inspecting and revising them. His illustrative computer models, which build and manipulate their own internal models, show successes and failures comparable with those of his human subjects.

So far, so Marrian. Unlike physical optics, however, possible-worlds semantics – like theoretical semantics in general – is controversial. One would therefore not expect a psychology of reasoning based on theoretical semantics to be as persuasive as a psychology of low-level vision based on the principles of image-formation. Some of the nine constraints suggested by Johnson-Laird are independently questionable: thus we saw in Chapter 5 that the very existence of semantic primitives – never mind their specific nature – is disputed. The crucial concept of *representation* is likewise problematic; indeed, part of Johnson-Laird's aim is to develop a theory of what (natural) representations are like. It is hardly surprising, then, that some of his claims about the nature, typology, and principles of individuation of mental models are sketchy and/or not motivated in detail by the underlying semantic theory. However, his work is an interesting attempt to provide an abstractly grounded psychological theory in what Marr regarded as highly unpromising territory.

As an illustration of his approach, let us consider a simple syllogistic problem which, on Johnson-Laird's view, requires only one model for its solution. He asked people to say what conclusions (if any) follow from these two premises:

All of the artists are beekeepers [first premise].
All of the chemists are beekeepers [second premise].

Half of his subjects drew one or more of the following conclusions, each of which is erroneous: (1) all of the artists are chemists; (2) all of the chemists are artists; (3) some of the artists are chemists; and (4) some of the chemists are artists. Only 50 percent of subjects replied – correctly – that there is no valid conclusion interrelating the artists and chemists.

Johnson-Laird sees all syllogistic problem-solving as having three stages: (i) a mental model of the first premise is constructed; (ii) the information in the second premise is added to the mental model of the first premise, *taking into account the different ways in which this can be done;* (iii) a conclusion is formulated which expresses the relation, if any, between the end-terms (those terms which occur only in a single premise), and which holds in all the models of the premises. If the italicized portion of stage (ii) has not been thoroughly done, then stage (iii) is likely to produce conclusions whose truth (given the truth of the premises) is *not* guaranteed. This schema covers a wide range of reasoning procedures, and Johnson-Laird provides computer models of many of them.

His explanation of the experimental results noted above follows this three-stage schema. Each subject starts by forming a mental model satisfying the first premise, "All of the artists are beekeepers." This could conceivably be done in many different ways (including the two Euler circles shown in Figure 6.3a), which differ in the nature and complexity of the model itself, the procedures required to use it, or both. Johnson-Laird suggests that the first premise "is naturally modelled by imagining an arbitrary but finite number of artists and labelling each of them as a beekeeper" [1981, p. 140].

What counts as an "arbitrary" number? Johnson-Laird's gloss on this word claims that the (competent) subject, like the corresponding computer programs for constructing and manipulating models, chooses some number or other, *already knowing* that the number of entities depicted is irrelevant to any syllogistic (though not to any numerical or proportional) inference that is drawn. This gloss allows for the unpredictability of the number actually chosen, but it does not exclude certain rogue numbers. For instance, the number 1 is presumably inappropriate, since a model denoting only one artist-labelled-as-beekeeper would be better suited to represent the sentence "There is an artist who is a beekeeper"; 2,281,896 would be unusable by people; perhaps it must be more than 1 but no more than "the magical number seven, plus or minus two" [Miller, 1956] (although even 7, associated as it is with cabbalistic mysteries, might sometimes be more distracting than helpful).

One example of a model of the first premise that might be constructed by "imagining an arbitrary but finite number of artists and labelling each of them as a beekeeper", says Johnson-Laird, is the symbolic tableau:

$a = b$
$a = b$
$a = b$

This model could lead one to infer (by means of a relatively simple procedure) that all of the beekeepers are artists, which may or may not be so. People do sometimes take it that "All B's are A's", given that "All A's are B's": if their mental model is like this one, such a conclusion would be natural. An alternative model of the first premise, which would guard against this implication while still leaving it open as a possibility, is:

$a = b$
$a = b$
$a = b$
  (b)
  (b)
  (b)

The brackets around the items in the bottom half of this tableau symbolize the fact that beekeepers-who-are-not-artists may or may not exist. Someone doing syllogistic reasoning would be better served by the latter representation, because this explicitly allows for a set of possible worlds implicitly excluded by the former.

Next, the subject must form a model of the second premise, "All of the chemists are beekeepers." The model of the second premise is sometimes constrained by the model already constructed to represent the first premise; for instance, some syllogisms require that the *same* number of items be used to represent the middle term in both premise-models. In the case being illustrated, let us assume that a model of the second premise is formed in the way just described for the first premise, thus:

$c = b$
$c = b$
$c = b$
  (b)
  (b)
  (b)

The next step is somehow to combine the information in the second premise with that in the first. That is, the models representing the two premises must be integrated. (This could be done in various ways, as we shall see.) Then, the problem-solver must use the resulting integrated model to formulate a putative conclusion, subsequent testing of which may prompt revision of the model. The initial constraints on this conclusion are that it be true of the current integrated model and that it interrelate the two end-terms: "artists" and "chemists". However, depending on the nature of the model, the inference may or may not be valid.

For example, one premise-integration model that could easily – though inadvisably – be constructed by a very simple procedure (given that the number of artist-tokens happens to be the same as the number of chemist-tokens) is this:

a = b = c
a = b = c
a = b = c
   (b)
   (b)
   (b)

(Notice that the sets of bracketed b-tokens have been conflated.) Such a model would allow one to infer, invalidly: *all of the artists are chemists,* and/ or *all of the chemists are artists.* Johnson-Laird believes that people some-times do construct a model of this general type, since (as noted with respect to items (1) and (2) above) some of his subjects did draw these faulty conclusions.

A different way of combining the second premise with the first would be:

a = b = c
a = b = c
a = b
    b = c
   (b)
   (b)

A model like this one could be constructed from the two premises by way of a clearly definable token-matching procedure, directing the removal of one pair of brackets and the matching of the newly unbracketed b-token with one of the c-tokens. Some such procedure may be already available to the experienced reasoner; but Johnson-Laird specifies a computational procedure by which the second integrated model could be constructed as a result of testing and modifying the first [1983, p.132]. This second model, unlike the first, would not enable one to make the invalid inferences (1) and (2). But it also is unsatisfactory, because it would allow the unaccept-able "conclusions" (3) and/or (4) above (*some of the artists are chemists* and/or *some of the chemists are artists*).

About half the experimental subjects said – correctly – that *no* conclusion linking the artists and the chemists can validly be drawn from the two premises. Johnson-Laird [1981,p.141] suggests that, "fortunately for the rational reputation of the human race", their final model was something like this:

a = b
a = b
a = b
    b = c
    b = c
    b = c

Again, a procedure can be clearly defined for producing this model by combining the two premise-models (the bracketed b-tokens are here not conflated but dropped). None of the four commonly drawn invalid inferences, (1) to (4) above, is enabled by such a model.

The rational reputation of the human race notwithstanding, this last tableau would seem naturally (*sic*) to support the invalid inferences *None of the artists are chemists* and *None of the chemists are artists*. Certainly, the rules of tableau-interpretation may be specified so as to preclude these invalid inferences. But they seem *prima facie* to be naturally available. This raises the question of what is meant by a natural representation and a natural use (interpretation) of one.

Johnson-Laird regards mental models as *natural* in two broad senses. First, their origins and usefulness lie in our perceptual abilities. Much as some connectionists hope to explain the solution of logical–mathematical problems in terms of our powers of pattern-matching, so Johnson-Laird sees mental models as being generated and explored with the help of our powers of perception and imagination. This should not be taken too literally: the term "imagining" in the recipe "imagining an arbitrary but finite number of artists and labelling each of them as a beekeeper" does not imply that the problem-solver must form any mental pictures of artists (though this may happen). Rather, *some inner symbol or other* is set up to represent each artist, each of which tokens is somehow linked to some symbol representing a beekeeper – and the tokens and links (and thus the overall structure of the model) are manipulable by operations of a broadly *perceptual* nature.

The second feature of a natural mental model of discourse, according to Johnson-Laird, is that its structure "corresponds directly to the structure of the state of affairs that the discourse describes" [1983, p. 125]. This is why, despite his basic emphasis on quasi-perceptual operations, he sometimes recommends discrete representations in preference to continuous ones. Thus his approach to syllogistic reasoning depends on his belief that, in general, models mapping one finite set of individual tokens onto another (like the various tableaux shown above) are more natural than representations (such as Euler circles or Venn diagrams) which map finite sets of individuals onto infinities of points. (This is not to say that non-natural representations are never useful: if the previous example were represented

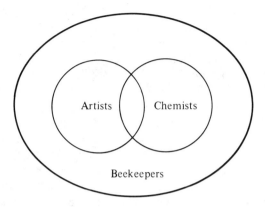

Fig. 6.4.

by the diagram in Figure 6.4, we should not be tempted – as we are by Johnson-Laird's preferred tableau shown above – to infer either *None of the artists are chemists* or *None of the chemists are artists.*)

Mental models, on Johnson-Laird's view, should not be seen as the poor man's way of doing things that could be better done by way of abstract principles. They are not a second-best to logic. On the contrary, he argues that mental models often enable us to make valid inferences – and to understand language – where logic does not.

For instance, he suggests a simple spatial model for representing the meaning of "to the left of" which allows us to infer (validly) *both* that if A is immediately to the left of B, and B of C, then A is to the left of C, *and* that if A is to the left of B, and B of C, and . . . Y of Z, then A is *not* necessarily to the left of Z. Thus, according to this model, "to the left of" acts as a transitive relation over short chains, but not necessarily over long ones. This may sound like nonsense. But Johnson-Laird reminds us of a circular dinner-table: Mary may be to the left of Joan, and Joan of Sally, and . . . of Ann – but Ann may be *to the right of* Mary. (What counts as a short chain is relative, and we must be able to construct models representing tables of different sizes: if the table is tiny, compared with the size of the people sitting round it, even Sally may not be to the left of Mary, but rather *opposite* her.) The phrase "to the left of" will probably be understood in a strictly transitive way by all concerned whenever *transitivity* is being discussed by logicians, or Piagetians. But people can, and do, interpret this phrase differently (by means of distinct mental models) in different contexts, and this variability of the ordinary-language phrase has to be allowed for in explaining how we can reason with it.

The thought-processes involved in commonsense reasoning and adventurous thinking are generally acknowledged to be even more elusive than those needed for cryptarithmetic or syllogisms. *A fortiori,* in Johnson-

Laird's view, they are not amenable to purely formal accounts of reasoning. (Thus he is sceptical of the work done by AI-researchers on *nonmonotonic reasoning,* in which the current representation has to be revised because new information is discovered to be inconsistent with it [Doyle, 1979; McDermott & Doyle, 1980; Davis, 1980; McCarthy, 1980; 1986].) Informal models and analogies are crucial to everyday reasoning, and the psychologist must attempt to describe how they work.

But Johnson-Laird faces an even greater challenge with respect to these phenomena than most psychologists do, because of his claim (noted above) that the structure of mental models corresponds directly to the structure of the state of affairs they represent. A psychology of mental models which satisfied this criterion would be a theory not only of the mind, but of the world (and all possible worlds) too. For to be able to identify the structure of the state of affairs in general, one would need answers to the fundamental questions of philosophical semantics, ontology, and metaphysics. If Johnson-Laird's typology of mental models (described briefly below) is both sketchy and controversial, this is due not least to the difficulty of these highly abstract questions.

In an attempt to provide the groundwork for dealing with all of human reasoning in a systematic way, Johnson-Laird outlines a provisional (and, he allows, very likely incomplete) typology of mental models. These are broadly classified as *physical* and *conceptual,* representing physical and abstract domains respectively (but conceptual models can represent the physical world too). Each class and sub-class involves specific computational primitives, operations, and constraints.

He defines six intrinsically different types of physical model (though does not exemplify them in detail), each of which is said to be somehow isomorphic with the physical structures it represents. These are hierarchically ordered, in that each model-type is defined in terms of the preceding one. The basic member of the hierarchy is a *relational* model, which is a static "frame" consisting of a finite set of tokens (with a finite set of properties) representing a finite set of physical entities (and properties), and a finite set of relations between the tokens representing physical relations between the entities. Building on this base, Johnson-Laird defines what he terms *spatial, temporal, kinematic,* and *dynamic* models, and *images.* A spatial model is a relational model in which the only relations are spatial, and tokens are located within a (symbolic) 2D- or 3D-space. A temporal model is a sequence of spatial models in time (not necessarily real time: an evolutionist can think of the first cavemen only a split second after thinking of the last dinosaurs). A kinematic model is a temporal model (which may or may not run in real time) that represents change as continuous. A dynamic model is a kinematic model with causal relations represented in it. Finally, an image (which Johnson-Laird likens to Marr's 2½D-Sketch) represents the visible characteristics of a 3D spatial or kinematic model.

Johnson-Laird's discussion of *conceptual* models (which depends heavily on his procedural semantics) likewise attempts a principled classification, as opposed to a collection of theoretically unrelated examples. Each of the four types of conceptual model is constructed from its parts according to constraints which, he claims, result in its being usable in specific semantically coherent ways. The most basic conceptual model is *monadic,* and is used in representing assertions about individuals, their properties, and identities between them. A monadic model is constructed out of: a finite number of tokens representing individuals and properties; the two binary relations of identity and non-identity (of individuals or of properties); and a notation (like the brackets in the syllogism-tableaux, above) indicating that the existence of a particular sort of entity is uncertain. A *relational* model has, in addition, a finite number of relations between the tokens. This enables the representation not only of problems involving predicates like "father of", but also of problems posed in terms of definite descriptions (such as "the present King of France") and various quantifiers (such as "more than"). The *meta-linguistic* models contain tokens which correspond to linguistic expressions and to relations between expressions and models. This recursiveness in principle enables one to reason about one's own reasoning, and about propositional attitudes (including goals and beliefs) generally. Finally, *set-theoretic* models contain tokens which represent sets (as opposed to individuals), and *the members of those sets must be specified before the set-theoretic model is formed.*

Johnson-Laird's detailed justifications of his model-typology have a Marrian flavour. For example, the set-theoretic constraint italicized above is not based on experimental studies of model-construction in subjects solving problems about sets. Rather, it is included specifically to prevent the thinker from generating the inconsistencies associated with Russell's paradox. (Consider the set of all sets that are not members of themselves. Is *this* set a member of itself or not? If it is, it isn't – and if it isn't, it is.) Johnson-Laird is not reporting a contingent fact, but arguing *a priori* that the avoidance of paradoxical contradictions requires such a constraint, since without it rationality would not be possible. Similarly, his claims that certain forms of model are in principle adequate to represent particular logical connectives, quantifiers, and definite or indefinite descriptions rest not on experimental results but on abstract argument. And his assessment of the varying difficulty of distinct syllogisms stems from his theory about the computational adequacy of the relevant models; the role of his experiments involving syllogisms is to test these predictions.

This is not to say that his supposed justifications are always acceptable. For instance, even if everyday thinking is usually constrained by the condition on set-theoretic models cited above, *not all* rational thought can be so bounded; Lord Russell deliberately ignored any such limitation when formulating his paradox for the technical purposes of set-theory. Strict proofs as to the computational adequacy of a given model (or set of models) for solving a problem can be provided only for relatively well-understood problems. Johnson-Laird's work on syllogistic reasoning has not gone unchallenged [Rips, 1986], and (as he admits) his hierarchical categorization of mental models is sketchy and incomplete, and its philosophical foundations are shaky. The bounds on useful representations, and the basic concept of *representation* itself, are obscure (other computationally informed discussions include Amarel, 1968; Hayes, 1974; and Sloman, 1978, 1985, and in preparation). Finally, much as vision may often involve theoretically messy short-cut procedures acquired by learning or evolution, so reasoning also may often rely on short-cut measures (including useful but unsystematic analogies); a theory adequate to *guarantee* successful reasoning may not explain all the true conclusions actually reached by people – not to mention all the inconsistencies or mistakes. Nevertheless, Johnson-Laird has made an interesting attempt to develop a principled answer to the question how everyday reasoning is *possible.*

Theories of reasoning, especially if they posit improvement due to error-detection, typically have implications for the psychology of learning. Thus Johnson-Laird discusses not only the building of mental models, but their revision; and Newell and Simon believe that their theories can illuminate learning as well as problem-solving. Let us turn, then, to discuss computational approaches to learning and development.

7 Learning and development

Few computer models of learning or development achieve a significant match to human behaviour (and even technological learning programs are less impressive than other results in artificial intelligence). Some would say that this is because learning and development involve processes of a type which cannot be modelled using current computer technology. Others (some of whom share the view just mentioned) would say that it is because our theoretical understanding of these psychological phenomena is weaker in the first place.

Do we know, for example, what is the theoretical distinction between *learning* and *development* – or even whether there is one? Do we have any clear notions as to what abstractly definable task or tasks might underlie them, at what D. Marr called the computational level? Are there any useful mathematical results about learning or development which psychologists should bear in mind? Is learning a genuine class (what philosophers call a *natural kind*), such that at least some common principles underlie every instance? Or are there fundamentally different types of learning (for instance, concept-learning and skill-learning), for which utterly distinct theories are appropriate? Is there a radical theoretical distinction between piecemeal incremental learning and holistic behavioural change (such as Piagetian developmental stages)? Must any adequate theory of learning or development posit psychological processes of a type that can be modelled only in computers more brainlike than von Neumann machines? If so, do we have any ideas about the specific computational constraints and potential involved? If self-organizing systems are able to learn things without being taught, is task-analysis unnecessary in explaining learning? And what of empiricism and rationalism: Can one learn starting from a *tabula rasa,* or must the mind already possess a rich computational structure if it is to be able to learn anything new?

The poverty of empiricism

With respect to the last of these questions, many early researchers in artificial intelligence shared A. M. Turing's broadly empiricist assumption: "Presumably the child brain is something like a notebook as one buys it from the stationer's. Rather little mechanism and lots of blank sheets. . . . Our hope is that there is so little mechanism in the child brain that something like it can be easily programmed" [Turing, 1950, p. 31]. Accordingly, they hoped that learning might be possible in self-organizing systems with minimal prior content or structure.

However, subsequent theoretical work on the computational prerequisites of learning has shown this hope, at least in its extreme form, to be illusory. (So, too, has empirical research in developmental psychology: babies have more inbuilt psychological structure than empiricism allows.) Unstructured self-organizing systems can learn little of any interest; as we shall see later, they are *in principle* incapable of acquiring even some concepts that one would expect to fall within their competence. More generally, it has become increasingly evident that psychologists must adopt the "Kantian" position (see Chapter 2) that learning involves prior interpretative processes, some of which are innate and/or not open to conscious control. To seek a theory of learning within a computational psychology is necessarily to accept that every learning system possesses some inbuilt computational structure and elementary meanings.

The learning programs that will be described provide some illustrative examples, but the point has been argued in abstract terms by J. A. Fodor [1976], who (while not discussing any specific computer models) saw computer science as providing the clearest account of computation. He pointed out that the notion of computation *presupposes* some system of representation: some descriptive language capable of coding discriminations, and a set of symbolic transformations that preserve semantic properties such as truth and reference. As he put it, "no computation without representation". (The term "computational" carries the implications just listed even if, as suggested in Chapter 3, not all computational processes are of the formal-syntactic type characteristic of von Neumann machines which Fodor had in mind.)

Indeed, Fodor's anti-empiricist argument went much further than this. He claimed also that human beings must be born already possessing a representational system capable of expressing the content of all the concepts learnt throughout infancy and adult life, from "cat" through "curry" to "computer". Contrary to what we normally assume, concept-learning does not result in new conceptual, or semantic, content. In Fodor's words, "You cannot learn a language whose terms express semantic properties not expressed by the terms of some language you are already able to use" [p. 61]. There must therefore be an innate language of thought ("mentalese"), a species-specific psychological universal comparable with N. Chomsky's linguistic universals.

Fodor arrives at his highly counterintuitive conclusion by arguing that only one coherent kind of psychological theory for concept-learning has ever been proposed, or is even conceivable. This treats concept-learning as a process of inductive extrapolation: the formation and subsequent confirmation of hypotheses. The learner therefore must have a language, or representational system, that is capable of expressing the hypothesis *prior* to learning. Fodor adds that new predicates (concepts) can be generated only by way of explicit definitions in terms of existing predicates. This entails that learning cannot add semantic content. In principle, all concepts reduce to (are translatable into) combinations of elementary concepts that are not, and cannot be, learnt – and which are therefore innate.

The weak point in Fodor's argument is his assumption that the meaning of new concepts can be given only by explicit definitions in terms of previously existing ones (ultimately, of the elementary predicates). There is an alternative account of meaning, originally developed within the philosophy of science (a theory Fodor actually recommends later in his book). Theoretical concepts in science denote unobservable entities. So, although they must be rooted in observation-statements, they are not directly definable in observational terms. They can however be *implicitly* defined by "meaning-postulates": sets of axioms (theories) in which the new concepts are mentioned [Carnap, 1956]. These axioms, together with the inferential network linking them to other theoretical axioms and to observation-statements, provide a *partial* definition of the new terms – much as geometrical axioms partially define "point" and "line". The term's meaning can be indefinitely enriched or refined by adding further axioms, some of which will contain still newer theoretical terms. It follows, *pace* Fodor, that new concepts can be added to a language without having to be translatable into the elementary terms of that language.

But if Fodor's extreme nativism must be rejected, his more modest version stands. He is correct when he argues that *some* fairly complex representational system must be presupposed by a computational psychology. This implies that simulating a child's mind will be less easy than Turing hoped. For all programs capable of learning must start out with significant computational structures and expectations.

This is true, for instance, of the pioneering computer models of learning – one a "concept-learner" and the other a "skill-learner" – developed by P. H. Winston [1975] and D. A. Waterman [1970] respectively.

Winston's concept-learning program (which I have elsewhere described at length [Boden, 1987, chap. 10]) used examples, and counterexamples, to learn simple structural concepts such as *arch*, *table*, and the like. Its success depended on having small sample-sets, carefully ordered to minimize the differences between current concept and current sample. That is, the counterexamples presented by Winston were near-misses, having as few differences as possible (preferably, only one) from the learner's current concept. (For the present, we may ignore the fact, whose general significance will be discussed later, that Winston's account of *just what* his program could learn was misleading.)

As the first version of its concept of "arch", it used its description of the first positive example it encountered. This description might note (for example) that an arch has two blocks supporting another block. Thereafter, on being shown further samples (of non-arches as well as arches), it could modify its current concept in two ways. Either it could generalize the concept by substituting a superordinate for a subordinate term (which allows both "slabs" and "pyramids" to be the top "object" in an arch), or it could make the concept more specific by marking a previously listed property as necessary rather than merely permissible (which captures the fact that the inner sides of the two supporting blocks must not touch each other). It did not make concepts more specific by substituting a subordinate for a superordinate term, because its initial description was couched at the lowest hierarchical level (so a slab would be described as a "slab", not as an "object").

This concept-learner was far from a *tabula rasa*. All the concepts it learned had to be defined in terms of a previously specified set of properties and relations. Moreover, its methods of comparing samples, so as to arrive at a coherent concept covering all and only the positive instances, were provided by the programmer. It relied on inbuilt "comparison-notes" for representing logically distinct differences between current concept and current sample. These determined the concept-modifications, such as hierarchical generalization and the addition of "must" or "must-not" labels to particular properties or relations. In short, it knew *all and only* the relevant properties before its learning started, and it knew *what* conceptual modifications to apply *when*. In light of the anti-empiricist point made above, the pre-primed nature of Winston's program is no accident.

Insofar as Winston's model had psychological relevance, his methods of example-comparison and concept-modification were reminiscent of the type of concept-learning that had been experimentally investigated some years earlier by J. S. Bruner and colleagues [Bruner, Goodnow & Austin, 1956]. In these tasks, the concepts are arbitrarily defined by the experimenter in terms of conjunctions of distinct observable properties (like colour, relative size, and geometrical shape), which are the only salient properties present in the test-material. On the basis of his experimental data, Bruner had defined certain general "strategies" for sample-selection and concept-modification, noting the distinct informational conditions in which they were used by his subjects. And he had produced a logical analysis of the experimental tasks (similar to that informing Winston's model), which showed that these sampling strategies were often optimal, thus making concept-modification relatively efficient. But whereas Winston's program could deal with hierarchical concepts, Bruner's logically simpler learning-strategies could not, because he did not define his concepts in terms of hiearchically related properties (thus "red" was not subdivided into "scarlet" and "crimson").

Among the psychological studies prompted by Bruner's example were a series of experiments and computer models directed by E. B. Hunt [Hunt, Marin & Stone, 1966]. Although he studied the learning of naturally occurring concepts as well as newly defined ones, Hunt shared Bruner's and Winston's basic assumption that concepts can be thought of as sets of rules. (Fodor accepted this assumption too, as we shall see; but some philosophers deny it and reject psychological accounts of learning and development based on it [Geach, 1957; Hamlyn, 1978].) On this view, people possess a set of concepts (C1, C2, . . . Cn) and rules (R1, R2, . . . Rn) about when to apply them. Three such rules might be: "If a thing has properties *a, b,* and *c,* it is a C1"; "If a thing has properties *x, y,* and *z* – but not *q* – it is a C2"; and "If a thing has property *r,* it is *not* a C3."

One of the conditions Hunt investigated was naturalistic concept-learning, in which the learner is told not only *whether* each sample is an example or counterexample, but also *why* (the properties responsible for its classification are explicitly identified). He found that, even when this discriminatory information is provided, it is not always easy for the learner to arrive at an explicit definition of the concept concerned. Nor is it easy for the teacher to define the concept, if asked to do so. For, where naturally occurring concepts are concerned, many of the rules are tacit, being made explicit only when the person is required to say what are the properties of *particular examples* (classified as C1, or C2) which make one classification appropriate and another inappropriate. Moreover, the rules are often given as a ragbag, not as a systematically constructed concept. Some of them may even be mutually contradictory.

According to this psychological approach, concept-learning is discovering both which properties to look for and how best to look for them. Hunt and his colleagues outlined a number of tree-search techniques to describe their subjects' behaviour, and discussed their comparative efficiency. Some of these techniques were embodied in their domain-independent General Enquirer program, which could be used by social scientists to carry out a crude type of content-analysis on textual materials. And their work on learning strategies was later developed by J. R. Quinlan [1979; 1982; 1983] as the ID3 algorithm, an inductive concept-learner whose technological applications include various purpose-built AI-programs and expert-system shells.

Quinlan's concept-learning algorithm is more powerful than Winston's in a number of ways. It is domain-independent. It can cope with much larger sets of examples, presented in any order. It can learn from experience which properties to look for first (although in the last analysis it can seek only those properties already specified to it). It can provide the programmer with a better representation of the concept being learnt than was given to it in the first place. It can find the most efficient method of classification in a given domain if it is provided with a representative sample of the range of real-world cases. And it sometimes discovers useful regularities of a fairly complex kind, previously unknown to human experts – such as new rules for chess end-games.

Like Winston's program, however, the ID3 algorithm is no *tabula rasa*. It has built-in computational assumptions about how hierarchical classificatory information should be organized, which enable it to analyse its input sensibly. Given a set of rules having the simple logical form described above, ID3 can identify any inconsistencies. As well as this logical tidying, it learns from experience. From a large collection of input-examples (each described to it by one or more rules), it extracts an overall classification-rule in the form of a decision-tree. (The input-description usually mentions only properties known to be relevant. But, provided that it can tell whether an example falls into the relevant class, ID3 can assess a property's relevance itself. Thus it used seemingly irrelevant board-descriptions as the basis of its identification of previously unknown winning-patterns for chess end-games.)

The individual decisions are ordered by their position in the decision-tree. The algorithm is *guaranteed* to find the shortest tree-search by which to classify the examples given to it. That is, it learns to ask the right questions in the right order, so as to decide as quickly as possible whether something is an example of C1 or C2, or . . . Cn. Suppose, for instance, that having property q is a sufficient condition for something's falling under the concept C1. Even if it is just as easy to check for q as for any other property (which in practice may not be true), it does not follow that the most efficient decision-procedure will start by looking for it. For property q may be possessed by only a tiny percentage of the exemplars of C1. Even if property q were a *necessary* condition of C1, it might sometimes be sensible to consider other properties first – for instance, if examples of C1 were comparatively rare within the corpus.

Despite its psychological origin (in Hunt's work), Quinlan's algorithm is not psychologically realistic. Lacking our short-term-memory limitations, it can search much larger example-sets than we can (including sets so large that not all examples can be considered in its fast memory simultaneously). It does not model human difficulties in processing negative or disjunctive information, which influence subjects' learning even of logically simple concepts [Bruner *et al.*, 1956]. And it ignores the fact that, in practice, some relevant properties are more difficult to identify, less salient, than others. But this does not make it psychologically irrelevant. It tells us that a theory of concept-learning positing hierarchical discrimination-trees and mental computations equivalent to those of ID3, albeit limited by short-term-memory considerations, could in principle explain successful performance in a wide variety of cases. And it offers a structure within which to explore different weightings of relevant properties with varying perceptual salience.

Skills and task-analysis

Concept-learning is one thing, skill-learning another – at least, so it appears at first sight. The second pioneering model of learning mentioned above (and there described as a skill-learner) was Waterman's poker-player, which improves its poker-skill by modifying its heuristics for betting. It can learn both "explicitly" (where a "trainer" supplies explicit information about the ways in which a bet is sensible or risky) and "implicitly" (where the program has to work this out for itself in the course of playing). Even in the latter case, it learns to play as well as an experienced (non-professional) person.

But, like Winston's model, it does not do so in a computational vacuum. The evaluations and alterations of the program's betting strategy are guided by the abstract constraints on poker-play. These include not only the rules of the game (whereby a Royal Flush beats a Full House), but also general "axioms" (such as "*If* you-bet-high or you-bet-low *then* you-keep-betting", and "*If* you-bet-high and opponent's-hand-is-higher-than-your-hand *then* you-bluff-opponent") and ways of classifying the program's hand as "excellent", "good", "fair", or "poor" (by assigning quantitative values to the various cards). These constraints inform the program's changing hypotheses about why it won or lost. Thus the heuristics it learns take into account the quality of the program's hand, the size of the pot, the size of the last bet, and the opponent's general style of play. (For example: if your hand is poor, bet high if the pot is small, the opponent's last bet is small, and the opponent is conservative and can be easily bluffed; if your hand is fair, bet high if the pot is not large, the opponent has just replaced one card, and either the opponent is easily bluffed or his last bet is small.)

In addition to highly task-specific knowledge about poker, Waterman's program is supplied with ways of recognizing the need for various types of rule-change and ways of effecting them. The changes made by the poker-learner are primarily *generalization* of rules found to be over-specific, *specialization* of rules that are over-general, and *pruning* of redundant rules (though in the explicit training mode, the program can also *insert* new rules suggested to it by the trainer). These modifications are carried out by heuristics (ordered for priority by Waterman) for altering heuristics. One such learning heuristic is the generalization of an existing action-rule by enlarging the set(s) defined by one or more of the symbolic values in the rule. Another is the sort of generalization that makes one or more variables in the rule irrelevant (this is applicable only in the implicit training mode, because the trainer will not have drawn attention to an irrelevant feature).

The priority-ordering of heuristics (both for playing and for learning) solves – or, rather, avoids – the problem of conflict-resolution in selecting heuristics. All the heuristics are coded as condition–action productions, which (unlike the productions described in Chapter 6) are placed on an ordered list. During play, the program searches the list of play-heuristics from top to bottom, until it finds one whose left-hand condition is matched. Any heuristics elsewhere (below) in the list whose conditions are also matched will not fire, because they will not be found: after a production has been triggered, the program starts at the top of the list again. The priority-ordering itself can be modified, so that learning involves not only transforming the content of productions (generalizing or specializing their conditions) but also altering the priority-relations within the ordered list.

Waterman's was one of the first models of skill-learning to be based on production-systems. This methodology has since been widely used by experimental psychologists (many, like Waterman himself, students of A. Newell and H. A. Simon) to model the acquisition of skills. One example is P. Langley's [1982] model of language-acquisition, in which the linguistic rules are incrementally improved by recovery from errors – not, as in Waterman's model, from both successes and failures. Since the focus is on the role of negative examples in learning, Langley's model relies on the discrimination (not generalization) of rules. Another (which has implications for the design not only of man–machine interfaces but of time-sharing computer systems in general) is an experimentally based model of how people learn to use a word-processor, in which the learner's skill is represented at a number of levels, down to the individual finger-movements involved in typing [Card, Moran & Newell, 1983].

A prime reason for the popularity of production-systems is that, because of the independence of the individual rules, they can represent *gradual* learning. It might seem *prima facie* that this theoretical strength carries with it a complementary weakness: perhaps production-system models of skill-learning can allow *only* for the incremental addition of new forms of behaviour, *not* for overall behavioural change? However, this is to underestimate the generality of the representation, or logical form, concerned. This is evident, for instance, in the production-systems written by J. H. Larkin [1979; Larkin *et al.*, 1980] to model the acquisition of problem-solving expertise in physics.

Experiments show a holistic change in people's skill: novices and experts differ less in their physical knowledge than in how they access and use it. They have distinct strategies for selecting potentially relevant principles from long-term memory; and where a novice carries out several distinct steps (writing an equation, binding the variables in it, and then solving it), the expert gives the result immediately. Larkin and her colleagues model novice and expert by *means–end* and *knowledge-development* strategies respectively. Means–end analysis uses top-down problem-solving ("backward-chaining"): it notes the *desired* physical quantity or variable, searches for any equations including that quantity, and then works backwards – marking as "desired" any unbound variable needed to solve the equations on the way. The knowledge-development method, which requires the execution of only half as many productions as means–end analysis does, works bottom-up (by "forward-chaining"). It begins with the *known* quantities in the problem statement, and applies appropriate equations to derive new quantities from them until the desired quantity is reached. Since this strategy only selects a physical principle for use when it knows that all but one of the quantities mentioned in it are known, it can be modelled by "collapsed" productions, whereby a principle is both selected and applied in only one step. Larkin and her colleagues give rules for the identification and collapse of principles, by means of which the system's observed form of behaviour is changed.

In effect, then, the knowledge of physics which initially was stored as separate facts becomes converted to a procedural form. Many computational psychologists believe that expertise in general, from tying one's shoe-laces to doing physics, involves automatization of this sort. Such a change in knowledge-representation could explain why information that is consciously accessed while a skill is being learnt comes to be ignored (and may even be inaccessible) once the skill has been acquired. Our initial verbal representations about what to do gradually give way to unverbalized (possibly even unverbalizable) habits of action.

The development of declarative knowledge-that into procedural knowledge-how relates to the philosophical question of what counts as a *basic action* [Boden, 1973]. If a basic action is defined as an action that requires no special conscious attention, then some basic actions – such as the expert's selection and application of a principle of physics – start out as non-basic ones. But if defined as an action that requires no special attention and is *also* a gift, *at no time* compounded of more elementary actions, then raising one's arm is a basic action, but applying one's knowledge of physics is not. (Since even paradigm-cases of basic action are skills not possessed by newborn babies, psychologists should explain sensorimotor development in terms of elemental motor-procedures identified at a much finer level of detail than the philosopher's basic actions. Marr's early psychophysiological work outlined a computational theory of cerebellar development that might account for the increasing smoothness and co-ordination of the baby's arm-raising [Marr, 1969].)

The automatization view of skill-learning informs J. R. Anderson's [1983] ambitious ACT* system, a model of cognition in which, as in Larkin's model, task-knowledge initially stored in declarative form gradually comes to be procedurally compiled. (We saw in Chapter 6 that although ACT*'s procedural knowledge is represented as a production-system, its declarative knowledge is stored as a semantic network.) ACT*'s cognitive skills – which, as in the Larkin model, employ both backward and forward search – tackle tasks such as finding (simple) geometry-proofs, writing programs in the LISP programming language, and producing textbook-like translations of sentences from English to French.

ACT*'s problem-solving gets started by way of *general* interpretative productions, which take items of declarative knowledge as data and use them in various ways (depending on the task-environment). In solving geometry-problems, for instance, ACT* calls first on its store of geometrical facts (postulates, theorems, and definitions) and schematic examples of worked-through problems. These two sources of declarative knowledge about geometry are applied by skill-independent problem-solving procedures that embody no geometrical expertise.

Subsequent practice leads to learning, which involves both the reinforcement and the creation of production-rules. Rules are reinforced, or strengthened (their likelihood of being chosen increases) so long as they are not found to lead to errors. If they do result in errors, they are weakened (but no alternative rule is proposed unless the discrimination-process mentioned below can come into play).

New rules are created by three main processes: *proceduralization, composition,* and *tuning.* Proceduralization takes place when a declarative item has been used in a particular way several times: general learning processes create a new production, which omits the interpretative step and applies the knowledge directly. The declarative item remains in the semantic net, so that ACT* comes to possess multiple, logically redundant, representations of equivalent information. Composition produces one production where there were several before: so an oft-used sequence of steps (productions) is collapsed into one only. The initial productions remain in the system and continue to be active until the new rule has been successfully used, and reinforced, so often that it regularly takes priority over the older rules; consequently, learning is even more gradual than it would be if the addition of a new rule led immediately to its use whenever possible. And tuning enables ACT* to learn which problem-solving operators are more appropriate to specific task-features.

Tuning improves those rules which have already had some degree of success, as opposed to deleting or amending those rules which have been unsuccessful. This adaptive learning is modelled in four ways: by *analogy,* in which methods are chosen that have already succeeded on similar problem-statements (irrespective of their solutions); by *generalization,* which starts from two similar problem-solutions and produces a rule that applies to both the problems-with-solutions involved (basically, by replacing constants with variables in the rule-condition – but extra constraints need to be added to prevent over-generalization); by *discrimination,* in which errors (in the form of near-misses) lead the condition or the action of a rule to be restricted to make it more selective; and by *composition* (similar to that described above).

In justification of his model, Anderson appeals to the "sufficiency condition" for a psychological theory of skill-learning: that it should specify mechanisms powerful enough to produce the observed behaviour. The sufficiency condition is taken seriously by all computational psychologists, since a program's producing performance *p* proves beyond question that it is powerful enough to generate *p* (whereas a verbal theory's predicting *p* does not). And the *p* generated by Anderson's computer model of skill-learning does match his experimental data (mostly on students learning geometry or LISP-programming). To this extent, it is psychologically persuasive. But we noted in Chapter 2, with respect to S. M. Kosslyn's model of visual imagery, that even a very detailed match to experimental data may be achieved by essentially *ad hoc* means, leaving basic theoretical questions open. Various theoretical weaknesses of Anderson's approach to learning will be discussed in the following section.

It was noted above that production-systems are especially well suited to model gradual, experiential, learning (as opposed to highly structured and carefully ordered tutorials) – though this is not to deny that other forms of representation can model such phenomena. In recommending production-systems for this purpose, it is commonly said that any rule can easily be added at any time, and that individual rules can easily be identified for the purpose of evaluation and criticism.

This is true, to a large extent. The problems of credit-assignment (deciding which actions are useful or unhelpful) are lessened if the various actions or heuristics are individually expressed as distinct productions. (For an account – relevant to evolution as well as psychology – of how *sub-goals* might be rewarded even though the overall process fails, see Holland, 1984.) Moreover, because productions are logically independent, a new rule can always be added without rewriting any other. And, given a system-architecture (like that described in Chapter 6, but unlike Waterman's) in which rule-firing depends only on simultaneous pattern-matching of all conditions, the programmer does not have to worry about where to put the new rule.

However, the result will not necessarily be a useful or coherent system: there is nothing to stop one adding "if *p* then not-*q*" to a rule-base that already contains "If *p* then *q*". (Technological *expert systems* are bedevilled by unmanageable rule interactions, as extra productions are added to represent further details of the human expert's knowledge.) Simple architectural principles can ensure that something will always get done, even if contradictory rules co-exist. But, since "learning" implies not mere change but also improvement, content-neutral conventions cannot suffice for modelling learning.

In short, analysis of the learnt task is necessary in the production-system approach too. Whether or not there are any domain-independent principles of learning, the precise nature of the prior computational structures needed by a learner will depend on just what it is that is to be learnt.

The general theoretical importance of task-analysis was discussed in Chapter 3 in relation to the psychology of vision. In that context, we noted H. C. Longuet-Higgins' contribution to the theory of stereopsis; his theory of musical perception, drawing on his elaboration of the fundamental theory of harmony, was mentioned in Chapter 6; indeed, most of his work offers some abstract analysis of the task, not only an algorithm capable of performing it [Longuet-Higgins, 1987]. It is no accident, then, that he has inspired a psychologically motivated computer model of learning that highlights task-analysis as a theoretical priority [Power & Longuet-Higgins, 1978].

Longuet-Higgins' program learns the numerals, or number-names, in various natural languages. Its original input is a small sample of numerals in the language concerned, each identified as denoting a specific number. Eventually it becomes capable of generating a potentially infinite set of numerals, attached to the relevant numbers. If one then inputs a number, it will give the correct numeral. If one types in an incorrect number–numeral pair, it will identify the deliberate mistake (it realizes that "two dozen" cannot be the English numeral for 24).

The program's task can be stated more precisely: any given language has syntactic (surface-structure) rules for forming numerals, and it is these syntactic rules which the program must learn. It must do this despite the fact that the surface-structure rules in various languages differ considerably. The languages presented to the program were chosen for maximal surface-variation, and include (among others) French and biblical Welsh. The French name for 99 (in effect, "four twenty ten nine") may seem complicated to English readers, but it is simple in comparison with the biblical Welsh for 59 ("four on fifteen and two twenty") or 2,999 ("subtract one five twenty and nine hundred and two of thousand").

The "syntactic" rules for forming numerals in these languages cannot be stated without referring to *semantic* content: the arithmetical notions of sum, product, difference, and primitive number. (Primitive numbers are directly named by single words in the lexicon of the language concerned.) These concepts are needed in interpreting unfamiliar numerals, or in distinguishing well-formed from ill-formed numerals. It follows that the abstract computational constraints on the task of *learning* a numeral system are partly arithmetical. Although the names of the primitive numbers can – indeed, must – be learnt by rote, the other (infinitely many) number-names in the system can be learnt only if the learner already possesses concepts such as sum and product.

In addition to drawing on arithmetical knowledge, the learning-task is constrained by two abstract linguistic rules. Despite surface variations, the same two basic rules generate the numeral systems of every language examined so far. Longuet-Higgins argues that this surprising fact is, and must be, exploited in learning to count.

The first universal constraint underlies the inductive jump from "twenty-one" and "twenty-nine" to "twenty-five", and also to "ninety-seven" once "ninety" has been learnt by rote. It concerns expressions in which the (semantically) major term is a number rather than a product, and states that "if two such expressions, having the same major term and the same arithmetical operation, are both realized by a given syntactic form, then any expression involving the same major term, the same operation, and an intermediate value of the minor term, is well-formed, and is also realized by that form" [Power & Longuet-Higgins, 1978, p. 395].

The second constraint allows the program to induce the correct English expression for 513, having been told that the numeral for 113 is "one hundred and thirteen". This constraint applies to the syntactic forms of sums and differences in which the (semantically) major term is not a constant but a product. It is: "If a sum or difference has a product as its major term, then the syntactic form or forms by which it can be realized are left unchanged by replacing that product by any other product which is generated by the same formula."

These universal constraints function as very general inductive principles, which enable the program to interpret unfamiliar numerals correctly. For instance, it interprets "soixante-dix" (a compound of the primitives "soixante" and "dix") as the *sum* of 60 and 10 rather than their *product*, which would be named "six cent". By contrast, it recognizes "quatre-vingt" as the product of 4 and 20, not their sum. For the constraints allow it to assume that if a smaller number precedes a larger number, without a conjunction, then a *product* is in question (compare "quatre-vingt," "four hundred", "twenty-four" – and the "four *and* twenty" blackbirds baked in the pie).

The point of general psychological importance here is that these two linguistic universals *must* constrain the learning-task. In other words, they are analogous to Marr's physical constraints. They are not only true (of all examined languages) but also transcendental: without them, numeral-learning would be impossible. If *any* set of rules might underlie a given numeral system, a learning-mechanism would have scant chance of hypothesizing the right ones (and might have to start from scratch for every language acquired). Indeed, without taking it as axiomatic that the rules will not suddenly change at 24 ("two dozen"?), and again at 678, and so on, the learner could never stop. As in the case of vision, the learning-task is made computationally manageable by taking certain abstract constraints for granted. (To use Wittgenstein's terminology, our "forms of life" – including the way in which we count – are not only a biological inheritance but a computational necessity.)

Longuet-Higgins' theoretical analysis of the counting program is inconsistent with empiricism. Certainly, it does not imply the existence in brains of "hardwired" arithmetic operations, or innate linguistic rules specifically flagged for numbers. One does not have to be an ardent empiricist to find such claims implausible. But it does imply that there are very general principles of syntax and morphology, evolved for talking about things, such that the structure of the domain constrains the linguistic descriptions of it – *and the way in which those descriptions can be learnt.* The "things" can be numbers or anything else, but numerals are relatively amenable to study because the number-domain is so well understood.

A second example illustrating the general point that a psychological theory of how we acquire some ability should rest on a precise analysis of that ability is the "psycholexicology" of G. A. Miller and P. N. Johnson-Laird [1976]. Although psycholexicology is primarily concerned with word-meanings, it has implications for how we learn words and concepts. Being committed to a procedural semantics (described in Chapter 5), these authors define words in terms of the psychological processes involved in using them. In general, their approach grounds concepts in mechanisms evolved for the perception of properties, relations, and motions in the physical (including the animate) world. Word-meanings can therefore be learnt only if specific (innate or previously learnt) perceptual procedures are available and can be put together in the appropriate ways.

Miller and Johnson-Laird define a wide variety of words in terms of specific computational procedures, many of which are not only complex but also recursive and/or heterarchical. All are based on primitive perceptual routines (chosen in the light of psychological and physiological evidence) which test for predicates denoting (for instance) spatial, temporal, causal, and intentional properties and relations.

Fodor [1978, 1979; Johnson-Laird, 1978; Wilks, 1982] has derided their procedural semantics as being, in essence, mere out-dated verificationism [Fodor, 1978]. But Fodor is making the same mistake here that underlies his nativist views on learning, criticized above. That is, he is ignoring the possibility that meaning can be *partially* defined, by meaning-postulates (axioms or procedures) mentioning terms only some of which are suited to direct observational test. Miller and Johnson-Laird do not claim that all conceptual meaning can be directly identified in terms of perceptual predicates, nor precisely translated into such predicates. Rather, they claim that the psychological procedures that define meanings (however abstract) are ultimately grounded in perceptual routines, that this is how theoretical networks get linked to the world. For instance, they argue that the concept of hierarchical class-inclusion (and hierarchical memory-search) is derived from the psychologically more primitive concept of spatial inclusion. Computational modelling and, not least, the use of recursion enable them to offer definitions of significant scope and complexity.

The primitive perceptual routines are computationally primitive with respect to the semantic procedures built out of them. But they need be neither computationally unanalysable nor innate. Miller and Johnson-Laird allow, for instance, that the acquisition of some routines requires movement in and action on the material world. They cite evidence showing that infants learn the word "in" before they learn "on", and both before "under" and "at", and they point out that the child's understanding of such locative terms appears to depend on the availability of bodily action schemata. (If it is physically possible to put *x* in *y*, then a twenty-month-old child asked to put *x* on *y* will instead put it inside *y*, while if it is possible to put *x* on *y*, then a child asked to put *x* *under* *y* will place *x* on top of *y* instead.) Their explanation of why children learn the word "at" later still is that its meaning is more complex: it involves the abstract notion of *region* and (when fully developed) concepts of size, salience, and mobility.

Concepts like these are involved not only in language (and much animal behaviour), but also in the reasoning abilities that would be needed by an intelligent robot. Some relevant research is being done within artificial intelligence, including work by P. J. Hayes [1979; 1985] (see also the 1984 special volume of *Artificial Intelligence*). Hayes' "naive physics" is not composed of physicists' equations, nor is it even fully consistent with them. Rather, it aims to represent our everyday intuitions about *weight, support, velocity, height, inside/outside, next to, boundary, path, entrance, obstacle, fluid*, and *cause*. Since most of these concepts were used by Miller and Johnson-Laird in defining perceptual primitives, work on naive physics might eventually contribute to the abstract analysis that will be needed in explaining how everyday physical knowledge is acquired.

Meta-epistemology and general principles of learning

Hayes' work on naive physics, like his discussion "Some Philosophical Problems from the Standpoint of Artificial Intelligence" [McCarthy and Hayes, 1969], is a contribution to what his co-author J. McCarthy calls *meta-epistemology*. The aim of meta-epistemology is to identify general representational or computational constraints on the sorts of mechanisms that are in principle capable of computing particular notions. These constraints are relevant to the computer-modelling of learning because, as McCarthy [1968] has remarked, one cannot make a machine learn something unless the machine is capable of representing what it is that is learnt.

Within AI in general, meta-epistemology is still in a primitive state. Principled comparisons of distinct computational procedures and representations are regularly made within theoretical computer science, but relatively little effort in AI has focussed on such theoretical analysis.

Accordingly, the meta-epistemology of learning is under-developed too. Most computerized learning depends on programs constructed in *ad hoc* ways. Too often, there is no clear statement of just what range of performance the program can learn, and no attempt to analyse the underlying principles that account for its power and limitations. Sometimes descriptions of what a program can do are positively misleading, because *just what it does* is not clearly understood even by the programmer. Nevertheless, there have been a few theoretically rigorous – and surprising – results in this area.

Some of the earliest examples of such results concern a simple type of connectionist system (perceptrons); these will be discussed in the final section of the chapter. Perhaps the first meta-epistemological result relating to non-connectionist models of learning was one (partly inspired by psychological work) which not only proved that Winston's program had unsuspected limitations but also explained its successes in a principled way [Young, Plotkin & Linz, 1977]. Young and his co-authors' powerful concept-learning algorithm was a generalization of a strategy earlier identified by Bruner. Unlike Bruner's, their "focussing strategy" could deal with hierarchically structured concepts, such as those learnt by Winston's program. Indeed, it could be seen as a generalization of Winston's technique. It dealt uniformly with descriptive features (such as predicates, relations, and multi-valued dimensions) which Winston had treated as special cases; it functioned irrespective of the order of presentation of samples; and it explained the logical role of near-misses, whose importance Winston had recognized intuitively.

The essential advance they made was to represent a conceptual hypothesis not (like Winston) by one node in the hierarchical description-space concerned, but by two. The "lower" node describes the specific instances already known to fall under the concept, and the "upper" node contains the most general description known to be possible, given the instances encountered so far. So the two nodes set boundaries (identifying sufficient and necessary conditions respectively) to the search-space within which the concept must lie, and an efficient learning strategy shifts these boundaries until they meet. (The near-misses, and negative information generally, play a role in adjusting the upper node, but not the lower.)

Young and associates' focussing strategy can be thought of as the logical core of a recently acclaimed technique for computerized learning: the method of "version spaces". This method is the heart of the LEX program, which learns the mathematical skill of symbolic integration [Mitchell, Utgoff & Banerji, 1983].

Like someone learning from experience, LEX does not know exactly what it is trying to learn. The initial task-knowledge possessed by the program, as by a human student learning how to integrate, includes very general knowledge of the sorts of mathematical operators that might be useful, and the ability to tell whether a proposed solution of an integration problem really is a solution or not. On the basis of its practice on a large number of example-problems, LEX defines heuristics (in the form of IF–THEN rules) for selecting the appropriate mathematical operators in various problem-situations.

LEX does not have to make a yes–no decision at every point, but can reserve judgment to some extent. It can represent the fact that a heuristic is only *partially* learnt, and it can estimate the degree of applicability of such a heuristic at each point in the problem-search. It does this by way of a version-space representation, wherein each partially learnt heuristic is represented by the *range* of all alternative plausible descriptions of it, given the evidence available so far. A description is plausible if it applies to all the known positive instances and none of the known negative instances. As more instances are considered, the range of what LEX deems plausible decreases. Eventually, the range is narrowed down to one description only.

The version-space representation of the heuristic does not list all possible alternatives, as there are too many for this to be feasible. Rather, it makes explicit only the maximally specific and minimally specific descriptions of it. As more instances are examined, the former description becomes more general and the latter becomes more specific (the heuristic being learnt becomes gradually more well defined) until they coincide. It is as though there is a grey area between two black areas, one of which contains what is known about what the heuristic *must* be like, while the other contains what is known about what it *cannot* be like. The two black areas grow incrementally, encroaching on the grey area until eventually there is no grey left. LEX is guaranteed to succeed, given enough examples, because the two initial descriptions sweep out the entire search-space as they move towards one another.

For each problem it attempts to solve, LEX uses the heuristics it already knows about, criticizes the resulting putative solution, and then modifies the relevant heuristics. Next, it chooses another problem in the light of what it has learnt so far. This "propose–solve–criticize–generalize cycle" is repeated until determinate definitions of all the relevant heuristics have been achieved (at which point there are no grey areas left).

In the Problem-Solving phase, operators are chosen at each step (each node in the search-space) by reference to the heuristic which matches the node best. Both black and grey areas of the heuristic's version-space can be considered here, because LEX can estimate the *degree* of match of a partially defined heuristic. (This is defined as the proportion of the members of the heuristic's version-space that are applicable at the relevant point in the problem-solving search.)

The role of the next module, the Critic, is credit-assignment: it examines the record of the search-tree generated in solving the problem, so as to decide (not always correctly) which individual steps were helpful in leading to the overall solution and which were not. It labels these steps as positive and negative instances respectively, and passes them on to the Generalizer.

The Generalizer defines the version-space for each heuristic by computing the two black areas which (on the evidence so far) delimit its plausibility. For each positive instance, the Generalizer identifies the current heuristic whose version-space includes it (if none exists, it proposes a new heuristic defined in terms of this particular instance). If necessary, it generalizes the current maximally specific description (a black area) so as to include the positive instance. Conversely, a negative instance may lead it to make the minimally specific definition (the other black area) more restrictive. In general, then, it improves the definition of the heuristic, so as to exclude any description that is inconsistent with the instance concerned. This new definition is now available for use in the next cycle, and may be further refined by the Generalizer next time around.

The most recent definitions influence the selection of the problem to be used for the next cycle, for the problems on which LEX practises are generated by the program itself. In proposing a problem likely to lead to the refinement of an existing heuristic, it generates one which corresponds as closely as possible to the positive instance it considered last. In proposing a problem likely to lead to a new heuristic, it looks for two operators with similar preconditions, neither of which are mentioned in any existing heuristic (so that there is as yet no way of deciding which to apply when). So it is able to focus on practice-problems that are likely to be fruitful, given the partially defined heuristics developed so far.

(Whereas the original LEX learnt by induction from large numbers of examples, a more recent extension of it, LEX2, learns new mathematical concepts or heuristics by constructing "justifiable generalizations" drawn from *single* examples [Mitchell & Keller, 1983]. These generalizations, which are tested on further examples of a similar type, attempt to identify the properties of the examples that were useful in reaching the solution, so as to provide a set of specific heuristic procedures suited to varying conditions. The power of this goal-directed learning depends crucially on abstract task-definition, because the generalizations are based on LEX2's abstract formal definitions of what it is to lie on a solution-path in this domain.)

The similarity between LEX and the earlier two-node representation was not widely recognized (Young and associates had reported their results in a one-page abstract) but has recently been remarked by A. M. Bundy and colleagues in a third meta-epistemological discussion of learning [Bundy, 1984; Bundy, Silver & Plummer, 1985]. Bundy shows that the Young focussing algorithm is in fact a very powerful technique. It subsumes not only Winston's program and the method of version-spaces, but also many other learning procedures developed to model superficially different types of learning.

Computer models of learning, such as those mentioned above, apparently differ greatly. Some deal with concept-learning, some with skills. Some are production-systems, others are not. Some rely on discrimination, some use both discrimination and generalization, and some employ version-spaces. Some are guaranteed to reach a solution, while others are not. – But are these differences really fundamental? Do they reflect radically distinct forms of learning, in principle requiring distinct psychological theories? How can we be sure? These are among the meta-epistemological questions addressed by Bundy.

He remarks, for instance, that there need be no radical distinction between models of concept-learning and of skill-learning. If concepts are modelled as sets of rules (which many psychologists take them to be, as we have seen), and if skills are likewise modelled as sets of rules, then we should rather speak of models of "rule-learning". To put the point another way: although Waterman's program is generally described as a skill-learner, one could just as well say that it learns *the concept of a good poker-bet;* similarly, one could describe Quinlan's ID3 concept-learner as learning *classification-skills.*

One dimension on which Bundy compares superficially diverse models of learning is the way in which rules are modified in light of negative and/or positive information (including far-misses, in which there is more than one difference between the sample and the current rule). He points out that rule-learning programs consist of two main parts: a *critic* for identifying faults, and a *modifier* for correcting them. (The first skill-learner to embody a module explicitly labelled "Critic" was G. J. Sussman's [1975], described at length in Boden, 1987 [chap. 10].) Faults in rules may concern matters of fact (inappropriate heuristics) or of control (sub-optimal ordering of appropriate heuristics), and one might expect different correction-techniques to be suitable in either case. At present, however, most techniques can be applied equally to both, because most current rule-learning models include control-information within the rules (instead of representing it separately at a higher level, as in Bundy's own model of mathematical reasoning [Bundy, 1983]).

In general, Bundy complains (as did Marr) that too many people discuss computer models in terms of *behaviour* (or *performance*) rather than abstractly definable *competence.* He does not take the (excessively stern) Marrian view that the computer-modelling of learning is a waste of time without prior answers to basic questions such as those listed at the outset of this chapter. He allows that (as with vision, or language) apparently premature attempts to program learning may teach us something useful. But this will be so only to the extent that exploratory work leads on to theoretical analysis. If it does not, any general lessons learnt in the exploration will be superficial and ill-understood, and may be positively misleading.

A candidate general lesson that would be psychologically significant, if sound, has considered by Bundy in a further theoretical paper [Bundy, 1984]. He puts forward – only to reject – a putative theoretical principle comprising three claims found in the literature on computer-learning (the first two of which were made by Langley, in light of experience with his language-learning program):

(i) A generalization-based rule-learner will arrive at the correct form of a complex rule before arriving at the correct form of a simple rule;
(ii) for a discrimination-based rule-learner the opposite is the case;
(iii) for a rule-learner using version spaces, the rate of arriving at the correct form of a rule is independent of the complexity of the rule.

This putative law, based on observations of the performance of a sample of learning programs rather than on theoretical analysis, is described by Bundy as "both superficial and misleading" [p. 21].

The first two claims within the law are superficial because, insofar as they are true, their truth can be explained in terms of the computational analysis which proves that the version-space approach must terminate. The same analysis shows them to be misleading, because they apply only to conjunctive concepts and because they do not make clear that a pure discriminatory method can never be certain that it has arrived at the correct definition of a concept, even when it has done so. The final claim is superficial likewise: Bundy explains it by pointing out that, because the maximally and minimally specific definitions have to meet, there is indeed a sense in which a version-space model will learn concepts at a rate that is independent of their complexity. However, because the rate of learning in each case depends on the order of presentation of instances, this sense is a probabilistic one, which cannot be precisely defined – so the third claim is misleading also.

Bundy's prime concern is with technological matters. In analysing the theoretical principles that underlie various learning models, he wants to improve AI-practice and teaching, and to relate its underlying scientific principles to general computer science. But his work has a psychological relevance, because abstract theoretical results about learning algorithms can be used as standards in assessing psychological theories of learning.

Anderson's ACT*-model of skill-learning, for instance, has been criticized in light of the sorts of meta-epistemological issues highlighted by Bundy. T. O'Shea [personal communication] has remarked a number of ways in which ACT* is less powerful than current AI learning programs. For example, its credit-assignment is very crude compared with LEX's, because ACT* makes no distinction between rules tried unsuccessfully and rules not tried at all. Moreover, unlike Mitchell's system, it has no ideal solution, no theory of good performance against which a solution can be carefully measured. This is why it strengthens rules indiscriminately, provided only that they have been used without running into trouble. Again, unlike Quinlan's program, ACT* does not minimize search or aim at maximal efficiency. And unlike some AI-programs (such as D. B. Lenat's AM, mentioned below), it can handle only one goal at a time, it has no metrics for the *interest* of alternative solution-paths, and its analogy-matching is unconstrained so that *any* similarity is taken as relevant.

Anderson might counter that he is a psychologist, not a technologist, so that these comparisons are irrelevant. In particular, the inefficiency of ACT* reflects his belief that parsimony is not a feature of the human mind. But O'Shea's point is that it is highly doubtful whether Anderson has a clear understanding of *just what his system can and cannot do,* and *why.* Without this theoretical grasp of the principles underlying the program, Anderson is not in a good position to compare it with human learning (whether efficient or not) or to make it better. The system's various incarnations as it evolved over the years from ACT into ACT* were not motivated in a principled way, but were suggested *ad hoc* by comparisons between ACT*'s performance and experimental data.

An adequate meta-epistemology would include a general classification of at least some types of error (although, for reasons explained below, we cannot expect a principled theory of all errors). Error-correction is used by many learning programs, as we have seen. In some (such as ACT*, just noted) the error-discriminations are relatively crude, because the model has no built-in theory of what might constitute error. But a number of computer modellers, including some whose interest in learning is psychologically motivated, have tried to approach errors more systematically–often via the computer scientist's notion of "bug".

A bug is a mistake, but not just any mistake: a false factual assumption is not a bug, nor is a momentary slip in executing some procedure, nor the choice of a procedure that is wholly inappropriate to the goal. Bugs might feature in the meta-epistemology of learning, because a bug is a precisely definable and relatively systematic erroneous variation of a correct procedure. With respect to learning and teaching, then, "bug" is an optimistic notion: it implies that elements of the correct procedure or skill are already possessed by the thinker, and that what is wrong is a precisely definable error that could be identified and fixed.

An early classification of learning bugs was made by Sussman [1975]. He showed how a self-modifying program could diagnose bugs so as to criticize and repair its own problem-solving procedures (by way of his error-correcting Critic, mentioned above). Sussman's bug-definitions cited highly general teleological notions such as *goal, brother-goals,* and *prerequisites* of goal-directed action. A similarly general concept of bug was used, and applied to psychological (educational) problems, by S. Papert [1980]. Papert argued that bug-sensitive programming using the LOGO programming language could help children to improve their own thinking abilities, and raise their self-confidence generally–the defeatist "I'm no good at this" giving way to "How can I make myself better at it?" Although early psychological studies provided some support for Papert's claims [Howe, O'Shea & Plane, 1980], recent research suggests that the educational effect of the LOGO-environment is neither so strong nor so generalizable as he expected [Pea & Kurland, 1984; Kurland *et al.,* 1986; Pea, Kurland & Hawkins, in press]. (Papert's suggestion that the Piagetian stage-progressions might be re-ordered in children growing up in a computer culture is even more speculative.)

Other bug-classifications used in the study of learning (and teaching) are more task-specific. One example, drawn up with educational applications in mind, is an analysis of a large sample of children's subtraction-errors in terms of the deletion or over-general application of individual rules such as the "borrowing" rule [O'Shea & Young, 1978]. Another, also concerned with subtraction, is J. S. Brown's notation, which provides a precisely defined (and programmed) diagnostic tool for identifying errors in students' work [Brown & Burton, 1978; Brown & VanLehn, 1980; Burton, 1982]. (Brown expects to produce similar notations for arithmetic, algebra, and calculus, and perhaps for operating computer systems or controlling air-traffic.)

Bugs in human minds are conceptualized by Brown as "patches" (a term drawn from computer-programming) that arise from the subject's attempts to repair a procedure that has encountered an impasse. He defines various repair-heuristics and critics, and claims that the method of repair is theoretically independent of why the procedure was incorrect in the first place. This claim underlies his explanation of the observable error-pattern he calls bug-migration, wherein a subject shows a different bug on two identical tests given only a few days apart. Since only certain bugs migrate into each other, and since they seem to travel both ways, Brown suggests that two bugs will migrate relative to each other only if they can be derived by different repairs to the same impasse.

Brown's main aim is to develop a "generative theory of bugs": a set of formal principles that can be applied to a particular correct procedural skill so as to generate all the bugs actually observed during learning, and no others. Such a theory would lie at Marr's first (computational) level, furthering the explanation of learning by defining all possible bug-driven learning episodes, at least with respect to a given domain.

A comprehensive generative theory (or many domain-specific theories) of *bugs* may be in principle possible. For bugs are defined as precisely definable, relatively systematic, variations of a correct procedure. Indeed, some learning programs (such as LEX) derive their power largely from an implicit or explicit classification of the possible bugs in the relevant problem-domain.

But a computational-level theory of all possible *errors* – including not only (quasi-rational) bugs but mere unprincipled errors too – is another matter. Even in highly constrained tasks like those mentioned by Brown, it is probably not psychologically realistic to hope for this. A generative classification of all errors is attainable only if random (trial and) error never takes place, if momentary slips never occur for reasons essentially unconnected with the task, and if adaptive responses to the environment are all constrained at the computational level. (Although unsystematic errors could not be predicted from first principles, they might be represented *post hoc* in a computer model, such as a Newell–Simon production-system.) Of course, a fully comprehensive error-classification is not strictly necessary for learning theorists, who need consider only those errors from which we can learn. A Marrian theory covering all error-driven learning is possible only if we never make unprincipled errors or if, having made them, we cannot learn from them.

Error, whether principled or not, has been seen by many theoretical psychologists as the prime, or even only, source of learning. I have argued elsewhere that this is not so [Boden, 1984]. Error is a normative notion, definable only with respect to some goal. Failure to achieve a goal can indeed be a spur to learning (and triggers discrimination-mechanisms in many computer models of learning, as we have seen). No less important, however, is a relatively undirected *exploration,* not only of the environment but also of the searcher's mental structures. Admittedly, one might say that this exploration is really goal-directed, since it aims (for example) to identify, and to shift, the current constraints on thinking. But the highly general, epistemological, goals of creative exploration are very different from specific goals defined within the accepted constraints.

Largely because of the difficulty in defining the exploratory task, or goals, very little computational work has been done on learning by exploration. Those learning programs which employ generalization could be thought of as embodying a very simple form of exploration; some recent models of scientific discovery developed by Simon and his students draw on experimental and historical evidence in simulating the search for definable types of mathematical function [Langley *et al.,* 1987]; and there has been some discussion of adaptive processes within relatively ill-defined systems [Selfridge, Rissland & Arbib, 1984]. But the examples most relevant to exploratory learning are found in Lenat's work, in particular his Automatic Mathematician (AM) [Lenat, 1982; 1983a; 1983b; Lenat & Brown, 1984].

This program starts with a collection of primitive mathematical (set-theoretical) concepts, and some transformational rules (*heuristics*) which it uses to explore the space potentially defined by the primitive concepts. It generates and then explores concepts and hypotheses about number theory, guided by its hunches about which are likely to be the most interesting. Like human hunches, the program's judgments of what ideas are most promising are sometimes wrong. But it has come up with some mathematically powerful ideas, including primes, square roots, addition, and multiplication – which it notices can be performed in four different ways, itself a mathematically interesting fact. It has also originated one minor theorem (about the class of *maximally divisible* numbers).

Since exploration lies at the core of creativity, one might ask whether this improvement in the program's mathematical performance should be attributed to creativity rather than learning. Against this, it should be said that it was Lenat who provided the basic concepts and heuristic rules used by AM, that these rules do not change in any way (although Lenat's later programs embody *meta-heuristics* for changing heuristics), and that some of AM's heuristics are suspiciously specific (the rule generating its "discovery" of prime numbers was used nowhere else [Ritchie & Hanna, 1984]). We need not decide on an answer here, since for present purposes the distinction between learning and creativity is not crucial [cf. Boden, in preparation].

Is development different?

The distinction – or lack of it – between learning and development is more to the point. Many psychologists believe that learning and development differ significantly at the theoretical level. This is so even though both are widely regarded as types of adaptive change, brought about largely by interaction with the environment. In particular, learning is often said to be gradual and piecemeal; development, non-incremental and holistic. Piaget, for instance, saw development as an equilibratory process involving a succession of underlying and pervasive structural changes, each of which causes a sudden qualitative alteration in the child's behaviour across a wide range of tasks. (Piaget's notion of equilibration is admittedly very vague; even so, it touches upon questions which computational psychology must eventually address [Boden, 1979, chap. 7; 1982a].)

This notion that development is due to non-incremental structural change has been challenged by R. M. Young [1976], whose argument draws on his studies (including computer-modelling) of seriation.

Seriation is a typical Piagetian experimental task, in which the subject is asked (for example) to put seven blocks in order so as to build a staircase [Piaget, 1952; Inhelder & Piaget, 1964]. Piaget described three main *stages* of seriation, which are observationally distinct. At first, the child may build one or two short sequences, but cannot integrate them; next, the child can use trial-and-error methods to build a perfect sevenfold staircase; finally, the child builds the staircase rationally, starting with the shortest or longest block and successively adding the correct neighbour. According to Piaget, the qualitatively different types of seriation are structurally discontinuous at the deeper psychological level (corresponding to "pre-operational", "concrete operational", and "formal operational" stages).

Young's computer models of seriation are production-systems in the Newell–Simon paradigm (see Chapter 6, above). As such, they rely both on experimental protocols and on logical analysis of the task. Taking into account idiosyncratic details (such as touching a block that is not picked up, or double-tapping one block with a finger moving along the staircase), Young models a superficially chaotic range of finely distinguished seriation-behaviours. Each of these is represented by a different set of production-rules. But they are unified by a theoretical matrix defining a three-dimensional "space"of seriation skills.

As either rule-inspection or abstract task-analysis can show, some individual rules concern general *episode-structure* (the basic cycle of getting blocks and adding them to the staircase, together with the special case of the first block of all). Such rules have to be included if the model is to perform anything classifiable as seriation at all. Other rules concern *selection* of the next block, *evaluation* of the portion of the staircase built so far, or *placement and correction* of blocks. The last three categories provide the theoretical dimensions by reference to which any experimental subject can be located. Young claims that most of the rules are "surprisingly independent", in the sense that given the basic episode-cycle, "almost any collection of the rules . . . yields a psychologically plausible production system for seriation" [p. 198]. Different regions of the skill-space represent distinctive types of seriation-behaviour, and a child's specific location represents her characteristic performance, the problems she can or cannot solve, and the nature of her errors. No matter how it is attained (whether by incremental learning or not), seriation must fit one of these possible profiles.

Young explicitly rejects Piaget's explanation in terms of underlying developmental stage-discontinuities. We noted above that a single rule added to Larkin's production-system can give an overall improvement in physics problem-solving. Similarly, adding just one rule to Young's model produces a qualitative change in performance comparable to what Piaget would term a stage-progression.

For example, consider the production-system represented in Figure 7.1 (read it from the bottom upwards: when you find a rule whose condition is satisfied, assume that the specified action is taken and then start again at the bottom of the list). Figure 7.1 models a particular "concrete operational" child who can build a perfect staircase, but who cannot be relied on to pick up a block of suitable size *unless* he is picking the first block of all (rule B2); otherwise, he picks the nearest block (rule S1).

Now consider a new rule, S2:

S2: IF you want to add a block to the staircase THEN decide that you want to get a suitable one from the pool, that is, one of about the right size.

Suppose that rule S2 is added to the system shown in Figure 7.1 and given priority over (placed immediately underneath) rule S1. The system now represents a second "concrete operational" child, able likewise to produce a perfect staircase, but whose behaviour is phenomenologically different: *this* child always picks up a block of about the required size, though not necessarily the correct one. (Provided that S2 is given priority, S1 need not be deleted: though still present, it is functionally forgotten.) In fact, these two children are one and the same child, at earlier and later experimental

T1: IF you want to seriate the blocks THEN decide that you want to add a block to the staircase.

S1: IF you want to add a block to the staircase THEN pick up the nearest block.

P1: IF you want to place a block in the staircase THEN position it at the right-hand end.

P2: IF you want to place a block in the staircase, and a block has just been examined and found unsuitable THEN return it to the pool.

P3: IF you want to place a block in the staircase, and there are just two blocks in it already, similar in size but the wrong way round THEN rotate the two blocks.

PG1: IF you want to place a block in the staircase, and the staircase has just been rearranged THEN examine it.

PG2: IF you want to place a block in the staircase, and you have just examined that block and found it to be one or two units smaller than its neighbour THEN accept it (leave it where it is in the staircase).

B1: IF you have just undertaken the task of seriating the blocks THEN decide that you want to put the first one in the staircase.

B2: IF you want to put the first block in the staircase THEN get a big one.

B3: IF you want to put the first block in the staircase, and you've just got a block THEN put it at the far left of the space you'll be building in, and leave it there.

Fig. 7.1. Productions for seriation. (N.B. Read from the bottom upwards.) (Adapted from R. M. Young [1976], *Seriation by Children: An Artificial Intelligence Analysis of a Piagetian Task.* Basel: Birkhauser. P. 78.)

sessions. (Young assumes that, somehow, the child learnt the equivalent of rule S2, giving it priority because of its usefulness.) Young's work thus counts as a study of *micro-development:* the detailed changes in a child's behaviour and cognitive resources over a relatively short time, not only between experimental sessions but within them too.

An even more striking change in performance would result if a new rule (S3), to "pick the *biggest* block", were to be added and given priority over all other selection-rules (placed immediately below rule S2). This one item would shift the system into "formal operational" seriation.

A Piagetian might object here that development is holistic in a sense stronger than that allowed by Young, on the ground that equivalent stage-changes can be observed in many different domains simultaneously. For example, visual and tactile seriation seem to develop together. Young does not discuss this issue at length, although he does consider the generalization of seriation from blocks to discs. However, he does offer an explanation of *horizontal decalage,* in which (for instance) seriation by weight lags behind seriation by length. The abstract task-constraints of seriation, in whatever domain, assume that perceptual (or other) routines are available to test for *equality;* since more complex procedures are required to recognize equal weights than are normally needed to compare lengths, it is not surprising that weight-seriation appears later. If seriation appears simultaneously in various domains, this is because the requisite perceptual tests are already available, to be put to the service of abstract ordering constraints once these arise.

Young's is one of the few computer models of developmental processes (most of which are also production-systems [Baylor & Gascon, 1974; Baylor & Lemoyne, 1975]). Indeed, specifically computational treatments of developmental psychology are still uncommon. But work on micro-development is increasing, and is being done by computationally informed psychologists who focus on the precise procedural details of thinking. Some of this work explicitly questions the assumption of a distinction of principle between learning and development [Thornton, 1982, forthcoming]. And some aims to use the psychological changes that occur in childhood to illuminate the nature of skill-acquisiton in adults: thus A. Karmiloff-Smith [1979; 1986; 1987; Karmiloff-Smith & Inhelder, 1975] conceptualizes *consciousness* in general in terms of four levels of (meta)-representation, citing extensive micro-developmental evidence (on language, spatial maps, and object-drawing) in arguing that the flexible voluntary control of skilled behaviour is made possible by these "reiterated representational redescriptions" of the basic performance-procedures.

The computational approach suggests one way in which there might, indeed, be a radical difference between learning and development. Bearing in mind the distinction (introduced in Chapter 2) between the *architecture* and the *program* (*rules*) of a computational system, it may be that development involves architectural change (caused by physical maturation of the nervous system) whereas learning does not. However, to say that development is at base architectural is not to say *which* psychological changes are the developmental ones. Still less is it to specify the particular architectural alterations involved. Some explanations of developmental change suggested by non-computational psychologists are relevant here. For example, P. E. Bryant's [1974] attack on Piaget focusses on the changing limits of the young child's short-term memory – which is one of the eight architectural features listed by Newell and Simon (see Chapter 6). As yet, however, computational psychologists have said very little in detail about how one might map developmental adaptations onto architectural change.

Connectionist approaches to learning

The concept of mental architecture is relevant also in distinguishing between various theoretical approaches to *learning*. For it is sometimes suggested that learning may require psychological processes of a type that cannot, in practice, be modelled (except as toy systems for purposes of illustration) using a von Neumann architecture. Indeed, von Neumann himself [1958] believed this, remarking – prophetically, as we shall see – that thermodynamics might be a better model of computation than formal logic. Although most work has been done using traditional computing techniques, there are now an increasing number of computational studies of learning based on (simulated) parallel architectures [Rumelhart & Mc-Clelland, 1986a].

In the early 1950s, D. O. Hebb's [1949] neurophysiological ideas on the synaptic changes leading to the formation of "cell-assemblies" prompted various models of parallel learning networks, in which representations were embodied as a specific set of weights, and pattern of excitation, in the connections between network-units. Although some of these involved simple, randomly connected, parallel architectures (such as M. L. Minsky's Heath Robinson machine made with aircraft-components and soldering iron [Bernstein, 1981]), most were simulated on digital computers. Influential examples included F. Rosenblatt's self-organizing perceptrons [Rosenblatt, 1962], and the versions of O. G. Selfridge's [1959] Pandemonium machine which showed simple learning behaviour (such as L. Uhr and C. Vossler's feature-learning machine of 1961, described in Chapter 2).

This pioneering connectionist work was typically done with mathematical questions in mind about what these systems were in principle capable of doing – and of learning. Some of the earliest meta-epistemological results on learning concerned a primitive type of connectionist system known as a *perceptron* – abstractly defined as a single-layer neural net of linear threshold-units, without any loops or feedback paths. Rosenblatt's [1962] "perceptron convergence theorem" proved that a particular learning algorithm (a rule specifying how to adjust the weights on unit-connections) was *guaranteed* to find the correct set of weights for any pattern that is in principle learnable by a perceptron.

Not surprisingly, some people were led to hope that perceptrons would function as self-organizing systems that could learn a usefully wide range of concepts by experience, without requiring any prior knowledge or specific tuition.

However, a series of counterintuitive mathematical proofs soon showed that these simple networks cannot compute some discriminations which might seem *prima facie* to fall within their competence. For example, an early paper by Minsky and Selfridge [1961] on learning in random nets showed that perceptrons cannot compute parity: even though they can inspect every part of an image to say whether or not it contains a dot, they cannot tell whether the image contains an odd or even number of dots overall. These arguments were later developed in a lengthy discussion by Minsky and S. Papert [1969]; among their additional examples was a demonstration that although perceptrons can recognize convexity, they are in principle incapable of computing spatial connectedness. It follows that a simple perceptron will never learn to discriminate connectedness or to recognize that the number of apples on a dish is odd – for what they can never compute, they can never learn to compute.

Naturally, neural nets of a more complex kind than single-layer perceptrons have greater learning potential. As early as the 1940s, W. S. McCulloch and W. H. Pitts had proved that multi-layered nets of linear threshold-units are in principle capable of computing *any* function expressible in the terms used to define the propositional calculus. However, this meta-epistemological proof was more an encouragement than a practically usable result, since no *general* learning algorithm was (or is yet) known which will enable multi-layered networks to compute such logical functions. This situation is comparable to the more recent case of Boltzmann machines (discussed below), where knowing that a certain type of learning is in principle possible does not guarantee that it is possible in practice.

Ironically, one of the first people to attempt to build a parallel learning machine was largely responsible for the relative decline in connectionist research after the mid 1960s. Minsky's meta-epistemological critique of perceptrons led all but a few stalwarts to abandon research on parallel learning systems. This fact is doubly ironic, because the surprising limitations on computational power identified by Minsky and Papert referred only to parallelist systems of a very simple kind: the reaction against network-models in general was hence unjustified. During the late 1960s and the 1970s, most psychologically and technologically motivated computer models of learning (including those discussed earlier in this chapter) were sequential in conception as well as implementation.

To be sure, some research on parallelist models went on throughout this period. Rosenblatt [1962] continued his studies of perceptual learning and more complex types of perceptron. Cognitive psychologists such as D. A. Norman, D. E. Rumelhart, J. R. Anderson, and G. H. Bower provided a number of associationist models of perception, language, and (long-term, short-term, and semantic) memory [e.g. Norman & Rumelhart, 1970; Anderson & Bower, 1973; Norman, 1976]. With respect to computer-modelling in general, however, parallelism was a minority-taste.

Marr, at this time, was using parallelist ideas to address a problem of neurological learning: how the cerebellum – considered as a piece of biological hardware – comes to control skilled movement [Blomfield & Marr, 1970]. He defined a connectionist algorithm whereby neural contexts (originating in cortical impulses, and mediated by the mossy and parallel fibres of the cerebellum) could be learnt, and then reproduced, by the Purkinje cells. Although the algorithm as Marr defined it was later proved to be faulty (it would eventually lead to a state in which all the weights are at a maximum value [Sejnowski, 1977]), it was an ancestor of some connectionist processes that are now current. Marr's shift to what he later promulgated as the *computational* approach occurred after he gave a seminar on his ideas about the cerebellum at MIT, at which Minsky remarked from the floor that we have to think about "the [abstract] problem of motor-control" before we can ask the right questions about the cerebellar hardware. Marr moved to Minsky's laboratory at MIT, where (influenced by B. K. P. Horn and others) he decided to consider "the problem of *vision*" instead [Poggio, personal communication].

The current renaissance in connectionist (PDP) computer models of learning owes much to the successes in parallel processing for vision achieved in the late 1970s. Although there has been no clear pendulum-swing for learning, as there has for vision, there is now an increasing interest in updated versions of ideas about learning that were dominant at the very outset of computer-modelling.

Those cognitive psychologists (listed above) who showed a continuing commitment to parallelism throughout the 1960s and 1970s were an influential force in the mid 1980s. Learning models inspired by them include Rumelhart's studies of feature-acquisition [Rumelhart & Zipser, 1985]; and others (including a model of the child's acquisition of verb-morphology, discussed below) are described in Rumelhart & McClelland, 1986a. Minsky [1980, 1986] has sketched a theory of "K-Lines", whereby learning and memory are explained in terms of the activation (and partial re-activation) of sets of simple neural units working in parallel. And Rosenblatt's pioneering attempts to provide mathematical analyses of various types of learning system have a new, and appreciative, audience.

This audience includes G. E. Hinton and T. J. Sejnowski, whose analysis of learning in *Boltzmann machines* (like Hinton's work described in Chapter 3) is within the same general tradition as Rosenblatt's work on perceptrons [Hinton & Sejnowski, 1983; Ackley, Hinton & Sejnowski, 1985; Hinton & Sejnowski, 1986]. Not all Boltzmann machines are learning machines: the basic definition of a Boltzmann machine is of an equilibrium-seeking connectionist system. But, as we shall see, Hinton and Sejnowski have defined a learning algorithm that enables a Boltzmann machine to learn by changing the weights on the various connections.

Hinton's recent work, with Sejnowski, on connectionism assumes the individual elements in the system to be *binary* (*on/off*) and *stochastic*. In terms of the classroom-analogy used in Chapter 3 to illustrate different forms of connectionism, we have here a fourth type: Classroom D. Each child in Classroom D either speaks her message or does not; there is no whispering or shouting, as there was in Hinton's early connectionist architecture. The class-decision of Classroom D is reached by convergence to an optimal *probability-distribution,* not to a particular equilibrium-state. This is because the Boltzmann child, though usually responding strictly on the basis of the evidence being passed to her by her neighbours, occasionally speaks up – or keeps silent – irrespective of it. By contrast, each element in

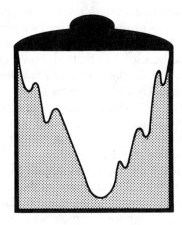

Fig. 7.2. (Adapted from D. E. Rumelhart & J. L. McClelland (eds.) [1986a], *Parallel Distributed Processing,* Vol. 1. Cambridge, Mass.: MIT Press. P. 287.)

Hinton's early models (each child in Classroom C) was rational in that its response depended entirely on the evidence it was receiving at the time.

This seems strange: Hinton and Sejnowski appear to prefer a less discriminating, less rational, system. Their explanation is twofold. First, if one treats the units as binary (which admittedly real neurones are not), one can make use of mathematical techniques that already exist for describing self-equilibrating systems. And second, a stochastic co-operative network is in principle – though not necessarily in practice – more likely than a deterministic one to reach the best solution (the optimal equilibrium-state), because it can avoid getting stuck in locally attractive but globally sub-optimal solutions. (It is perhaps no accident that biologically evolved nervous systems contain noise, or stochastic nervous activity.)

To illustrate the advantage of stochastic systems, Hinton considers the problem of how to shake a box of marbles whose inner surface contains hills and valleys of varying depths so that all the marbles eventually end up at the bottom of the box (see Figure 7.2). If the box is shaken too hard, the marbles will never settle into equilibrium, for some will jump from valley to valley at every shake. If the box is shaken too gently, the marbles will reach equilibrium; but they will not all be available at the bottom of the box, since some will be lodged in the higher valleys. Only if the box is shaken moderately will they all eventually reach the bottom.

Specifically, the box must be shaken with just enough force to make marbles jump out of even the deepest of the higher valleys, but not enough to make them jump back into any higher valley from the bottom one. What counts as just enough force in any case will depend on the heights and distribution of the valleys. If we knew beforehand just how strong our shaking should be, we could be confident of getting (almost) all the marbles to the bottom. But we would not need this prior knowledge if we could see where the marbles are after each shake, for then we could continually adjust our shaking ourselves. It would be useful to be told, however, that the best strategy is to begin with energetic shaking and then gradually calm down. For the early shaking would quickly dislodge even those marbles lying in the deeper valleys, whereas the final shaking would not cause any high jumps. (Although some awkward boxes could have hills and valleys shaped in such a way that there is in practice no way of shaking them which guaranteess success, the principle would still hold.)

The mathematics needed to solve problems like this is already available: the Boltzmann equations of thermodynamics. These represent the temperature of a large volume of gas as an overall energy-equilibrium obtained by (binary) energy-transfer between pairs of neighbouring molecules. Thermodynamics deals with stochastic systems: the energy-states of an individual molecule are not predictable, but the energy-distributions of large collections of molecules are. (As I remarked at the beginning of Chapter 1, von Neumann predicted in the 1950s that ideas from thermodynamics might be needed in understanding – and modelling – human psychology.) Accordingly, Hinton and Sejnowski use thermodynamic equations in defining Boltzmann machines and also in defining and justifying a learning algorithm that could be used by such machines.

A Boltzmann machine is a system of stochastic binary units in which the computational processes are *iterative* and *local* (that is, they concern the *repeated* mutual adjustments of *neighbouring* units). The behaviour of an individual unit is partly stochastic and partly determined by its weighted connections with its neighbours. (Likewise, a marble will jump unpredictably if it is shaken, but it will roll downwards at a fixed acceleration when it can.) In the basic Boltzmann machine (as also in Hinton's connectionist system described in Chapter 3), the excitatory/inhibitory weights on the various connections are *fixed*. An optimal global equilibrium-state (more accurately: an optimal probability-distribution, made up of the probabilities of co-excitation of many pairs of neighbouring units) is attained by a process comparable to that of minimizing the global energy of a physical system. For equilibrium is reached in Boltzmann machines by a method called simulated annealing. Annealing is a method commonly used for cooling metals, in which energy-equilibrium is reached more quickly by starting at a high temperature and cooling down gradually. (This corresponds to the general strategy described above, of shaking the marble-box forcefully at first and more gently later.)

A Boltzmann machine could be used to generate a representation of a visual scene, for instance, if its fixed weights were determined in accordance with the physical constraints on image-formation that were discussed in Chapter 3. That is, the weights would have been chosen in advance so that optimal equilibrium was most likely when the correct interpretation had been reached. The system as a whole would include both basic receptor-units and units sensitive to interpretative connections dealing with edges, and the like. The receptor-units would in effect be "clamped" into certain on–off states by the input-stimulus. The system would then reach equilibrium (its representation of the scene) by a process of simulated annealing, in which the stochastic binary units would be subjected to decreasingly many random changes (they would be more agitated at first and less agitated later).

To enable a Boltzmann machine to *learn*, one must give it some way of changing the weights on its connections so as to make them more appropriate (more likely to lead to an optimal probability-distribution). This process requires feedback, based on the comparative evaluation of successive decisions about equilibrium-probabilities. It is this feedback which, in effect, tells the system which direction (which changing of weights) is "downhill". So a Boltzmann learning algorithm must be able to measure and compare the probability of neighbouring units' being co-excited in two equilibrium-situations: (1) with the environmental input present and (2) in the free-running state where there is no environmental input. Hinton and Sejnowski's learning algorithm defines the relevant measures.

(These measures are taken at equilibria, each of which is reached by simulated annealing, as described above. In principle, the *learning* in Boltzmann machines could also exploit simulated annealing, in that the *changes* to the weights would be large at first and get smaller as time goes on. In practice, however, this is not yet possible. When the current toy-implementation of Hinton and Sejnowski's learning algorithm escapes from local minima, it does so primarily thanks to the noise, or inaccuracy, in the measures of the probabilities of unit-co-excitation.)

Hinton and Sejnowski's learning algorithm is domain-independent, since – thanks to continual feedback of estimates of global equilibrium – it does not need prior information about what the ideal weights are. It might account for the relatively speedy re-learning (even of apparently unrelated words) that occurs in recovery from brain-damage, since a portion of a familiar equilibrium-state suffices to seed the reconstitution of that entire state – by "holistic" regeneration as opposed to piecemeal inference [Hinton & Sejnowski, 1986]. And it is *guaranteed* to learn the optimal solution (thermodynamics guarantees equilibrium too: a snowball in hell might last a long time, but it could not last for ever).

The latter point is striking indeed. Seemingly, the problem of modelling learning is solved: all we have to do is to build a Boltzmann machine and say (*après* Leibniz), "Come, let it equilibrate!" However, we must be wary. There is no proof that a pure Boltzmann machine as defined by Hinton and Sejnowski could learn anything of interest within a finite period, such as an hour or a human lifetime. Nor is it intuitively obvious that, or how, the machine could be practically useful. Hinton and Sejnowski's current implementation of Boltzmann learning (simulated on von Neumann hardware) works only on toy-problems; not only does it model a tiny number of interconnected units, but it does not actually vary the weight-changes. Extensive empirical explorations of Boltzmann machines have not been carried out, because truly parallel hardware is only just becoming available. Hinton and Sejnowski do not even claim to possess any feel for what network-size and time-scales might be appropriate to different learning tasks. Indeed, they have concluded that Boltzmann machines are not a practical proposition for a general learning mechanism, because the time that would typically be required (in typically noisy conditions) would be excessive.

But this is not to say that their analysis is psychologically irrelevant. Turing's proof about the computational powers of universal Turing machines (which cannot exist, since their tape is infinitely long) was useful in showing that certain computations are in principle possible. It remained for computer engineers, including Turing himself, to answer the largely empirical question of whether, and how, one could build approximations to universal Turing machines that would do anything interesting. Analogously, these mathematical arguments about Boltzmann machines suggest that certain ways of learning are in principle possible – ways that are not well suited to digital computers, but which bear interesting analogies to the architecture (and stochastic nature) of the brain. Similar remarks apply to connectionist theories in general, especially those offering mathematical analyses of the computational power of various models [Rumelhart & McClelland, 1986a].

Finally, what of task-analysis? Given domain-independent learning algorithms and self-equilibrating connectionist systems, does task-analysis become redundant? This question cannot wait for an answer until the day when we have an all-singing, all-dancing, Boltzmann machine. For some computer models already exist whose performance, *prima facie,* might suggest that task-analysis is unnecessary.

Consider, for example, a recent connectionist model which learns the past tenses of English verbs, and whose performance closely resembles that of young children *in very detailed ways that were not explicitly programmed into it* [Rumelhart & McClelland, 1986b].

English-speaking children go through three broad stages in learning the past tense. At first, they use only a few verbs in the past tense, and generally employ the correct form; these verbs are very familiar and many are also irregular (such as "go/went", "come/came", "take/took", and "have/got"). Next, they use the correct past tense of indefinitely many regular verbs (including non-existent forms like "glitch/glitched") but often produce regularized, or over-generalized, forms of irregular verbs which previously they had used correctly (now saying "goed" instead of "went", for instance). Finally, they use both regular and irregular forms correctly.

More specific changes occur also as the infant's language develops. For example, early in the second stage there are many "base + ed" errors (such as "goed"); later, there are more "past + ed" errors (like "wented"). Other detailed changes in the child's speech relate to the fact that irregular verbs are not wholly irregular, or random: they can be classified into nine types, each of which forms the past tense in a different way. Some simply change the final phoneme (as in "build/built"); others change some internal vowel ("give/gave", "sting/stung"), perhaps also altering the final phoneme ("feel/felt", "bring/brought"). Children's error-patterns show that they learn these distinct classes of irregular verb-forms at differential rates.

Many of these childlike phenomena (including some very detailed speech-patterns) characterize the performance of the Rumelhart–McClelland connectionist model. The continual *training* provided to the system is an incremental set of verb-pairs. The first member of each pair is a representation of the phonological structure of the root-form, while the second member gives the phonological structure of the appropriate past tense. The model's output in trials wherein the only input is the root-form (of real or non-existent words) shows a striking similarity to the developing speech of infants: not only the three broad stages described above, but more detailed changes too (including some which have not yet been investigated in children).

The core of the connectionist system involved is a "pattern associator" network which learns the associations between the root-forms and the past-tense verbs. This network consists of a "pool" of units representing the various phonological features of the root-forms, and a second pool of units representing the phonological features of the past tense. Each unit corresponds to a different feature, and the weights of the excitatory/inhibitory connections between them are modifiable (broadly as described in Chapter 3). Initially, all weights are zero: the network knows what phonological features to look for but has no expectations of any specific feature-association or rule.

Each *training input* (a pair of root/past forms, described in terms of their constituent features) clamps the connections between the relevant units in the two pools, whose joint excitation causes equilibratory processes across the whole network in the sort of way previously described. The weights, or associative strengths, of the various interconnections are thus continually modified so as to reflect not only the current training pair but all previous pairs too. In the case of a *test-input*, only the units in the root-form pool are clamped: the units in the past-tense pool are left free to settle into equilibrium according to the connection-weights previously developed in the network. Finally, this equilibrium-state is decoded into a phonological output which reflects those units in the second pool which are most strongly activated.

Without going into detail, one can see why the three broad stages of learning described above are reproduced in this computer model. At first, while the set of training pairs is still small, most of the commonest verbs are irregular – which is to say that each learnt pair is in effect isolated from the influence of all others, with which it has little in common. At this stage, the system reproduces "go/went" just as easily as "talk/talked". As the input-corpus increases, the overwhelming majority of training pairs come to be regular. Consequently, the regular associations increase in strength so that they dominate the still-existing irregular connections. Now the model produces over-generalizations such as "goed". Finally, with the continual increase in the number of times any particular irregular pair has been presented to the network, the relevant association is gradually strengthened and is eventually able to outweigh the regular ones.

Clearly, this connectionist model does not learn by being provided beforehand with a program specifying the relevant phono-morphological rules. Nor does it generate any explicit rules itself. Rather, it gradually develops its own *implicit* associative rules. Although its behaviour can, at least to a good approximation, be described in terms of a sequence of sets of explicit rules, it is not a result of any such rules. (The qualification here is necessary because there are many intermediate stages where its behaviour, like that of children, does not perfectly correspond to a manageably finite set of exceptionless rules.)

This computerized verb-learner is regarded by its creators as a challenge to Chomsky's claims that there must be an innate Language Acquisition Device (LAD) specifying the possible categories of linguistic rules, and that the child's task is to discern the rules of the relevant linguistic community and to form internal (explicit but inaccessible) representations of them which can then be used in generating speech. The fact that Chomsky was unable to suggest how the child might induce linguistic rules from its input, they argue, does not mean that there is no way of doing so. They see their PDP-model as an existence-proof that such induction can occur, and that it need not involve the explicit representation of linguistic rules. (In Chomsky's terminology, their claim is that the phonological rules governing the morphology of the past tense in English are "descriptively" but not "explanatorily" adequate.)

The Rumelhart–McClelland model, like connectionist systems in general, does show that apparently rule-governed behaviour may be generated by implicit rules rather than explicit ones (a contrast discussed further in Chapter 8). But it does not prove that there is no innate LAD constraining the form or content of the relevant rules, nor does it tell us how the child learns to handle *sentences* of indefinite complexity. These points are relevant to the topic of task-analysis, with which this particular discussion opened.

It is noteworthy that all the verb-pairs input while training the model are already articulated in phonological terms, and that each individual unit in the network stands for (is excited by input of) a particular phonological feature. In other words, the task of inducing past-tense morphology had been analysed before the network was set up. Admittedly, no specific rules about morphological changes were programmed into it. But the (phonetic) categories in which any such rules would have to be expressed were specified in each input-pair, and their recognition was built into the functioning of the network-units. That is, the network had an innate disposition to look for associative patterns between *these* features rather than any others. (This is not psychologically implausible, in view of the apparent universality of basic phonological distinctions across all human languages.)

Moreover, a system of this type is in principle capable of nothing more than associative pattern-matching. It the learning task is to induce the grammatical structure of sentences, for example, the learner needs not merely to *associate* "noun-phrase" with "verb-phrase", or "determiner" with "adjective" and "noun", but to understand the role of these syntactic categories in building hierarchically structured sentences (with the possibility of nesting on several levels). How could a simple pattern-matcher represent the fact that a determiner can be followed directly by a noun, *or* by one or more (perhaps many more) adjectives and then a noun, *or* by adjectives separated by a conjunction, followed by a noun? If it could not, then it could not learn to generate or understand sentences like "The rich but miserly man asked the tall beautiful woman to pay." This is not to say that no connectionist system could do this: the brain does, after all. But simple pattern-matching is not enough: a connectionist grammarian would have to embody a virtual machine capable of representing the relevant hierarchical and recursive structures. That is, as already suggested in Chapter 6, some of the computational properties of von Neumann computers may need to be simulated by connectionist systems if such systems are to model the whole range of human thought. And for this sort of virtual–von-Neumann connectionist system to be modelled and applied to a specific task-domain (such as language-understanding), the modeller needs to have done the relevant (syntactic) task-analysis beforehand.

But what if we left some huge randomly connected perceptron to run in the corner of the living room for five years, and its performance eventually showed that it had learned to speak by itself? We should be none the wiser, except in the most general sense. All this experiment would show is that language can be learnt by a connectionist *tabula rasa*. It would not tell us how the learning took place, nor even what had been learnt. We still should not know just how the past tense in English differs from the future tense in Russian – in other words, what distinctions any system must be able to make in order to be able to generate the relevant words. Nor should we know whether – and why – people (and perceptrons) who cannot speak English cannot speak Russian either. If we had no theory of phono-morphology, or of grammar, we could say nothing about the general conditions satisfied by good equilibrium-states within this hypothetical machine. All we could say of it is: "It speaks." But psychologists already know that some five-year-old connectionist systems, including some to be found in their own living rooms, can speak. The theoretical problem is to explain this.

In short, task-analysis is needed for theories of learning, whether connectionist or not. To explain how systems learn to do *x*, we must understand both *what counts* as *x*-ing and what it is *necessary* to be able to do in order to be able to do *x*. There is no painless road to the explanation of learning.

8   Is computational psychology possible?

Bertrand Russell once said of mathematics that it was the subject in which nobody knows what they are talking about. He meant not that mathematicians are incompetent, but that the subject-matter of mathematics is philosophically problematic. Had he been writing today, he might have said, "one of the *two* subjects in which nobody knows what they are talking about". For computational psychology, also, is philosophically ill defined.

The general characterization of *computational psychologists* given in Chapter 1 identifies them as theorists who draw on the concepts of computer science in formulating theories about what the mind is and how it works. Hence the three criteria of computational psychology, broadly defined: a functionalism that seeks to explain psychological phenomena in terms of effective procedures; a commitment to psychology as the study of representations, and transformations thereof; and a generally computational approach to neuroscience, wherein not what the brain is made of but what it is doing – and how – is the focus of interest. In short, computational psychology characteristically compares mental processes with the sorts of information-processing carried out by computers.

But what is "information"? Doesn't it have something to do with meaning, and with understanding? Can a computer mean, or understand – or even represent – anything at all? How do we do such things? And what does "compare" mean here? Is it a merely metaphorical comparison? If so, is the basis of the comparison reasonably clear, or so vague as to be capable of evading every empirical test on the grounds that "*that* feature isn't relevant to the metaphor"? Or is the comparison a literal one, a theoretical claim that psychological processes *really are* computations, in precisely the same sense in which (some? all?) computer processes are? – And what are *computations,* anyway? (It would not have helped to reply to Russell, "Mathematics is about numbers" – for what are numbers?)

Computational psychologists differ over such questions. Nor can we find uncontroversial answers in the philosophy of mind. Functionalism itself, though increasingly popular, is not unproblematic (especially with respect to its account of experience-as-such, or what are technically termed *qualia* [P. M. Churchland & Churchland, 1982]). Moreover, functionalists disagree among themselves about the analysis of concepts such as *computation, representation,* and *intentionality,* about whether psychological predicates should be interpreted in a *realist* or an *instrumentalist* way, and about whether the familiar categories of folk-psychology (such as *belief* and *inten-*

tion) can be expected to play any theoretical role in a scientific psychology. Fundamental disagreements such as these are related to, and largely responsible for, the theoretical and methodological differences among the case-studies of psychological research already discussed.

As well as the broad definition mentioned above, there are at least two more restrictive definitions of computational psychology, each of which has figured in the preceding chapters. We may call these the *mathematical* sense and the *formalist* sense.

Competence and task-definition

The *mathematical* sense covers explanations of psychological competence rather than performance, theories focussing on abstract task-analysis rather than on process or algorithm. What is done – and how it must be done if it is to be done at all – is the focus of interest, not how it happens to be done in a particular case. There is thus a methodological analogy with pure mathematics, which deals with abstractly conceived relations of a timeless nature as opposed to the temporal processes by which those relations can be exhibited or discovered.

The suggestion that a scientific psychology requires a level of explanation termed computational (understood in the mathematical sense) was made by D. Marr, in relation to his work on vision (discussed in Chapter 3). But, as we have seen, the psychological insight expressed by it had been stressed some years earlier by A. Newell and H. A. Simon (with respect to *task-analysis* in problem-solving) and by N. Chomsky (with respect to linguistic *competence*).

All these workers recognized that an appropriate abstract task-identification can engender fruitful theoretical questions. Indeed, they all held that it gives us a clearer understanding of what the relevant psychological phenomenon, or domain, really is. That is, it helps us to identify what the *natural kinds* of psychology are – which may or may not coincide neatly with the categories of everyday folk-psychology, or of non-computational psychological theories. The question whether chimps can learn *language,* for instance, is today taken to depend not on their producing humanoid speech-sounds (which they cannot) or new meaningful symbol-strings (which they can), but on their ability to make syntactic discriminations (which has not yet been satisfactorily demonstrated). The shift in interpretation of this question is largely due to Chomsky's insistence that grammatical competence is essential to language as such.

It is perhaps unfortunate that Marr introduced the term "computational" to denote explanations concerning what earlier writers had called task-analysis or competence. For the mathematical sense of this term is psychologically maverick – and so potentially confusing. Whereas most psychologists use "computational" in referring to processes, Marr's usage specifically excludes questions about temporal process. Psychologists in general are interested not only in *what tasks* the mind can master but in *what goes on* in the mind, *how,* and *when.* So Newell and Simon (as we saw in Chapter 6) try to detail the moment-to-moment control of information-processing; and M. Marcus suggests processing algorithms (described in Chapter 4) that can both exploit the abstract constraints on parsing defined by Chomsky and account for various performance-factors (which Chomsky deliberately ignored). Marr was no exception, of course: he too wanted to know how vision happens, as well as what vision is. But it is what he termed the algorithmic level of explanation which identifies what most other psychologists would call computational processes. Even if a mathematically computational analysis of a given domain is necessary, then, it is not sufficient for psychological purposes.

It is not clear, however, that a computational theory (in the mathematical sense) is always necessary, or even possible. To put the same point in another way, it is not clear that Marr's distinction between "Type 1" and "Type 2" theories [Marr, 1977] covers *all conceivable* scientific explanations: there may be a third option. A Type 1 theory is computational in the sense just described, providing an abstract identification of the task concerned. A Type 2 theory, by contrast, applies if and when information-processing is carried out by "the simultaneous action of a considerable number of processes, *whose interaction is its own simplest description*" [p. 38]. In other words, a Type 2 explanation would be nothing less than a complete description of all the processes responsible for a given phenomenon. What happens, happens: in an explanation of *why* it happens, there is no more – and, crucially, no less – that can be said.

Others before Marr had suggested that some psychological phenomena might be of the second kind. For example, J. von Neumann himself had argued that "it is futile to look for a precise logical concept, that is, for a precise verbal description, of 'visual analogy'. It is possible that the connection pattern of the visual brain itself is the simplest logical expression of this principle" [1960, p. 2091]. But Marr went further, for he implied that there is no possibility of scientific explanation in psychology other than by Type 1 or Type 2 theories – the latter very likely being, in practice, impossibly difficult to achieve.

To decree (with Marr) that a scientific psychology must be built upon a theory that is computational in this mathematical sense is to reject virtually all psychological theories, including many that are commonly termed computational because they fit the broad methodological definition given above. "So much the worse for them!" one might say. But this assumes that all psychological phenomena, if they can be scientifically explained at all (short of a Type 2 theory), *can* be adequately represented by an abstract theory of this kind.

In Chapter 3, and in successive chapters also, we questioned this assumption. It is challenged also by M. L. Minsky [1986], according to whom the mind is a "society" of many interacting processors that have evolved and/or developed largely independently of each other. There are reasons for thinking that evolution and/or individual learning have provided us with a number of "quick and dirty" methods of making inferences or interpretations of various kinds. Examples include the phrasal lexicon in language-understanding, the use of familiar cues in high-level visual processes, and piecemeal experiential learning (of a type which, in principle, might be appropriately represented by a production-system). Such methods are valuable if they often lead to the correct judgment or appropriate behaviour; they do not need to do so always, still less necessarily. Nor are they beyond the reach of a psychological science. Although they cannot, in principle, be discovered *a priori,* they can be discovered by empirical research. Moreover, their usefulness and limitations can be systematically investigated – in part, by comparing them with *ideal types* abstractly defined at the computational level.

The degree to which a given range of phenomena actually can be captured by a Type 1, competence, theory is an empirical question. Experimental research is required to discover which, if any, short-cut processes complicate the theoretical picture.

Low-level vision, parsing, and musical perception (as we have seen) are to a significant extent amenable to computational analysis in the mathematical sense. Many highly specific details of these phenomena are explicable in terms of an abstract task-analysis. Even certain aspects of semantics and pragmatics may be specifiable in abstract terms, although these are more controversial. We can hope for an abstract computational theory of (certain aspects of) conversation, for example, only if we have a coherent underlying theory of speech-acts as opposed to a rag-bag list of intuitively based categories. Some computer models have been discussed, above, which attempt analysis of the tasks involved in mapping a word-string onto a semantic representation, mapping an extended text onto its thematic representation, or interpreting (and generating) conversations in which a word-string may have very different meanings according to the beliefs and intentions of the speakers.

By contrast, it was argued in Chapter 6 that the higher mental processes (such as reasoning, belief-fixation, and memory) are for various reasons intrinsically less well suited to a competence-model – but that explanations of high-level thinking are nonetheless available, insofar as they identify generative structures within the mind that make possible the richly various performance phenomena. Despite his rejection of Newell and Simon's detailed work on problem-solving, Marr himself allowed that relatively coarse concepts such as R. C. Schank's "primitive actions", or Minsky's "frames", may be heuristically useful in highlighting the memory-access required to solve specific information-processing problems [1977, p. 44]. (Whether all phenomena traditionally studied by psychologists are analysable as distinct tasks is another question: social psychologists offer theories of attitude-change and personality-development, but it is most unlikely that these are natural kinds.)

In short, while it is undoubtedly salutary to try to achieve a theory that is computational in the mathematical sense of the term, this is not a *sine qua non* of any respectable psychological research.

Formalism: for and against

The *formalist* sense of computational psychology is more common than the mathematical sense. It covers those theories which hold that mental processes are, and/or are to be explained in terms of, the sorts of formal computations that are studied in traditional computer science and symbolic logic. These disciplines define "computation" as *the formal manipulation of abstract symbols, by the application of formal rules*. That is, the criteria for effecting one symbol-manipulation rather than another, and also for distinguishing the various transformations that are possible, are purely syntactic.

(Here I leave open two questions, both of which will be addressed later. First, whether a computer program has only syntactic properties, or whether it has intrinsic semantic properties too; we shall see that there is reason to doubt the programs-are-pure-syntax view. Second, whether all computation is of the formalist kind; below, I shall argue in relation to connectionism that a strictly formalist understanding of "computation" is over-restrictive.)

Many psychologists who adopt the methodology of computer-modelling have accepted this formalist definition of "computation". Accordingly, they assimilate mental processes to the symbol-manipulations specified by programs for von Neumann computers.

Sometimes the assimilation is merely metaphorical. Formalist computational concepts are then taken to be useful in formulating hypotheses about psychological function, even though it is allowed that mental processes may not really be computations. This non-committal approach is not inherently unscientific. Metaphors are commonly used in developing scientific theories – Rutherford's planetary model of the atom is just one example. Moreover, the explanation of one domain in terms of concepts drawn from another domain is not an evasion of the issue: on the contrary, it is a necessary aspect of the logic of explanation [Boden, 1962]. However, to use a metaphor in science is implicitly to promise to specify, at least after the exploratory period is past, where the metaphor breaks down. Devotees of the computational metaphor in psychology rarely attempt to identify its limits precisely.

Sometimes, however, the theoretical assimilation involved is much stronger – for some psychologists interpret formalist computational theories realistically, not metaphorically. They hold that minds literally perform computations, where computations are understood to be the sorts of formal operations which effect transformations of symbol-strings in digital computers. In short, they identify cognition and thinking in general with formal computation over formally specified representations.

One such theorist is Z. W. Pylyshyn [1984], whose views on imagery and belief-fixation were discussed in Chapters 2 and 6. He spurns the computational *metaphor,* saying that it removes the need to be rigorous in using one's model to explain behaviour. On the contrary, he holds that a computer model might do *the very same things* as the mind does, *in the very same way.* To specify the level of comparison at which such a claim might intelligibly be made, Pylyshyn borrows concepts from computer science in defining *strong equivalence:* a computer program and a cognitive process are strongly equivalent if they can both be represented by the same program in some theoretically specified virtual machine. (As we saw in Chapter 6, the virtual machine is the machine which the programmer can think is being used.) For Pylyshyn, representations having semantic content are physically instantiated in the brain, which has a functional architecture in just the same sense that a computer does. And mental processes, on his view, *really are* computations, that is, formal transformations defined over representations.

Pylyshyn was not the first computational psychologist to make a strongly realist commitment to formalism: his position owes much to the prior influence of Newell and Simon. Newell and Simon's theoretical work, likewise, had assumed the physical instantiation of mental representations in the brain. They too distinguished between the basic information-processing mechanisms provided by the functional architecture and the higher-level computational rules (what Pylyshyn terms the representation-governed processes) implemented by means of those mechanisms. Like Pylyshyn, they ascribed meaning, or semantic content, to representations while offering a *formalistic* definition of "computation". And they, also, held that certain information-processes in minds and computers are literally identical. For example, we saw in Chapter 6 that their theory of problem-solving allows only syntactic constraints to determine what can count as a match between patterns: purely *formal* matching suffices to fire individual rules, or productions, and thus to control (non-perceptual) information-processing in the human mind. This is not a methodological artefact due to their use of digital computers to model thinking but an expression of their commitment to a literally formalist psychology.

Indeed, Newell and Simon's account of *physical symbol systems* [Newell & Simon, 1972, pp. 21–26; Newell, 1980] – which they claim are both necessary and sufficient for intelligence in general – explicitly includes both digital computers and brains, and implies that human intelligence involves information-processing essentially similar to that which can occur in von Neumann computers. They define a physical symbol system as a set of entities called symbols, where a symbol is a physical pattern, in some natural or artefactual physical machine, which can be physically related to other such patterns in various ways (such as juxtaposition) to form compound symbol-structures, or "expressions".

In any physical symbol system, by definition, various computational processes exist that can build, modify, and compare expressions. In a particular case of symbol-manipulation, such processes operate on one expression – consisting of tokens, or instances, of various symbol-types (patterns) – to form a different expression. These processes are realized by physical means, whose precise nature will depend on the material of which the physical symbol system is made. Provided that a particular chemical substrate is physically capable of generating expression-patterns, so defined (which the inorganic materials used in computer-engineering undoubtedly are), it is in principle capable of implementing symbols, so defined.

Although all physical symbol systems are in fact physical things, Newell and Simon stress that they need not always be described as such. For psychological purposes, symbols, expressions, and the processes that operate on them are best described at a non-physical, information-processing, level. This level, say Newell and Simon, requires that one use the concepts of *designation* and *interpretation*. Their definitions of these terms imply an essentially *causal* theory of semantics: "An expression designates an object if, given the expression, the system can either affect the object itself or behave in ways depending on the object; and the system can interpret an expression if the expression designates a process and if, given the expression, the system can carry out the process." That is, the meaning of a symbol is the set of changes which the symbol enables the information-processing system to effect, either *to* or *in response to* some object or process. The object or process may exist in the external world, or it may be internal to the information-processing system itself.

Formalist computational psychology, typified by Newell and Simon's theory of physical symbol systems, has not gone unchallenged. As one might expect, its intellectual enemies attack it fiercely. J. R. Searle, for example, argues that it is fundamentally irrelevant to an understanding of the mind. What is more surprising, some of its *allies* – such as J. A. Fodor – also deem it incapable of explaining how our mental representations mediate our behaviour. Below, we shall consider both Searle's hostile critique and Fodor's more ambivalent position.

First, however, I must mention two criticisms from an ally who questions the form, if not the spirit, of the Newell–Simon definition of physical symbol systems. A. Sloman [1986b; in preparation] disputes their materialist assumption that physical instantiation is *necessary* to symbols. In principle, a digital-formalist symbolic representation could be instantiated by a bevy of immaterial angels jumping on and off immaterial pin-heads (and a connectionist representation could consist of classrooms of angels in telepathic communication). For present purposes, this criticism is not crucial. Our immediate concern is not with angels but with terrestrial beings, and there is no suggestion that the symbols in biological and electronic systems are not physically based.

Sloman's second criticism is more important, although even this does not reject the Newell–Simon enterprise at heart. Sloman faults Newell and Simon for defining symbols in a way that mentions only the physical, not the virtual, machine. Symbols, and representations, are structures which may be physical *or* abstract. Abstract symbols (or representations) include virtual symbols (or representations) in a virtual machine, such as the symbols defined at successive levels of the visual system by Marr. We saw in Chapter 3 that Marr posits (and instantiates within his own computer models) several layers of virtual machines, and that a symbol which is complex at level n may function as a primitive at level $n + 1$. What Marr terms computational and algorithmic questions may be raised at levels of representation far removed from the basic physical instantiation, which can in effect be ignored, or taken for granted. In other words (*pace* Newell and Simon, and Pylyshyn too), there is no such thing as "the" virtual machine of the human mind. Rather, there are several, or even many, such abstract machines or symbol-systems. Although the most fundamental of these are of course instantiated in the brain, most are not immediately constrained by neurophysiological details. While this criticism is theoretically and methodologically important (casting doubt on talk of "the" human virtual machine), it could readily be incorporated within the Newell–Simon definition. Sloman's point is that computational psychology is more complex than one might have thought, not that it is irrelevant or impossible.

Some other intellectual allies of Newell and Simon offer a friendship that is decidedly double-edged. Fodor [1980] surely counts as an ally, for (as we shall see) he has argued that computational psychology is the only theoretical psychology we can ever hope to achieve. Yet he believes that it is in principle incapable of addressing what many would regard as the prime question of psychology: how symbolic processes guide our perceptions of and actions in the world.

Computational psychology treats mental processes as operations defined in terms of formal manipulations of formally described representations. It follows, says Fodor, that it can view mental processes only as operations within an *uninterpreted* logical system. On this view, a computational psychology could distinguish among (for example) visual perception, visual illusion, and imagery only – if at all – by identifying *intrinsic* computational differences among distinct mental functions, not by relating such functions differentially to actual or possible worlds. So although computational theories can describe mental states and processes, they cannot have anything to say about how mental states map onto the world. Computational psychology, says Fodor, is committed to "methodological solipsism" (a phrase borrowed from H. Putnam [1975]). That is, there is no point in trying to discover any mappings between the mind and the world, because for the purposes of psychological research *how the world is makes no difference to one's mental states*.

This is not to deny that mental representations have meaning, nor to doubt that there is some interpretation of the formal system within the mind – though just how "meaning" and "interpretation" are to be analysed is a controversial question of philosophical semantics. Causal theories of meaning, as remarked above, stress the *causal processes* by which a representation is generated or which it helps to bring about – including (but not restricted to) changes occurring at the organism–environment interface. Non-causal accounts include model-theoretic semantics (mentioned in Chapters 5 and 6), which focusses on the *abstract isomorphism* between a representation and actual or possible worlds. There may well be causal processes (within the nervous system, including the sensory transducers) mediating between thought and action. The primitives and operations of the psychological calculus may indeed map onto some model, such as the environment and our activities in it (including the external memory and behavioural protocols investigated by Newell and Simon) and/or imaginary worlds of various kinds (like the imagined lighthouse-islands of Kosslyn's and of Pylyshyn's experiments, described in Chapter 2). But such matters, insists Fodor, lie outside the formal-syntactic concerns of a computational theory.

Fodor goes even further: he argues that no psychology will ever be able to map the semantic relations between our minds and the world. He is not indulging in a mere demarcation dispute between philosophy and psychology, forbidding the latter to say anything about semantic properties such as meaning. He grants that there could in principle be a *naturalistic psychology*: a scientific study of the causal links between mental representations and environment in which (according to the realist philosophical semantics which Fodor shares with Putnam [1975]) meaning is grounded. So, by implication, do Newell and Simon: their talk of causally defined designation and interpretation is germane to what Fodor terms *naturalistic,* not computational, psychology. Unlike Newell and Simon, however, Fodor believes that a naturalistic psychology can never be achieved in practice.

His pessimism rests on the fact that, in order to discover causal links between mental states and environmental conditions, we should have to be able to identify representations and their referents independently. This is in principle possible (given Fodor's realist semantics), but only if the relevant natural kinds, or real essences, have been identified – which identification can be effected only by science. So a comprehensive naturalistic psychology, capable of explaining how our mental representations affect thought and behaviour, would require the prior completion of physics.

Moreover, the physics would have to be systematically related to the mental representations. That is, a naturalistic psychology could explain only those psychological phenomena which are mediated by concepts denoting scientifically identifiable natural kinds. But many of our concepts are not scientifically projectible and so would not appear even in a completed physics. "Water", for instance, may refer to a natural kind (namely, what the chemist identifies as H_2O), but "pencil" surely does not, for indefinitely various objects with diverse physical properties could count as pencils. Since there can be no physics-of-pencils, there can be no psychological theories of how we choose, use, or even see pencils (although theories of 2D-to-3D mapping like those discussed in Chapter 3 could explain how we see *narrow octagonal cylinders with brightly coloured surfaces*). In general, phenomena identified in terms of unprojectible concepts are not amenable to scientific explanation.

We are not actually interested in having theories about how we relate to pencils, because we do not believe that anything of general psychological importance attaches to them. The same cannot be said of questions involving the concepts of everyday folk-psychology: how we attribute beliefs; how we execute intentions; how we converse; how we assert, question, reply, or promise; how we learn new skills; how we make decisions; how we solve problems; how we modify attitudes; how we adjust our beliefs, or cling to our prejudices, in the light of new evidence; how we assess personalities; how we recognize hostility or friendliness; . . .

Many psychologists, including some discussed in previous chapters, hope to find systematic answers to questions like these, because we normally assume that the concepts of folk-psychology have explanatory power. But these concepts must be scientifically projectible if they are to appear in a theoretical psychology. As we saw in Chapter 6, Fodor [1980] has argued that they are not projectible – also dismissing theoretical concepts that are similar in kind, such as those used in Schankian computer models of memory or text-processing. In Fodor's discussion of methodological solipsism, research on topics identified in folk-psychological terms is held to be scientifically valueless: the best we can hope for is to collect a number of intriguing (and occasionally, pragmatically useful) anecdotes about them.

Fodor's attitude to the scientific status of folk-psychology, so dismissive a few years ago, is radically different in his very recent work [in press]. Now, he argues that evolutionary pressures would have favoured creatures whose ideas about mind captured *real* properties of brains. This claim is highly persuasive. The philosopher J. L. Austin [1961] took an essentially similar position in arguing that the conceptual analysis of ordinary-language psychological terms is likely to be a fruitful first step in a philosophy, and even a science, of mind.

But, as Austin pointed out, it may not be the last step. Indeed, it cannot be, since (as is implied by all the previous chapters) a complete theoretical psychology would have to go further than the folk-psychological level. For example, even if one were prepared to accept "Because he understood the speaker to want the salt" as an explanation (in ordinary-language terms) of someone's behaviour (likewise identified in folk-psychological terms), one would still need to ask *how it is possible* for someone to understand a sentence (*a fortiori*, a non-interrogative sentence) as a question. Moreover, the categories of folk-psychology might be adjusted (at least for the purposes of a scientific psychology) in the process. The evolutionary considerations stressed by Austin and (recently) Fodor suggest only that ordinary-language words will identify natural kinds *broadly conceived*. As has already happened in physics, the scientific characterizations of the relevant natural kinds may not be precisely co-extensive with the equivalent ordinary-language terms (which in any event are not precisely definable themselves).

A willingness to include folk-psychology within one's psychological science is thus not incompatible with a computational approach. Nor is it necessarily inconsistent with the claim (part of Fodor's methodological solipsism) that a formalist computational psychology cannot explain our relation to the world. (Whether or not a computational theory can have a genuinely semantic aspect depends on one's theory of *meaning*.) But it is inconsistent with the claim that a computational psychology is the only scientific psychology we can ever hope to achieve. To that extent, Fodor's case for methodological solipsism is now much weaker.

Scepticism about whether theoretical psychology could ever explain phenomena identified in folk-psychological terms has been expressed not only by Fodor [1980] but by other writers too. Some of these say nothing one way or the other about computational theories, for the question whether the psychological concepts used in everyday life are scientifically projectible is logically independent of the status of the formalist approach. But some are staunch allies of computational psychology whose views have been significantly influenced by Fodor himself.

For instance, S. C. Stich [1983] agrees with Fodor that cognitive science must define mental states in purely formalist terms. He does not go so far as to say that any attempt to produce a naturalistic psychology is a waste of time. But he concurs with Fodor's judgment that formalism will not provide scientific status to folk-psychological concepts, it being doubtful whether such concepts can be mapped onto the categories of a formal-syntactic psychology – or onto neurophysiology either.

Stich reminds us that folk-psychology individuates propositional attitudes in terms of their semantic content: belief is *the belief that p*, desire is *the desire that q*, and so on for intentional terms in general. He argues that these content-based ascriptions are irremediably vague and highly dependent on the physical or cultural context, and that intentional ascriptions are therefore not scientifically projectible. The difficulties of ascribing, or denying, a specific belief or desire to a person are most obvious in regard to members of "primitive" cultures, infants, and senile or brain-damaged people. But Stich claims that similar problems, in principle, attend the ascription of beliefs and desires to normal adults of one's own culture.

He concludes that there may be no isolable causal process common to all cases in which we ascribe a particular belief or intention or expectation . . . to someone; there may not even be an approximate mapping, as there is between chemistry and rules of thumb in cooking. If we ever discover that no such isomorphism exists, we shall have shown that beliefs and intentions are no more real than phlogiston or witches, in which case the pseudo-explanatory vocabulary of folk-psychology will wither away. As to whether this radical change in our way of thinking about ourselves and other people will ever take place, Stich declares himself agnostic: "It is too early to say whether folk psychology has a future" [Stich, 1983, p. 242; cf. P. M. Churchland, 1981; Churchland & Churchland, 1982]. Irrespective of the eventual fate of everyday psychological concepts, Stich accepts Fodor's argument that theoretical psychology must be computational, describing mental processes in formal-syntactic terms alone.

According to Fodor's early defence of methodological solipsism, then, computational psychology is simultaneously important and impotent. Because we cannot discover systematic organism–environment causal relations, it is the only scientific psychology we can expect to achieve. But because its theories are expressed in purely formal terms, it cannot explain how our ideas enter into our lives. Is he right?

Fodor is correct in saying that the scope of a naturalistic psychology is limited. My discussion of the *mathematical* sense of "computational psychology" made a similar point: abstract task-analysis is possible only for tasks which are scientifically projectible. Whether its scope is so drastically limited as Fodor's methodological solipsism suggests is another question, whose answer requires not only abstract enquiry but experimental study too.

It is unnecessarily defeatist to assume that empirical investigation of the causal relations between organism and environment is a waste of time. Without such investigation, the *modules* that Fodor himself [1983] attributes to the mind (as we saw in Chapter 6) would never have been identified. We may (as was suggested earlier in this chapter) discover some psychological processes originally brought about by evolutionary accident, processes which contribute to the efficiency of perception, for example. And we may discover further psychologically relevant natural kinds, some of which may not be confined (as modules, on Fodor's definition, are) to peripheral, computationally encapsulated processing.

Concepts like *belief, intention, problem-solving, conformity, learning,* and *conversation* (and more technical terms, such as *dissonance, schema,* or *speech-act*) are descriptively useful, and most are *prima facie* explanatory. Some of them may indeed be non-projectible, and so unsuitable for inclusion–even as useful approximations–within a scientific psychology (whether computational or not). But it is not clear that all of them are, or that all psychologists who investigate such matters are doomed to be mere collectors of scientifically irrelevant anecdotes. It is too early to condemn all research into such matters, on pain of irrelevance to science. Even Stich allows that some aspects of folk-psychology may have a future. And, as noted above, Fodor himself (on persuasive evolutionary grounds) now accords a higher scientific status to ordinary-language psychological terms than he did in his paper on methodological solipsism.

Moreover, one does not need to be a champion of folk-psychology to regard naturalistic investigation as perfectly proper. Empirical study of the causal relations between mind and environment has already led to new theoretical concepts, scientifically superior to the more familiar categories of everyday language. The work on vision discussed in earlier chapters is a prime example. In short, Fodor's defence of methodological solipsism as a research strategy in psychology is unacceptable.

What of Fodor's claim that computational psychology is semantically empty, that it can say nothing about the world, because it conceives of the mind only as an uninterpreted formal calculus? This aspect of methodological solipsism is more commonly accepted (both within and outside the computationalist camp). But it, too, is problematic.

It is true that one can treat computational psychological theories (for example, Newell and Simon's rules for cryptarithmetic) as though they were part of formal logic, which defines symbols and operations in purely syntactic terms. But it is not obvious that this is how they should be treated. To be sure, Newell and Simon (as we noted in Chapter 6) based their theory of production-systems on the work of a formal logician, E. Post. However, they themselves were doing not logic, but psychology: they were talking about what goes on in a person's mind, about the control of internal and bodily actions. Moreover, they explicitly claim that the mental processes defined by a formalist psychology are literally identical with processes that could occur in a von Neumann computer. Their psychological theory should therefore be likened not to an uninterpreted logical calculus, but rather to a computer program.

It may seem that this answers our question–and in Fodor's favour, at that. For computer programs, also, can be treated for certain purposes as purely formal systems. Indeed, many would claim that they can be treated thus for all proper purposes. "Programs are pure syntax" is an assumption so widely made as to be almost a cliché. It is accepted not only by most proponents of computational psychology, but by its opponents too–who use it as a main weapon in their philosophical arsenal, as we shall see.

If programs are nothing but syntax, then computational psychology (ig-noring naturalistic research into causal processes) is indeed a solipsistic theory. It could not even express semantic relations between various repre-sentations and processes within the mind itself, never mind those between the organism and the external environment. However, some writers reject this common assumption, arguing that computer programs have an intrinsic causal-semantic aspect (to be distinguished from any abstract isomorphism there may be between programmed formalisms and actual or possible worlds). If they are right, computational psychology is not inherently solipsistic, and its enemies are largely disarmed.

The crucial assumption at issue here will be discussed – and rebutted – presently. First, let us see how it has been used by some enemies of the computational approach to mount a radical attack on this way of describing the mind.

Searle [1980] is no friend of computational psychology, but a deeply unsympathetic critic who regards computational theories as essentially worthless. He makes two main claims, the first of which takes for granted the programs-are-pure-syntax assumption mentioned above.

His first claim is that formalist accounts, appropriate in explaining the meaningless symbol-manipulations in computers, are unable to explain how human minds employ *symbols* properly so called. Intentionality can-not be explained in computational terms. Searle's point here is not that no machine can think. Humans can think, and humans, he allows, are ma-chines; he even adopts the materialist credo that only machines can think. Nor is he saying that humans and programs are utterly incommensurable. He grants that, at some highly abstract level of description, people (like everything else) are instantiations of digital computers. His point, rather, is that nothing can think, mean, or understand *solely* in virtue of its instantiat-ing a computer program.

To persuade us of this point, Searle employs an ingenious thought-experiment. He imagines himself locked in a room, in which there are various slips of paper with doodles on them; a window through which people can pass further doodle-papers to him, and through which he can pass papers out; and a book of rules (in English) telling him how to pair the doodles, which are always identified by their shape or form. Searle spends his time, while inside the room, manipulating the doodles according to the rules.

One rule, for example, instructs him that when *squiggle-squiggle* is passed in to him, he should give out *squoggle-squoggle*. The rule-book also provides for more complex sequences of doodle-pairing, where only the first and last steps mention the transfer of paper into or out of the room. Before finding any rule directly instructing him to give out a slip of paper, he may have to locate a *blongle* doodle and compare it with a *blungle* doodle – in which case, it is the result of this comparison which determines the nature of the doodle he passes out. Sometimes many such doodle–doodle comparisons and consequent doodle-selections have to be made by him inside the room before he finds a rule allowing him to pass anything out.

So far as Searle-in-the-room is concerned, the *squiggles* and *squoggles* are mere meaningless doodles. Unknown to him, however, they are Chinese characters. The people outside the room, being Chinese, interpret them as such. Moreover, the patterns passed in and out at the window are understood by them as *questions* and *answers* respectively: the rules happen to be such that most of the questions are paired, either directly or indirectly, with what they recognize as a sensible answer. But Searle himself (inside the room) knows nothing of this.

The point, says Searle, is that Searle-in-the-room is clearly instantiating a computer program. That is, he is performing purely formal manipulations of uninterpreted patterns: he is all syntax and no semantics. The doodle-pairing rules are equivalent to IF–THEN productions. Some of the internal doodle-comparisons could be equivalent to a Schankian script (for instance, the restaurant script mentioned in Chapter 5). In that case, Searle-in-the-room's paper-passing performance would be essentially comparable to the performance of a "question-answering" Schankian text-analysis program. But "question-answering" is not question-answering. Searle-in-the-room is not really *answering:* how could he, since he cannot understand the questions? Practice does not help (except perhaps in making the doodle-pairing swifter): if Searle-in-the-room ever escapes, he will be just as ignorant of Chinese as he was when he was first locked in.

Certainly, the Chinese people outside may find it useful to keep Searle-in-the-room fed and watered, much as in real life we are willing to spend large sums of money on computerized "advice" systems. But the fact that people who already possess understanding may use an intrinsically meaningless formalist computational system to provide what they interpret (*sic*) as questions, answers, designations, interpretations, or symbols is irrelevant. They can do this only if they can externally specify a mapping between the formalism and matters of interest to them. As remarked in Chapter 5, one and the same formalism might be mappable onto both dance-routines and tapestry-work, in which case it would be suitable for use (by people) in answering questions about either domain. In itself, however, it would be meaningless – as are the Chinese symbols from the point of view of Searle-in-the-room.

It follows, Searle argues, that no system can understand anything solely in virtue of its instantiating a computer program. For if it could, then Searle-in-the-room would understand Chinese. Hence, theoretical psychology cannot properly be grounded in computational concepts.

Searle's second claim concerns what a proper explanation of understanding would be like. According to him, it would acknowledge that meaningful symbols must be embodied in something having "the right causal powers" for generating understanding, or intentionality. Obviously, he says, brains do have such causal powers whereas computers do not. More precisely (since the brain's organization could be paralleled in a computer), neuro-protein does whereas metal and silicon do not: the biochemical properties of the brain-matter are crucial.

Newell and Simon's definition of physical symbol systems is rejected by Searle, because they demand merely that symbols be embodied in some material that can implement formalist computations – which computers, admittedly, can do. On Searle's view, no electronic computer can really manipulate symbols, nor really designate or interpret anything at all – *irrespective* of any causal dependencies linking its internal physical patterns to its behaviour. (This strongly realist view of intentionality contrasts with the instrumentalism of D. C. Dennett [1971; 1978]. For Dennett, an intentional system is one whose behaviour we can explain, predict, and control only by ascribing beliefs, goals, and rationality to it. On this criterion, some existing computer programs are intentional systems, and the hypothetical humanoids beloved of science-fiction would be intentional systems *a fortiori*.)

Intentionality, Searle declares, is a biological phenomenon. As such, it is just as dependent on the underlying biochemistry as are photosynthesis and lactation. He grants that neuroprotein may not be the only substance in the universe capable of supporting mental life, much as substances other than chlorophyll may be able (on Mars, perhaps) to catalyse the synthesis of carbohydrates. But he rejects metal or silicon as potential alternatives, even on Mars. He asks whether a computer made out of old beer-cans could possibly *understand* – a rhetorical question to which the expected answer is a resounding "No!" In short, Searle takes it to be intuitively obvious that the inorganic substances with which (today's) computers are manufactured are essentially incapable of supporting mental functions.

In assessing Searle's two-pronged critique of computational psychology, let us first consider his view that intentionality must be biologically grounded. One might be tempted to call this a positive claim, in contrast with his negative claim that purely formalist theories cannot explain mentality. However, this would be to grant it more than it deserves, for its explanatory power is illusory. The biological analogies mentioned by Searle are misleading, and the intuitions to which he appeals are unreliable.

The brain's production of intentionality, we are told, is comparable to photosynthesis – but is it, really? We can define the *products* of photosynthesis, clearly distinguishing various sugars and starches within the general class of carbohydrates, and showing how these differ from other biochemical products such as proteins. Moreover, we not only *know that* chlorophyll supports photosynthesis, we also *understand how* it does so (and *why* various other chemicals cannot). We know that it is a catalyst rather than a raw material; and we can specify the point at which, and the sub-atomic process by which, its catalytic function is exercised. With respect to brains and understanding, the case is very different.

Our theory of what intentionality is (never mind how it is generated) does not bear comparison with our knowledge of carbohydrates: just what intentionality *is* is still philosophically controversial. We cannot even be entirely confident that we can recognize it when we see it. It is generally agreed that the propositional attitudes are intentional, and that feelings and sensations are not; but there is no clear consensus about the intentionality of emotions.

Various attempts have been made to characterize intentionality and to distinguish its sub-species as distinct intentional states (beliefs, desires, hopes, intentions, and the like). Searle himself has made a number of relevant contributions, from his early work on speech-acts [1969] mentioned in Chapter 5 to his more recent account [1983] of intentionality in general. A commonly used criterion (adopted by Brentano in the nineteenth century and also by Searle) is a *psychological* one. In Brentano's words, intentional states direct the mind on an object; in Searle's, they have intrinsic representational capacity, or "aboutness"; in either case they relate the mind to the world, and to possible worlds. But some writers define intentionality in *logical* terms [Chisholm, 1967]. It is not even clear whether the logical and psychological definitions are precisely co-extensive [Boden, 1970]. In brief, no theory of intentionality is accepted as unproblematic, as the chemistry of carbohydrates is.

As for the brain's biochemical "synthesis" of intentionality, this is even more mysterious. We have very good reason to believe *that* neuroprotein supports intentionality, but we have hardly any idea how – *qua* neuroprotein – it is able to do so.

Insofar as we understand these matters at all, we focus on the neurochemical basis of certain *informational functions* – such as message-passing, facilitation, and inhibition – embodied in neurones and synapses; for example: how the sodium-pump at the cell-membrane enables an action potential to propagate along the axon; how electrochemical changes cause a neurone to enter into and recover from its refractory period; or how neuronal thresholds can be altered by neurotransmitters, such as acetylcholine. With respect to a visual cell, for instance, a crucial psychological question may be *whether it can function as a DOG-detector*. If the neurophysiologist can tell us which molecules enable it to do so, so much the better. But from the psychological point of view, it is not the biochemistry as such which matters but the information-bearing functions grounded in it. (Searle apparently admits this when he says, "The type of realizations that intentional states have in the brain may be describable at a much higher functional level than that of the specific biochemistry of the neurons involved" [1983, p. 272].)

Metal and silicon are undoubtedly able to support some of the abstract mathematical-computational functions necessary for 2D-to-3D mapping. Moreover, they can embody DOG-detectors, which seem to be involved in many biological visual systems (even though they are not necessary in absolute terms). Admittedly, it may be that metal and silicon cannot support all the functions involved in normal vision, or in understanding generally. Perhaps only neuroprotein can do so, so that only creatures with a terrestrial biology can enjoy intentionality. But we have no specific reason, at present, to think so. Most important in this context, any such reasons we might have in the future must be grounded in empirical discovery: intuitions will not help.

If one asks which mind–matter dependencies are intuitively plausible, the answer must be that none is. Nobody who was puzzled about intentionality (as opposed to action-potentials) ever exclaimed, "Sodium – of course!" Sodium-pumps are no less "obviously" absurd than silicon chips, electrical polarities no less "obviously" irrelevant than old beer-cans, acetylcholine hardly less surprising than beer. The fact that the first member of each of these three pairs is *scientifically* compelling does not make any of them *intuitively* intelligible: our initial surprise persists.

Our intuitions might change with the advance of science. Possibly we shall eventually see neuroprotein (and perhaps silicon too) as obviously capable of embodying mind, much as we now see biochemical substances in general (including chlorophyll) as obviously capable of producing other such substances – an intuition that was not obvious, even to chemists, prior to the synthesis of urea. At present, however, our intuitions have nothing useful to say about the material basis of intentionality. Searle's "positive" claim, his putative alternative explanation of intentionality, is at best a promissory note, at worst mere mystery-mongering.

Searle's negative claim, that formal-computational theories cannot explain understanding, is less quickly rebutted. My rebuttal will involve two parts: the first directly addressing his example of the Chinese room, the second dealing with his background assumption (on which his example depends) that computer programs are pure syntax.

The Chinese-room example has engendered much debate, both within and outside the community of cognitive science. Some criticisms were anticipated by Searle himself in his original paper, others appeared as the accompanying peer-commentary (together with his reply), and more have been published since. Here, I shall concentrate on only two points: what Searle calls the Robot reply, and what I shall call the English reply.

The Robot reply accepts that the only understanding of Chinese which exists in Searle's example is that enjoyed by the Chinese individuals outside the room. Searle-in-the-room's inability to connect Chinese characters with events in the outside world shows that he does not understand Chinese. Likewise, a Schankian teletyping computer that cannot recognize a restaurant, hand money to a waiter, or chew a morsel of food understands nothing of restaurants even if it can usefully "answer" some of our questions about them. But a robot, provided not only with a restaurant-script but also with camera-fed visual programs and limbs capable of walking and picking things up, would be another matter. If the input–output behaviour of such a robot were identical with that of human beings, it would demonstrably understand both restaurants and the natural language (Chinese perhaps) used by people to communicate with it.

Searle's first response to the Robot reply is to claim a victory already, since the reply concedes that cognition is not solely a matter of formal symbol-manipulation but requires in addition a set of causal relations with the outside world. (One may doubt whether his triumph is justified: even Fodor allows that a comprehensive psychology would be computational *and* naturalistic.) Second, Searle insists that to add perceptuomotor capacities to a computational system is not to add intentionality, or understanding.

He argues this point by imagining a robot which, instead of being provided with a computer program to make it work, has a miniaturized Searle inside it – in its skull, perhaps. Searle-in-the-robot, with the aid of a (new) rule-book, shuffles paper and passes *squiggles* and *squoggles* in and out, much as Searle-in-the-room did before him. But now some or all of the incoming Chinese characters are not handed in by Chinese people, but are triggered by causal processes in the cameras and audio-equipment in the robot's eyes and ears. And the outgoing Chinese characters are not received by Chinese hands, but by motors and levers attached to the robot's limbs, which are caused to move as a result. In short, this robot is apparently able not only to answer questions in Chinese but also to see and do things accordingly: it can recognize raw bean-sprouts and, if the recipe requires it, toss them into a wok as well as any of us can.

(The discussion of vision in Chapter 3 suggests that the vocabulary of Chinese would require considerable extension for this example to be carried through. And the account of language-processing in Chapters 4 and 5 suggests that the same could be said of the English required to express the rules in Searle's initial question-answering example. In either case, what Searle-in-the-room needs is not so much Chinese, or even English, as a programming language. We shall return to this point presently.)

Like his roombound predecessor, however, Searle-in-the-robot knows nothing of the wider context. He is just as ignorant of Chinese as he ever was, and has no more purchase on the outside world than he did in the original example. To him, bean-sprouts and woks are invisible and intangible: all Searle-in-the-robot can see and touch, besides the rule-book and the doodles, are his own body and the inside walls of the robot's skull.

Consequently, Searle argues, the robot cannot be credited with understanding of any of these worldly matters. In truth, it is not *seeing* or *doing* anything at all: it is "simply moving about as a result of its electrical wiring and its program", which latter is instantiated by the man inside it, who "has no intentional states of the relevant type" [1980, p. 420].

Searle's argument here is unacceptable as a rebuttal of the Robot reply, because it draws a false analogy between the imagined example and what is claimed by computational psychology.

Searle-in-the-robot is supposed by Searle to be performing the functions performed (according to computational theories) by the human brain. But, whereas most computationalists do not ascribe intentionality to the brain (and those who do, as we shall see presently, do so only in a very limited way), Searle characterizes Searle-in-the-robot as enjoying full-blooded intentionality, just as he does himself. Computational psychology does not credit the brain with *seeing bean-sprouts* or *understanding English:* intentional states such as these are properties of people, not of brains. In general, although representations and mental processes are assumed (by computationalists and Searle alike) to be embodied in the brain, the sensorimotor capacities and propositional attitudes which they make possible are ascribed to the person as a whole. So Searle's description of the system inside the robot's skull as one which can understand English does not truly parallel what computationalists say about the brain.

Indeed, the specific cerebral procedures hypothesized by computational psychologists, and embodied by them in computer models of the mind, are relatively stupid – and they become more and more stupid as one moves to increasingly basic theoretical levels [Dennett, 1978]. Consider the theories of natural-language parsing described in Chapter 4, for example: a parsing procedure that searches for a determiner does not understand English, nor does a procedure for locating the reference of a personal pronoun; only the person whose brain performs these interpretative processes, and many others associated with them, can do that. The capacity to understand English involves many interacting information-processes, each performing only a limited function but together providing capacity to take English sentences as input and give appropriate English sentences as output. Similar remarks apply to the individual components of the computational theories of vision, problem-solving, or learning described earlier. Precisely because psychologists wish to *explain* human language, vision, reasoning, and learning, they posit underlying processes which lack these capacities.

In short, Searle's description of the robot's pseudo-brain (that is, of Searle-in-the-robot) as understanding English involves a category-mistake comparable to treating the brain as the bearer, as opposed to the causal basis, of intelligence.

Someone might object here that I have contradicted myself by claiming that one cannot ascribe intentionality to brains and yet implicitly doing just that. For I spoke of the brain's effecting stupid component-procedures – but stupidity is virtually a species of intelligence. To be stupid is to be intelligent, but not very (a person or a fish can be stupid, but a stone or a river cannot).

My defence would be twofold. First, the most basic theoretical level of all would be at the neuroscientific equivalent of the machine-code, a level engineered by evolution. The facts that a certain light-sensitive cell can act as a DOG-detector and that one neurone can inhibit the firing of another are explicable by the biochemistry of the brain. The notion of stupidity, even in scare-quotes, is wholly inappropriate in discussing such facts. However, these very basic information-processing functions (DOG-detecting and synaptic inhibition) *could* properly be described as "very, very, very . . . stupid". This of course implies that intentional language, if only of a highly grudging and uncomplimentary type, is applicable to brain-processes after all – which prompts the second point in my defence. I did not say that intentionality cannot be ascribed to brains, but that full-blooded intentionality cannot. Nor did I say that brains or brain-processes cannot understand anything at all, in however limited a fashion, but that they cannot (for example) understand English. I even hinted, several paragraphs ago, that a few computationalists do ascribe some degree of intentionality to the brain (or to the computational processes going on in it). These two points will soon become less obscure, after we have considered the English reply and its bearing on Searle's background assumption that formal-syntactic computational theories are purely syntactic.

The crux of the English reply is that the instantiation of a computer program, whether by man or by manufactured machine, does involve understanding – at least of the rule-book. Searle's initial example depends critically on Searle-in-the-room's being able to understand the language in which the rules are written, namely English; similarly, without Searle-in-the-robot's familiarity with English, the robot's bean-sprouts would never get thrown into the wok. Moroever, as remarked above, the vocabulary of English (and, for Searle-in-the-robot, of Chinese too) would have to be significantly modified to make the example work.

An unknown language (whether Chinese or Linear B) can be dealt with only as an aesthetic object or a set of systematically related forms. Artificial languages can be designed and studied, by the logician or the pure mathematician, with only their structural properties in mind (although D. R. Hofstadter's [1979] example of the MU-game, mentioned in Chapter 6 above, shows that a psychologically compelling, and predictable, interpretation of a formal calculus may arise spontaneously). But one normally responds in a very different way to the symbols of one's native tongue; indeed, it is difficult to bracket (that is, ignore) the meanings of familiar words. The view defended in Chapter 5, that natural languages can be characterized in procedural terms, is relevant here: words, clauses, and sentences can be seen as mini-programs. The symbols in a natural language one understands initiate mental activity of various kinds. To learn a language is to set up the relevant causal connections, not only between words and the world ("cat" and the thing on the mat) but between words and the many non-introspectible procedures involved in interpreting them.

Moreover, we do not need to be told *ex hypothesi* (by Searle) that Searle-in-the-room understands English: his behaviour while in the room shows clearly that he does. Or, rather, it shows that he understands a *highly limited sub-set* of English.

Searle-in-the-room could be suffering from total amnesia with respect to 99 per cent of Searle's English vocabulary, and it would make no difference. The only grasp of English he needs is whatever is necessary to interpret (*sic*) the rule-book–which specifies how to accept, select, compare, and give out different patterns. Unlike Searle, Searle-in-the-room does not require words like "catalyse", "beer-can", "chlorophyll", and "restaurant". But he may need "find", "compare", "two", "triangular", and "window" (although his understanding of these words could be much less full than Searle's). He must understand conditional sentences, if any rule states that if he sees a *squoggle* he should give out a *squiggle*. Very likely, he must understand some way of expressing negation, temporal ordering, and (especially if he is to learn to do his job faster) generalization. If the rules he uses include some which parse the Chinese sentences, then he will need words for grammatical categories too. (He will not need explicit rules for parsing English sentences, such as the parsing procedures discussed in Chapter 4, because he already understands English.)

In short, Searle-in-the-room needs to understand only that sub-set of Searle's English which is equivalent to the programming language understood by a computer generating the same question-answering input–output behaviour at the window. Similarly, Searle-in-the-robot must be able to understand whatever sub-set of English is equivalent to the programming language understood by a fully computerized visuomotor robot.

The two preceding sentences may seem to beg the very question at issue. Indeed, to speak thus of the programming language understood by a computer is seemingly self-contradictory. For Searle's basic premise, which he assumes is accepted by all participants in the debate, is that a computer program is purely formal in nature: the computation it specifies is purely syntactic and has no intrinsic meaning or semantic content to be understood. If we accept this premise, the English reply sketched above can be dismissed forthwith for being an effort to draw a parallel where no parallel can properly be drawn. But if we do not, if–*pace* Searle (and Fodor, and Stich)–computer programs are not concerned only with syntax, then the English reply may be relevant after all. We must now turn to address this basic question.

Are programs pure syntax?

Certainly, one can for certain purposes think of a computer program as an uninterpreted logical calculus. For example, one might be able to prove, by purely formal means, that a particular well-formed formula is derivable from the program's data-structures and inferential rules. Moreover, it is true that a so-called interpreter program that could take as input the list-structure "(FATHER (MAGGIE))" and return "(LEONARD)" would do so on formal criteria alone, having no way of interpreting these patterns as possibly denoting real people. Likewise, as Searle points out, programs provided with restaurant-scripts are not thereby provided with knowledge of restaurants. The existence of a mapping between a formalism and a certain domain does not in itself provide the manipulator of the formalism with any understanding of that domain.

But what must not be forgotten is that a computer program is *a program for a computer:* when a program is run on suitable hardware, the machine *does* something as a result (hence the use in computer science of the words "instruction" and "obey"). At the level of the machine-code the effect of the program on the computer is direct, because the machine is engineered so that a given instruction elicits a unique operation (instructions in high-level languages must be converted into machine-code instructions before they can be obeyed). A programmed instruction, then, is not a mere formal pattern – nor even a declarative statement (although it may for some purposes be thought of under either of those descriptions). It is a procedure-specification that, given a suitable hardware-context, can cause the procedure in question to be executed.

One might put this by saying that a programming language is a medium not only for expressing *representations* (structures that can be written on a page or provided to a computer, some of which structures may be isomorphic with things that interest people) but also for bringing about the *representational activity* of certain machines. Indeed, one might even say that a representation *is* an activity rather than a structure.

Many philosophers and psychologists have supposed that mental representations are intrinsically active. Among the cognitive scientists who have recently argued for this view is Hofstadter [1985], who specifically criticizes Newell and Simon's account of *symbols* as manipulable formal tokens. In his words, "The brain itself does not 'manipulate symbols'; the brain is the medium in which the symbols are floating and in which they trigger each other" [p. 648]. Hofstadter expresses more sympathy for connectionist work – which as we have seen, is well suited to model cerebral representations, symbols, or concepts as dynamic processes. But it is not only connectionists who can view concepts as intrinsically active, and not only *cerebral* representations which can be thought of in this way: this claim has been generalized to cover traditional computer programs, specifically designed for von Neumann machines. The computer scientist B. C. Smith [1982; in press] argues that programmed representations, too, are inherently active – and that an adequate theory of the semantics of programming languages would recognize the fact.

At present, Smith claims, computer scientists have a radically inadequate understanding of such matters. He reminds us that as remarked above, there is no general agreement (either within or outside computer science) about what *intentionality* is, and there are deep unclarities about *representation* as well. Nor can unclarities be avoided by speaking more technically, in terms of *computation* and *formal symbol-manipulation*. For the computer scientist's understanding of what these phenomena really are is also largely intuitive. Smith's discussion of programming languages identifies some fundamental confusions within computer science. Especially relevant here is his claim that computer scientists commonly make too complete a theoretical separation between a program's control-functions and its nature as a formal-syntactic system.

The theoretical divide criticized by Smith is evident in the widespread *dual-calculus* approach to programming. The dual-calculus approach posits a sharp theoretical distinction between a declarative (or denotational) representational structure and the procedural language that interprets it when the program is run. Indeed, the knowledge-representation and the interpreter are sometimes written in two quite distinct formalisms (such as the predicate calculus and LISP, respectively). Often, however, they are both expressed in the same formalism; for example, LISP (an acronym for LISt-Processing language) allows facts and procedures to be expressed in formally similar ways, and so does PROLOG (PROgramming-in-LOGic). In such cases, the dual-calculus approach dictates that the single programming language concerned be theoretically described in two quite different ways.

To illustrate the distinction at issue here, suppose that we wanted a representation of family relationships which could be used to provide answers to questions about such matters. We might decide to employ a list-structure to represent such facts as that Leonard is the father of Maggie. Or we might prefer a frame-based representation, in which the relevant name-slots in the FATHER-frame could be simultaneously filled by "LEONARD" and "MAGGIE". Again, we might choose a formula of the predicate calculus, saying that there exist two people (namely, Leonard and Maggie), and Leonard is the father of Maggie. Last, we might employ the English sentence "Leonard is the father of Maggie."

Each of these four representations could be written/drawn on paper (as are the rules in the rule-book used by Searle-in-the-room), for us to interpret *if* we have learnt how to handle the relevant notation. Alternatively, they could be embodied in a computer data-base. But to make them usable by the computer, there has to be an interpreter-program which (for instance) can find the item "LEONARD" when we ask it who is the father of Maggie. No one with any sense would embody list-structures in a computer without providing it also with a *list-processing* facility, nor give it frames without a *slot-filling* mechanism, logical formulae without *rules of inference,* or English sentences without *parsing procedures.* (Analogously, people who knew that Searle speaks no Portuguese would not give Searle-in-the-room a Portuguese rule-book unless they were prepared to teach him the language first.)

Smith does not deny that there is an important distinction between the *denotational import* of an expression (broadly: what actual or possible worlds can be mapped onto it) and its *procedural consequence* (broadly: what it does, or makes happen). The fact that the expression "(FATHER (MAGGIE))" is isomorphic with a certain parental relationship between two actual people (and so might be mapped onto that relationship by us) is one thing. The fact that the expression "(FATHER (MAGGIE))" can cause a certain computer to locate "LEONARD" is quite another thing. Were it not so, the dual-calculus approach would not have developed. But he argues that, rather than persisting with the dual-calculus approach, it would be more elegant and less confusing to adopt a "unified" theory of programming languages, designed to cover both denotative and procedural aspects.

He shows that many basic terms on either side of the dual-calculus divide have deep theoretical commonalities, as well as significant differences. The notion of *variable,* for instance, is understood in somewhat similar fashion by the logician and the computer scientist: both allow that a variable can have different *values* assigned to it at different times. That being so, it is redundant to have two distinct theories of what a variable is. To some extent, however, logicians and computer scientists understand different things by this term: the value of a variable in the LISP programming language (for example) is another LISP-expression, whereas the value of a variable in logic is usually some object external to the formalism itself. These differences should be clarified, not least to avoid confusion when a system attempts to reason *about* variables by *using* variables. In short, we need a single definition of "variable", allowing both for its declarative use (in logic) and for its procedural use (in programming). Having shown that similar remarks apply to other basic computational terms, Smith outlines a unitary account of the semantics of LISP and describes a new calculus (MANTIQ) designed with the unified approach in mind.

As the example of using variables to reason about variables suggests, a unified theory of computation could illuminate how *reflective* knowledge is possible. For, given such a theory, a system's representations of data and of processes, including processes internal to the system itself, would be essentially comparable. This theoretical advantage has psychological relevance (and was a major motivation behind Smith's work).

For our present purposes, however, the crucial point is that a fundamental theory of *programs,* and of *computation,* should acknowledge that an essential function of a computer program is to make things happen. Whereas symbolic logic can be viewed as mere playing around with uninterpreted formal calculi (such as the predicate calculus), and computational logic can be seen as the study of abstract timeless relations in mathematically specified machines (such as Turing machines), computer science cannot properly be described in either of these ways.

It follows from Smith's argument that the familiar characterization of computer programs as all syntax and no semantics is mistaken. The inherent procedural consequences of any computer program give it a toehold in semantics, where the semantics in question is not denotational, but causal. The analogy is with Searle-in-the-room's understanding of English, not his understanding of Chinese.

This is implied also by A. Sloman's [1986a; 1986b] discussion of the sense in which programmed instructions and computer symbols must be thought of as having some semantics, however restricted. In a causal semantics, the meaning of a symbol (whether simple or complex) is to be sought by reference to its causal links with other phenomena. The central questions are "What causes the symbol to be built and/or activated?" and "What happens as a result of it?" The answers will sometimes mention external objects and events visible to an observer, and sometimes they will not.

If the system is a human, animal, or robot, it may have causal powers that enable it to refer to restaurants and bean-sprouts (the philosophical complexities of reference to external, including unobservable, objects may be ignored here, but are helpfully discussed by Sloman). But whatever the information-processing system concerned, the answers will sometimes describe purely *internal* computational processes – whereby other symbols are built, other instructions activated. Examples include the interpretative processes inside Searle-in-the-room's mind (comparable perhaps to the processes discussed in Chapters 4 and 5) that are elicited by English words, and the computational processes within a Schankian text-analysis program. Although such a program cannot use the symbol "restaurant" to mean *restaurant* (because it has no causal links with restaurants, food, and so forth), its internal symbols and procedures do embody some minimal understanding of certain other matters – of what it is to compare two formal structures, for example.

One may feel that the understanding involved in such a case is so minimal that this word should not be used at all. So be it. As Sloman makes clear, the important question is not "When does a machine understand something?" (a question which misleadingly implies that there is some clear cut-off point at which understanding ceases) but "What things does a machine (whether biological or not) need to be able to do in order to be able to understand?" This question is relevant not only to the *possibility* of a computational psychology but to its *content* also.

In sum, my discussion has shown Searle's attack on computational psychology to be ill founded. To view Searle-in-the-room as an instantiation of a computer program is not to say that he lacks all understanding. The formal-syntactic solipsism of Fodor and Stich can be dismissed likewise. Since (as remarked above) the theories of a formalist-computational psychology should be likened to computer programs rather than to logic, computational psychology is not in principle incapable of explaining how meaning attaches to mental processes.

Thus far, we have rejected two interpretations of formal-computational psychology which limit its scope to a lesser or a greater degree: Fodor's methodological solipsism and Searle's programs-are-pure-syntax attack. But a strictly formalist computational psychology must face other challenges besides these – not least, that of connectionism.

Computation and connectionism

The formalist definition of "computation" applies *par excellence* to information-processing in von Neumann machines, which involves the serial application of explicitly stored formal-syntactic rules to explicit, and localizable, symbolic representations. This type of processing underlies computer models that (like most of those discussed in previous chapters) are based on what J. Haugeland [1985] calls GOFAI: Good Old-Fashioned Artificial Intelligence. But as we have seen (especially in Chapters 3 and 7), the information-processes within connectionist models are radically dissimilar. If they are computations, they are computations of a very different kind from the formalist species.

Indeed, the differences are so great that the question arises whether the same theoretical vocabulary is admissible at all. Are non-sequential, cooperative, and equilibrium-seeking alterations of patterns of activity (as opposed to formally triggered syntactic transformations of symbolic forms) really *computations?* Are specifications of the progressive self-organization of a network of computational units, without any description of which rule to apply next, really *algorithms?* Are information-processing interdependencies that are implicit in the structure of excitatory and inhibitory (hard-wired or virtual) connections between units, rather than being explicitly defined as an instruction in a program, really *rules?* Are widely distributed excitation-patterns, as opposed to locatable (implementations of) formal symbols, embodiments of *symbols* – or even *representations?* In short, are connectionist theories and computer models really *examples* of computational psychology at all, or are they *competing alternatives* to it?

To put the same question in Kuhnian terms, are GOFAI and connectionism theoretical developments within the same scientific paradigm or not? If connectionist models were ever to be widely adopted by (psychological) scientists in preference to formalist ones, would this constitute what T. S. Kuhn [1962] describes as the overthrow of one paradigm by another? Or would it be an internal family matter, one intra-paradigmatic cousin taking over from another?

In the former case, computational psychology – properly so called – would have been abandoned as a dead-end. One could certainly say, in Popperian style, that the conjectures and (by hypothesis) the all-too-frequent refutations of formalist psychological modelling had provided much of the impetus for the development of connectionist models. This would be no mean accolade. Nevertheless, the refusal to categorize connectionist models as computational would (in this hypothetical situation) imply that the quest for a truly computational psychology had failed. In the latter case, the victory of connectionism would merely show that computational psychology can change and progress.

Certainly, if GOFAI and connectionism are in the same scientific family, they are not the closest of cousins – more like third cousins thrice removed. Connectionist systems are different, so different that they have been described as a "radical departure from the symbolic [formalist] paradigm" (and assigned to "the sub-symbolic paradigm" instead) [Smolensky, 1987, p. 101]. But radical departures can happen within a paradigm too. The descriptions of the double helix in the mid 1950s and of the genetic code a few years later both constituted radical departures from the way in which biochemical and genetic processes had been thought about before. They even spawned a new science: molecular biology. But molecular biology, like pre-1950s biology, studies living things as chemical systems. The truly fundamental paradigm-shift arguably occurred when physiological approaches replaced vitalism.

The "radical departure" of connectionism may best be thought of, likewise, as a change in some relatively basic ideas *within* the general computational approach. One of Kuhn's criteria for distinguishing paradigms is the use of distinct "exemplars": specific experiments regarded by the relevant scientific community as models of theoretical argument and methodological design. As we noted in Chapter 1, the speculations of W. S. McCulloch and W. H. Pitts [1943] about the logical properties potentially immanent in the nervous activity of the brain influenced both von Neumann's design of the digital computer and the pioneering connectionist work on neural nets (perceptrons) of people such as F. Rosenblatt. Arguably, it was McCulloch and Pitts who provided the schematic exemplar initiating computational psychology – and GOFAI-workers and connectionists, despite their undeniable differences, are thus working within the *same* general paradigm.

This is entirely consistent with D. A. Norman's claim that the PDP-models developed by his research-group "in no way can be interpreted as growing from our metaphor of the modern computer" and that they deal with a "new form of computation, one clearly based upon principles that have heretofore not had any counterpart in computers" [1986, p. 534]. Indeed, in arguing that computer science owes at least as much to psychology as computational psychology (whether connectionist or not) owes to computer science, he reminds us that the von Neumann computer was itself based on ideas about how the mind works. Among those seminal ideas, which (as we saw in Chapter 1) included work on cybernetics and cerebral models, the computational-mathematical arguments of McCulloch and Pitts were crucial.

Moreover, some leading connectionists insist that "it would be wrong to view distributed representations as an *alternative* to representational schemes like semantic networks or production systems that have been found useful in cognitive psychology and artificial intelligence" [Hinton, McClelland & Rumelhart, 1986, p. 78; italics in original]. They view PDP-networks rather as "one way of implementing these more abstract schemes in parallel networks", pointing out that their emergent properties (pattern-matching, content-addressable memory, and graceful degradation) provide powerful operations that can be regarded as primitives by psychologists considering more high-level theories implemented in more traditional ways. Thus we saw in Chapter 6 that Newell and Simon's theory of how production-rules get selected from moment to moment assumes powers of pattern-matching whose specific nature they do not address. We saw too that a connectionist pattern-matcher may have to *simulate* a von Neumann machine in order to do arithmetic. Just what the relations between formalist and connectionist approaches are is still unclear, and to set them in fundamental opposition to each other is quite likely a mistake [A. J. Clark, 1987].

If computational psychology is a paradigm, then, connectionism should probably be included as a particular development within it. However, it might be better to avoid the term "paradigm" altogether in this context. Kuhn provided a sociological criterion, according to which a *paradigm* enjoys the wide, and basically uncritical, acceptance of some entire scientific community. If the relevant community is psychologists at large, then computational psychology does not constitute a paradigm. Many more psychologists ignore, or even oppose, it than profess it. Not all of these are primarily concerned with issues such as psychotherapy or social psychology: some are interested in psychological phenomena to which one might expect the computational approach to be relevant, if it is relevant at all. Possibly, this may be a historically situated fact that will not long survive the passing of the twentieth century. For the moment, however, Kuhn's term "paradigm" seems inapplicable purely on sociological grounds.

If formalism and connectionism share a family relationship, this is seen by many as a family feud. Some long-standing critics of the formalist approach make no bones about their hope for an outright victory of connectionism, describing recent parallelist models as a potentially "devastating" challenge to conventional computational psychology [Dreyfus & Dreyfus, in press]. Likewise, some committed formalists regard connectionism as lying outside what they regard as computational psychology proper.

The formalists Newell and Simon (as we saw in Chapter 6) exclude basic perceptual processes, which they allow may involve massive parallelism, from the domain of phenomena to be explained by their psychological theory. And Pylyshyn doubts where the information-processes attributed by Marr to visual systems, or by G. E. Hinton and others to connectionist models in general, are truly "cognitive" or "representation-governed" – in which case, he claims, they are not *computations* [1984, pp. 214–215]. On his view, connectionist theories are concerned not with computation, or cognition, as such but with its *implementation:* they are "abstract models of the nervous system's instantiation of some operations of the functional architecture" [*ibid.*].

The reason Pylyshyn gives for denying computational status to connectionism is that the phenomena (so far) modelled by such processes are cognitively *impenetrable,* by which he means that they do not depend on semantic content (representations of beliefs and desires) and rationality, but are inflexible, automatic, and non-introspectible. However, his definition of *semantic content* (and of *representation*) in terms of the folk-psychological vocabulary of beliefs, desires, and rationality – in short, of everyday understanding – is tendentious. In considering the programs-are-pure-syntax position, we saw that meaning, or semantic content, is grounded in certain sorts of causal process. We saw, too, that understanding is not an all-or-none property, and that many interrelated information-processing capacities are required for understanding of the sort enjoyed by humans. The understanding of natural language evidently rests on mental procedures which enable beliefs and desires to be altered in the light of semantically relevant knowledge. This is why psychological experiments involving verbal instructions and/or verbally influenced imagination produce results (like those of Pylyshyn's experiments described in Chapter 2) that are cognitively penetrable. But semantic content, and representations, can exist at mental levels which are neither open to introspection nor capable of being altered by the specific cognitive content of the person's beliefs and desires.

The several levels of visual representation discussed in Chapter 3 provide examples. Theories about the construction of edges by DOG-detectors, for instance, or the generation of the 2½D-Sketch, are concerned not with physical implementation but with *computation* and *representation*. There is no good reason (*pace* Pylyshyn) to refuse to use these words in characterizing these phenomena. We do not know what it is which makes some mental contents and processes non-introspectible while others are open to consciousness (although modularity-theorists have suggested plausible evolutionary reasons why certain basic sensory procedures should be computationally encapsulated). Nor do we know, though Pylyshyn apparently assumes, that this distinction has a theoretical rationale so important that the terms "computation" and "representation" should be used on only one side of the psychological divide. Only if a connectionist system were intended as a model of specific neural circuitry and synaptic interactions (as described by neuroscience) would it be a model of implementation. Since the connectionist models considered in this book are concerned not with neurophysiology but with information-processes, words like "computation" and "representation" are appropriate.

A strictly formalist definition of computation is unnecessarily restrictive. Such a definition would exclude connectionist computer models and theories from the field of computational psychology. But connectionist systems are concerned with information-processing (not implementation), and they satisfy the *general* criteria of computationalism identified above – albeit in ways which differ from more traditional computer models.

Connectionist systems are not von Neumann machines, in which information-processing rules are explicitly coded within and accessed by the program. But as we have seen, they are designed so as to follow rigorous rules in passing from one state to another and in seeking an equilibrium. These rules ensure that the patterns of excitation and inhibition in the system vary in a way which reflects significant informational constraints (such as 2D-to-3D mapping). Such rules differ from von Neumann algorithms in that they are implicit (in a sense explained below) in the system and in that they do not enable one to specify precisely what will happen next from moment to moment. But their function in determining the information-processing within the system justifies their being regarded as a (different) type of algorithm.

Likewise, by means of varying weights and excitation-states, "non-von" machines manipulate symbols – of an unusual kind. In so doing, they may be said to perform computations, for their passage from one symbolic state to another can be mapped onto logical-semantic relations of various kinds (even Pylyshyn speaks of "computations" and "inferences" occurring within connectionist models). Certainly, the representations in a connectionist system are implemented very differently from those in a von Neumann computer, and are not hardware-independent in the same way. No individual unit implements any identifiable symbol or meaning, for meaningful representations exist only at the level of networks made up of many units. But such distributed representations, too, have properties that can be mapped onto abstract relationships of various kinds. And they, too, are able to mediate causal connections with the world, and with other representations and processes internal to the system itself, which (as argued above) are essential to semantic content, or meaning.

Moreover, there is no reason to believe, what Pylyshyn seems to suggest, that connectionist systems are intrinsically limited to the modelling of low-level sensory phenomena. (The more seriously one takes their analogy to the brain, the less reason one has to doubt their potential for modelling the higher mental processes also.) But no computer model, connectionist or otherwise, can embody a psychological theory unless such a theory exists to be embodied. For reasons elaborated in the preceding chapters, theories of (for example) 2D-to-3D mapping are less elusive than theories regarding beliefs and intentions. So it is hardly surprising that connectionists have thus far concentrated more on domains such as low-level vision or simple word-recognition than on phenomena (like belief-fixation) having indefinitely many degrees of freedom.

Connectionist models, then, do fall within the broad genre of *computational psychology*. Although they do not fit the strictly formalist definition, they satisfy the general characteristics of computational psychology identified in Chapter 1. They are the modern successors of the early perceptrons described in Chapter 2, and as we have seen, their success is largely based on theoretical insights (about the importance of detailed domain-knowledge) which originated within work of a more traditionalist kind.

Despite the many present uncertainties about their computational potential, connectionist systems have some advantages over traditional models [McClelland, Rumelhart & Hinton, 1986; Norman, 1986; Smolensky, 1987]. Their parallelism is better suited to many psychological phenomena than is the serialism of von Neumann machines. They need not be bound to strictly binary (on–off) decisions, since their mode of representation employs patterns of activity distributed over large cell-networks (and the individual units in some connectionist systems are themselves capable of continuously varying activity). Largely because of this, they are more capable of graceful degradation and approximate matching than are traditional computer models. And, not least, their reliance on distributed, co-operative processing enables the connectionist to counter an objection very commonly raised (e.g., Dreyfus, 1979; Dreyfus & Dreyfus, 1987) against computer-modelling in psychology: that thought cannot comprise only explicit representations.

In an attempt to clarify this widely held intuition, Dennett [1983] has distinguished *explicit* representations from *implicit* and *tacit* ones.

On his analysis, information is represented *explicitly* if there is in the system a physically structured object which is a formula in a language for which there is a semantics, and if there is also a mechanism for parsing the formula (this applies to computer models of the traditional, von Neumann, kind). It is represented *implicitly* (in Dennett's usage of this term) if it is logically implied by something that is stored explicitly.

(Information that is implicit in this sense may or may not be potentially explicit in a given information-processing system. Consider, for example, the discussion of zero-crossings in Chapter 3. We saw there that Marr, citing Logan's theorem, suggested that orientation is implicit in zero-crossings. If Marr was right in claiming that there are mechanisms that can compute orientation from zero-crossings *and* that orientation is then coded explicitly in the visual system, then it is potentially explicit also. As regards higher mental processes such as belief, it is unclear just how much of the implicit information is potentially explicit for the human subject concerned. Moreover, since people do not actually draw all the inferences of which they are potentially capable, they do not believe all the logical implications of their beliefs; hence the difficulty, stressed by Stich [1983], of individuating beliefs. A computational model of belief should take this fact into account, and some workers have attempted to do so [Haas, 1986].)

Last, information termed *tacit* by Dennett is built in to the system in some fashion that does not require the manipulation of explicit rules. Tacit information, in this sense, covers what previous chapters of this book have referred to as implicit representations or rules. It is the most basic, because the manipulation of explicit representations itself requires it. This definition is reminiscent of what G. Ryle [1949] called *knowledge how* (and Dennett argues for the existence of tacit information by a Rylean argument against infinite regress in mental process).

A von Neumann computationalist could point out that the instructions of the machine-code in a traditional computer embody tacit information in the sense just defined. Indeed, this fact underlies the rebuttal (above) of the programs-are-pure-syntax view. Why, then, is tacit knowledge so often assumed to be utterly alien to formalist-computational models? The reason is that the von Neumann traditionalist assumes that virtually all mental computations of interest to theoretical psychology lie above this level and involve explicit representation (although, as we saw in Chapter 6, some formalists allow that highly complex cerebral mechanisms may underlie the *virtual* machine posited by their theories).

The formalist-computational attempt to construct a thoroughly rule-following psychology on a minimal tacit base sits easily with the assumption that the biggest merely tacit knowers within the human being are relatively small cell-groups. This minimalist assumption may not be correct: some tacit representation in the brain may involve large cell-systems and relatively high-level knowledge. What counts as "large", of course, is problematic: the network (described in Chapter 7) that learns the past tense of English verbs is a relatively simple system, but both pools contain a unit for each and every distinct phonological feature relevant to this learning task.

Ryle writes as though the largest tacit knowers are whole people. Interpreted as an empirical claim – as opposed to the Wittgensteinian point that we normally ascribe "know" and cognate terms to persons, not to components of persons or of their bodies – this is an implausible view, given the considerable evidence (for example, the extraordinarily wide variety of clinical aphasias) for largely independent psychological functions within the mind. Dennett, while he acknowledges this Rylean possibility, leaves the empirical question open. His definition of "tacit" offers no idea of how large tacit representational systems might be, or of how they are possible. By contrast, connectionist computer models of psychological processes embody suggested answers to such questions.

For example, Hinton's work (discussed in Chapter 3) shows how it is possible for a relatively high-level representation, of 3D-shape, to be embodied over an entire network of cells; he even provides mathematical arguments showing that cell-assemblies of a specific size would suffice to compute certain spatial properties. In connectionist networks, there are no explicit rules of 2D-to-3D mapping, as there are in traditional scene-analysis programs such as those described in Chapter 2. Rather, there are implicit rules embodied as built-in connections engineered in such a way that they will effect this mapping tacitly. In addition, connectionist systems develop patterns of associative weights which may cause the system to behave *as though* it were following rules of a type which could be (and often are) made explicit in a von Neumann machine. The verb-learner described in Chapter 7 is one example: its final behaviour can be described in terms of the rules of English past-tense morphology, but these rules are neither programmed into it nor explicitly represented in it as a result of its learning.

The engineering of visual systems or speech-systems (for instance) in computers, whether in dedicated or general-purpose machines, is done by people. The engineering in the brain is due to evolution, which has produced visual and acoustic/phonetic machinery dedicated to various information-processing tasks involved in our causal commerce with the world. (An interesting philosophical discussion of how intentionality in general might have evolved has been provided by Dennett [1969].)

This chapter has asked whether computational psychology is possible *in principle*. Interpreted in what I have called the mathematical sense, the answer must be "Yes", although the scope of computational psychology (so understood) is still unclear. Interpreted in the formalist sense, computational psychology is possible likewise. Neither methodological solipsism nor the programs-are-pure-syntax attack shows it to be unattainable. Nor is it threatened by the recent development of connectionism, for connectionist models themselves are examples of computational psychology, broadly conceived. The next, final, chapter summarizes what it has achieved *in practice* and asks what we may expect of it in the future.

9   Conclusion

The advent of computational models grounded in artificial intelligence has been described by the cognitive psychologist D. A. Allport as the "single most important development in the history of psychology" [1980, p. 31]. Bearing in mind the many unanswered questions identified in the preceding pages, this judgment may seem to smack of hubris. What could lead someone in possession of his senses to say such a thing?

Allport's answer is significant, and in my view basically sound. Endorsing A. Newell's [1973] argument that "you can't play twenty questions with nature and win", Allport refers us not to lists of newly discovered empirical data but to a new manner of speaking. He blames the previously "chaotic" state of cognitive psychology, in which myriad experimental results jostled for our attention without any unifying theory, on the "lack of an adequate theoretical notation in which to formulate questions about mental process". And he predicts that "artificial intelligence will ultimately come to play the role *vis-à-vis* the psychological and social sciences that mathematics, from the seventeenth century on, has done for the physical sciences " [1980, p. 31].

Twentieth-century psychologists are even more justified in saying such a thing about the language of computation than were their seventeenth-century counterparts with respect to mathematics. Galileo Galilei gave good reason to suspect that as he put it, "mathematics is the language of God". But Alan Turing, three centuries later, *proved* that a language capable of defining "effective procedures" suffices, in principle, to solve any computable problem. If a psychological science is possible at all, it must be capable of being expressed in computational terms. (If a scientific psychology is not possible, the computational approach is not the only loser: all attempts to develop a science of the mind would be doomed to failure.)

It does not follow that the specific computational terms which will be required in practice are those developed by Turing, any more than post-Galilean physics had to rely solely on Galileo's mathematics. Turing's insight is not essentially confined to von Neumann machines. Just as mathematics has evolved in ways unpredictable by seventeenth-century scientists, so computer science will inevitably generate concepts different from those with which we are familiar today.

The universal Turing machine described in Turing's epoch-making paper is a theoretical ideal, to which actual computers running actual computer

259

language approximate in various ways. The notion of the Turing machine, together with the McCulloch–Pitts theorems about neural nets, soon led to the von Neumann digital computer – on which most computer-modelling has been based. Previous chapters detailed a number of ways in which the substantive content of psychological theory has been influenced by ideas drawn from this particular form of computer technology. In addition, they showed how some recent psychological theories are grounded in computational systems of a significantly different type, namely, connectionist models.

Furthermore, we may expect other types to emerge in the future: the space of computational possibilities has hardly been entered, never mind fully explored or satisfactorily mapped. Nor is there any question of our having exhausted the representational possibilities, even though much research in computer-modelling (formalist and otherwise) seeks to develop new types of representation, less limited in certain ways than those already available.

It is too early, therefore, to predict the success of the computational approach in general. We do not know the full potential of the von Neumann machine, and we are even more in the dark as regards the likely success of connectionist modelling. From the theoretical psychologist's point of view, as we have seen (in Chapters 3, 7, and 8), such models have some advantages over the von Neumann variety. But we have seen also that despite some attempts to provide abstract proofs about the computational potential and limitations of specific types of connectionist systems (Boltzmann machines, for instance), the computational potential of connectionism – of which there are already several different varieties – is still largely obscure.

Moreover, we have hardly touched upon the possibilities of exploiting scientific knowledge about the brain. Formalist models ignore such issues, and even current connectionist models are based only on general knowledge about cerebral function. No account is taken of the complexity of single neurones, or of the detailed anatomy of neural circuits in the brain [P.S. Churchland, 1986; Crick & Asanuma, 1986]. Neuroscientists sometimes suggest methods of representation that differ significantly from current ideas in computational modelling. For instance, recent neuroanatomical work has outlined ways in which spatial properties, and visuomotor co-ordination appropriate to those properties, might be computed relatively directly by suitably engineered (that is, evolved) projections between identifiable sheets of cells in the cerebral or cerebellar cortices [Pellionisz & Llinas, 1979; 1985]. The "tensor network theory" developed in the context of this work is thought by some to have the potential to explain mental processing in general [P. M. Churchland, 1986; P. S. Churchland, 1986, chap. 10].

This does not mean that computational psychologists should try to integrate all the discoveries of neuroscience into their theories and computer models. In general, neuroscientific work is significant to computational psychology only insofar as it relates to computational, information-processing, issues. Psychophysiological results suggesting, for example, that certain cells respond specifically to particular, and sometimes intuitively surprising, features of the outside world are relevant only if they illuminate how those features are recognized by the neural system. The key question for our purposes is not "Is there a grandmother cell, and if so which is it?" but, rather, "How does the brain manage to compute the judgment: 'That is Grandmother'?"

Neuroscientific research into the biological implementation of mental processes is increasingly guided by computational concerns – asking not merely "Where?" but also "How?" Thus studies of individual neurones in the chimp's temporal cortex that code, for instance, specific head-orientations, directions of gaze, or goal-oriented hand-movements, ask whether the neurones code what in Chapter 3 was distinguished as *viewer-centred* or *object-centred* representations [Perrett *et al.*, 1985; Perrett *et al.*, 1986]. Given that some cells appear to be involved in object-centred categorizations, the question arises how (and where) they or other cells in the chimp's visual system were able to compute head-orientation independently of the subject animal's varying viewpoint. Similarly, recent investigations of visuomotor co-ordination enquire not only which cerebral areas or cell-groups are involved but also what specific computations are required for the visually guided motor-activity of various organisms [Arbib, 1981]. And much as O. G. Selfridge's early ideas about perceptual "demons" led to the search for, and discovery of, feature-detectors in the frog's retina (see Chapter 2), so today's better-developed ideas about visual processing are contributing to the study of the neuroanatomical circuitry involved in low-level vision [Rolls, 1987].

The growing influence of computational ideas on neuroscience is one example that could be mentioned in answering the question "What has computational psychology achieved?" Other examples have been cited throughout this book. Sometimes, as in respect of low-level vision and parsing, one can point to clear scientific advance – not only in the asking of many detailed (and theoretically related) questions but in the answering of some such questions too. At other times – for instance in respect of learning – one can mention only some insights into very general constraints on theorizing in the domain concerned. These constraints must be recognized in future theorizing, and in computer-modelling of any type (formalist, connectionist, . . . ?).

The early days of computer simulation, when researchers were impressed by virtually any computer model whose performance remotely resembled the human case, are gone. Now, for reasons explored in the preceding pages, there is an increasing stress within computational psychology (and within technological artificial intelligence) on the abstract computational analysis of such matters. Computer output that can be admired but not understood heralds a performing toy, chic or otherwise, rather than a theoretical model.

Computational psychologists are accustomed to seeking a degree of precision, in the description even of highly complex mental processes, which (at worst) highlights theoretical lacunae and (at best) helps us to fill them. This attention to precise theoretical detail is not a passing fancy, a trendy fad born of a technological society and doomed to obsolescence, but an enduring contribution to psychological science. It has provided a standard of rigour and clarity which must make us permanently dissatisfied with less.

Many problems, of course, remain. Some have been identified, and a few discussed in detail, in previous chapters. Others have been conspicuous by their absence.

Little, for example, has been said about motivation and emotion. I have argued elsewhere that in principle, many aspects of these phenomena are intelligible in computational terms [Boden, 1972, chaps. 5–7]. (Hormonally based changes in mood, neutral with respect to specific cognitive content, are less amenable to a computationalist account [Haugeland, 1978; Gray, 1982].) However, they have not received much attention from computer modellers (although we saw in Chapter 5 that they are touched on in some work on text-understanding). The single-minded nature of virtually all current computer programs (despite an early exception [Reitman, 1965]) renders them fundamentally unsuited to the representation of psychodynamic matters. Many non-human animals appear to have diverse, potentially conflicting motives and emotions. The complexity of human purposes is even greater, because of the enormous representational potential provided by natural language and the variety of cultural influences on our beliefs and desires. To model such matters in a functioning system is at present beyond the state of the art; but some of these motivational complexities, and their relation to detailed scheduling and control within the mind, figured in an exploratory theoretical discussion by A. Sloman [Sloman & Croucher, 1981; Sloman, in press].

Nor have we specifically considered the application of computational ideas to animal (as opposed to human) psychology. The influence of behaviourism stifled theoretical enquiry into the nature of animal minds for two generations. Ethology was less open to this criticism than academic experimental psychology, but even so, it is only in very recent years that ethologists have deemed it scientifically respectable to revive these long-repressed questions. However, the questions are not always asked in the most fruitful terms. Even the self-styled cognitive ethologists tend to suffer from an ethological equivalent of the grandmother-cell syndrome in neurophysiology; that is, they concentrate too much on questions about *what* animals can do and not enough on questions about *how* they do it. As Sloman [1979] puts it, in commenting on recent–and, he admits, fascinating–studies of symbol-using in chimps: "In the long run we shall

all learn more if we spend a little less time collecting new curiosities and a little more time pondering the deeper questions. The best method I know of is to explore attempts to design *working* systems that display the abilities we are trying to understand" [p. 602]. By "*working* systems", of course, is meant computer models. Elsewhere, I have outlined some ways in which a computational approach might illuminate various issues within animal psychology [Boden, in press a].

A further topic only touched on in these pages is the potential for real-world psychological applications of computer-modelling – in psychiatry and education, for example. Psychiatric applications of computer technology are being explored by a few groups [Hand, 1985]. Most of these – for example, interactive programs used to give initial psychiatric interviews which are later discussed by the patient with the human psychiatrist – owe more to computer technology (in natural-language processing) than to psychological theory. Those computer models of psychopathology which do embody theoretical ideas (such as models of paranoid psychosis or of neurotic defence-mechanisms [Colby, 1981; Boden, 1987, chaps. 2, 3, and 5]) have no practical clinical use. Their interest is as putative existence-proofs or as teaching aids.

Many computer-based representations of some specific body of knowledge are useful as teaching aids. The expert systems of AI-technology are increasingly exploited in this way – to train medical students, for example, or budding lawyers. Such pedagogic uses rely little, if at all, on psychological theory. There are, however, some educational applications of theoretical ideas from computational psychology, some of which were mentioned in Chapter 7. Unlike trial-and-practice Skinner machines, the new forms of CAI (Computer-Assisted Instruction) focus on modelling the ways in which students represent a given knowledge-domain and the procedures they use to solve problems, and make mistakes, within it [Sleeman & Brown, 1982; O'Shea & Self, 1984]. As yet, only a few domains have been modelled in enough detail to be useful to pupils or teachers (one example is simple subtraction [Brown & Burton, 1978; Brown & VanLehn, 1980; Burton 1982]), but there is significant scope in principle for pedagogic applications in many different areas.

A number of groups are using AI-based LOGO programming environments (usually aiming not to teach domain-specific content but to improve children's thinking in general), and some encouraging results have been reported with both normal and handicapped children [Papert, 1980; Weir, 1987]. As was pointed out in Chapter 7, however, some optimistic neo-Piagetian claims for the educational potential of LOGO-programming are not yet clearly supported by the empirical evidence [Pea & Kurland, 1984; Kurland *et al.*, 1986; Pea *et al.*, in press].

One of the most important aspects of a scientific theory, and *a fortiori* of a theoretical psychology, is its influence on the social context as a whole.

Psychological theories (insofar as the public hears about them) can affect the way in which people think about themselves and about personal relationships – which because of the reflexive nature of human thought, has appreciable effects on social and personal behaviour. It was because the behaviourist B. F. Skinner was well aware of this that he devoted two books (*Walden Two* and *Beyond Freedom and Dignity*) to arguing that behaviourist psychology is compatible with those moral convictions and social practices which are worth saving – and incompatible with some he believed to be not only radically illusory but socially stultifying too. Whether his arguments are persuasive is not the point. The point, rather, is that psychologists should expect to be asked what implications their theories have for such matters, and should be prepared to answer.

Many people assume that a theoretical psychology based on computer models must necessarily be even more dehumanizing than one based on rats. This widespread assumption betrays a misunderstanding of the nature of such theories and of the complex systems (or theoretical machines) envisaged by them.

It is taken for granted that a computational psychology must be *mechanistic:* either denying any role at all to mental processes or describing them in a way which is fundamentally inappropriate. The first of these alternatives clearly misses the mark. Unlike behaviourists (and over-zealous physicalists of various kinds), computational psychologists believe that theories about internal mental processes are entirely admissible. Mentalistic concepts like *representation, inference,* and *intentionality* pervade computational theorizing, as we have seen. The second alternative – that these concepts are systematically misused by computationalists – is more controversial and has been a central topic of this book. The notion that computational psychology in general can have no place for intentionality was rebutted in Chapter 8. As for specific theories, we have seen that current computational approaches will very likely not suffice, and that different types of models will be developed in the future.

This reference to future efforts may bring to mind Dr Johnson's description of remarriage: "the triumph of hope over experience". We need not be similarly sceptical about the prospects for further computer-modelling in psychology. If some psychologists are turning to new entanglements, new forms of computer-modelling, that is hardly surprising. And if the excessive optimism of the honeymoon-period (thirty years ago) has been tempered by experience, that also was only to be expected. Despite the difficulties and disappointments, the past embrace of computational ideas by theoretical psychology has not been scientifically barren. Confidence, rather than mere hope, is the attitude appropriate to future partnerships of like kind. Just *what* their progeny will be of course remains to be seen. As with marriage, that uncertainty is part of the adventure.

References

Abelson, R. P. [1973] The Structure of Belief Systems. In R. C. Schank & K. M. Colby (eds.), *Computer Models of Thought and Language*. San Francisco: Freeman. Pp. 287–340.

Abelson, R. P. [1981] The Psychological Status of the Script Concept. *American Psychologist*, 36, 715–729.

Ackley, D. H., G. E. Hinton & T. J. Sejnowski. [1985] A Learning Algorithm for Boltzmann Machines. *Cognitive Science*, 9, 147–169.

Agin, G. J., & T. O. Binford. [1973] Computer Description of Curved Objects. *Proc. Third Int. Joint Conf. Artificial Intelligence*, Stanford, California, 629–640.

Allen, J. F., & C. R. Perrault. [1980] Analyzing Intention in Utterances. *Artificial Intelligence*, 15, 143–178.

Allport, D. A. [1980] Patterns and Actions. In G. Claxton (ed.), *Cognitive Psychology: New Directions*. London: Routledge & Kegan Paul. Pp. 26–64.

Allport, G. W. [1942] *The Use of Personal Documents in Psychological Science*. Social Science Research Council Bulletin 49. New York.

Amarel, S. [1968] On Representations of Problems of Reasoning About Actions. In D. Michie (ed.), *Machine Intelligence 3*. Edinburgh: Edinburgh University Press. Pp. 131–172.

Anderson, J. R. [1976] *Language, Memory, and Thought*. Hillsdale, N.J.: Erlbaum.

Anderson, J. R. [1979] Further Arguments Concerning Representations for Mental Imagery: A Response to Hayes-Roth and Pylyshyn. *Psychological Review*, 86, 395–406.

Anderson, J. R. [1980] *Cognitive Psychology and Its Implications*. San Francisco: Freeman.

Anderson, J. R. [1983] *The Architecture of Cognition*. Cambridge, Mass.: Harvard University Press.

Anderson, J. R., & G. H. Bower. [1973] *Human Associative Memory*. Washington, D.C.: Winston.

Arbib, M. [1981] Perceptual Structures and Distributed Motor Control. In V. B. Brooks (ed.), *Handbook of Physiology: The Nervous System II*. Bethesda, Md.: American Physiological Society. Pp. 1449–1480.

Austin, J. L. [1961] A Plea for Excuses. In J. L. Austin, *Philosophical Papers*. Oxford: Oxford University Press (Clarendon Press). Pp. 123–152.

Austin, J. L. [1962] *How to Do Things with Words*. Oxford: Oxford University Press.

Bach-y-Rita, P. [1984] The Relationship Between Motor Processes and Cognition in Tactile Visual Substitution. In W. Prinz & A. F. Sanders (eds.), *Cognition and Motor Processes*. Berlin: Springer-Verlag. Pp. 149–160.

Bainbridge, L. [1973] Review of Newell and Simon's *Human Problem Solving*. *Ergonomics*, 16, 892–899.

Ballard, D. H., & C. M. Brown (eds.). [1982] *Computer Vision*. Englewood Cliffs, N.J.: Prentice-Hall.

Bartlett, F. C. [1932] *Remembering: A Study in Experimental and Social Psychology*. Cambridge: Cambridge University Press.

Bartlett, F. C. [1958] *Thinking: An Experimental and Social Study*. London: Unwin University Books.

Barwise, J., & J. Perry. [1984] *Situations and Attitudes*. Cambridge, Mass.: MIT Press.

265

Baylor, G. W., & J. Gascon. [1974] An Information Processing Theory of the Development of Weight Seriation in Children. *Cognitive Psychology,* 6, 1–40.

Baylor, G. W., & G. Lemoyne. [1974] Experiments in Seriation with Children: Towards an Information Processing Explanation of the Horizontal Decalage. *Canadian J. Behavioral Science,* 7, 4–29.

Becker, J. D. [1973] A Model for the Encoding of Experiential Information. In R. C. Schank & K. M. Colby (eds.), *Computer Models of Thought and Language.* San Francisco: Freeman. Pp. 396–446.

Becker, J. D. [1975] The Phrasal Lexicon. *Theoretical Issues in Natural Language Processing,* Vol. 1. Cambridge, Mass.: BBN. Pp. 70–73.

Bernstein, J. [1981] Profile of Marvin Minsky. *New Yorker,* December 14, 50ff.

Bever, T. G., J. R. Lackner & R. Kirk. [1969] The Underlying Structures of Sentences Are the Primary Units of Immediate Speech Processing. *Perception and Psychophysics,* 5, 225–231.

Binford, T. O. [1971] Visual Perception by Computer. Paper given to the IEEE Conference on Systems and Control, Miami, December.

Binford, T. O. [1981] Inferring Surfaces from Images. *Artificial Intelligence,* 17, 205–245.

Black, J. B., & G. H. Bower. [1980] Story Understanding as Problem-Solving. *Poetics,* 9, 223–250.

Black, J. B., & R. Wilensky. [1979] An Evaluation of Story Grammars. *Cognitive Science,* 3, 213–230.

Block, N. (ed.). [1981] *Imagery.* Cambridge, Mass.: MIT Press.

Blomfield, S., & D. Marr. [1970] How the Cerebellum May Be Used. *Nature (London)* 227, 1224–1248.

Blum, H. [1973] Biological Shape and Visual Science, Part I. *J. Theoretical Biology,* 38, 205–287.

Boden, M. A. [1962] The Paradox of Explanation. *Proc. Aristotelian Soc.,* n.s., 62, 159–178. Reprinted in M. A. Boden [1981], *Minds and Mechanisms.* Ithaca, N.Y.: Cornell University Press. Pp. 113–132.

Boden, M. A. [1970] Intentionality and Physical Systems. *Philosophy of Science,* 37, 200–214. Reprinted in M. A. Boden [in press b], *Artificial Intelligence in Psychology: Interdisciplinary Essays.* London & Cambridge, Mass.: MIT Press.

Boden, M. A. [1972] *Purposive Explanation in Psychology.* Cambridge, Mass.: Harvard University Press.

Boden, M. A. [1973] The Structure of Intentions. *J. Theory of Social Behaviour,* 3, 23–46. Reprinted in M. A. Boden [1981], *Minds and Mechanisms.* Ithaca, N.Y.: Cornell University Press. Pp. 133–156.

Boden, M. A. [1979] *Piaget.* London: Collins Fontana.

Boden, M. A. [1980] Real-World Reasoning. In L. J. Cohen & M. B. Hesse (eds.), *Applications of Inductive Logic.* Oxford: Oxford University Press. Pp. 359–375. Reprinted in M. A. Boden [1981], *Minds and Mechanisms.* Ithaca, N.Y.: Cornell University Press. Pp. 157–173.

Boden, M. A. [1981] *Minds and Mechanisms.* Ithaca, N.Y.: Cornell University Press.

Boden, M. A. [1982a] Is Equilibration Important?: A View from Artificial Intelligence. *Brit. J. Psychology,* 73, 165–173. Reprinted in M. A. Boden [in press b], *Artificial Intelligence in Psychology: Interdisciplinary Essays.* London & Cambridge, Mass.: MIT Press.

Boden, M. A. [1982b] Implications of Language Studies for Human Nature. In R. J. Scholes & T. W. Simon (eds.), *Language, Mind, and Brain.* Hillsdale, N.J.: Erlbaum. Pp. 129–144. Reprinted in M. A. Boden [1981], *Minds and Mechanisms.* Ithaca, N.Y.: Cornell University Press. Pp. 174–191.

Boden, M. A. [1984] Failure Is Not the Spur. In O. G. Selfridge, E. L. Rissland & M. A. Arbib (eds.), *Adaptive Control in Ill-defined Systems.* New York: Plenum. Pp. 305–316.

Reprinted in M. A. Boden [in press b], *Artificial Intelligence in Psychology: Interdisciplinary Essays.* London & Cambridge, Mass.: MIT Press.

Boden, M. A. [1987] *Artificial Intelligence and Natural Man.* Second edn., expanded. London: MIT Press. (First edn., 1977. Hassocks, Sussex: Harvester Press.)

Boden, M. A. [In press a] Artificial Intelligence and Biological Intelligence. *J. Human Evolution,* 16. Reprinted in M. A. Boden [in press b], *Artificial Intelligence in Psychology: Interdisciplinary Essays.* London & Cambridge, Mass.: MIT Press.

Boden, M. A. [In press b] *Artificial Intelligence in Psychology: Interdisciplinary Essays.* London & Cambridge, Mass.: MIT Press.

Boden, M. A. [In preparation] *Mechanisms of Creativity.* To be published – London: Weidenfeld & Nicolson.

Bower, G. H. [1978] Experiments on Story Comprehension and Recall. *Discourse Processes,* 1, 211–231.

Bower, G. H. [1983] Affect and Cognition. *Phil. Trans. Royal Society London,* B, 302, 387–402.

Bower, G. H. [n.d.] Plans and Goals in Understanding Episodes. Unpublished manuscript.

Bransford, J. D., & M. K. Johnson. [1973] Considerations of Some Problems of Comprehension. In W. G. Chase (ed.), *Visual Information Processing.* New York: Academic Press. Pp. 383–438.

Brewer, W. F., & G. V. Nakamura. [1984] The Nature and Function of Schemas. In R. S. Wyer & T. K. Srull (eds.), *Handbook of Social Cognition,* Vol. 1. Hillsdale, N.J.: Erlbaum. Pp. 119–160.

Brewer, W. F., & J. R. Pani. [1983] The Structure of Human Memory. *Psychology of Learning and Motivation: Advances in Research and Theory,* 17, 1–38.

Brown, J. S., & R. R. Burton. [1978] Diagnostic Models for Procedural Bugs in Basic Mathematical Skills. *Cognitive Science,* 2, 155–192.

Brown, J. S., & K. VanLehn. [1980] Repair Theory: A Generative Theory of Bugs in Procedural Skills. *Cognitive Science,* 4, 379–426.

Bruner, J. S., J. Goodnow & G. Austin. [1956] *A Study of Thinking.* New York: Wiley.

Bryant, P. E. [1974] *Perception and Understanding in Young Children: An Experimental Approach.* London: Methuen.

Bundy, A. M. [1983] *The Computer Modelling of Mathematical Reasoning.* London: Academic Press.

Bundy, A. M. [1984] Superficial Principles: An Analysis of a Behavioural Law. *AISB Quarterly,* 49, 20–22.

Bundy, A. M., B. Silver & D. Plummer. [1985] An Analytical Comparison of Some Rule-Learning Programs. *Artificial Intelligence,* 27, 137–182.

Burton, R. R. [1982] Diagnosing Bugs in a Simple Procedural Skill. In D. Sleeman & J. S. Brown (eds.), *Intelligent Tutoring Systems.* London: Academic Press. Pp. 157–184.

Campbell, F. W. C., & J. Robson. [1968] Application of Fourier Analysis to the Visibility of Gratings. *J. Physiology (London),* 197, 551–566.

Carbonell, J. G. [1982a] Metaphor: An Inescapable Phenomenon in Natural-Language Comprehension. In W. G. Lehnert & M. H. Ringle (eds.), *Strategies for Natural Language Processing.* Hillsdale, N.J.: Erlbaum. Pp. 415–434.

Carbonell, J. G. [1982b] Experiential Learning in Analogical Problem Solving. *Proc. Amer. Assoc. Artificial Intelligence,* 2, 168–171.

Card, S. K., T. P. Moran & A. Newell. [1983] *The Psychology of Human–Computer Interaction.* Hillsdale, N.J.: Erlbaum.

Carnap, R. [1956] *Meaning and Necessity.* London: Phoenix Books.

Chisholm, R. M. [1967] Intentionality. In P. Edwards (ed.), *The Encyclopedia of Philosophy,* Vol. 4. New York: Macmillan. Pp. 201–204.

Chomsky, N. [1957] *Syntactic Structures.* The Hague: Mouton.

Chomsky, N. [1965] *Aspects of the Theory of Syntax*. Cambridge, Mass.: MIT Press.

Chomsky, N. [1980] Rules and Representations. *Behavioral and Brain Sciences*, 3, 1–15.

Chomsky, N., & G. A. Miller. [1958] Finite State Languages. *Information and Control*, 1, 91–112.

Churchland, P. M. [1979] *Scientific Realism and the Plasticity of Mind*. Cambridge: Cambridge University Press.

Churchland, P. M. [1981] Eliminative Materialism and the Propositional Attitudes. *J. Philosophy*, 78, 67–90.

Churchland, P. M. [1984] *Matter and Consciousness: A Contemporary Introduction to the Philosophy of Mind*. Cambridge, Mass.: MIT Press.

Churchland, P. M. [1986] Cognitive Neurobiology: A Computational Hypothesis for Laminar Cortex. *Biology and Philosophy*, 1, 25–51.

Churchland, P. M., & P. S. Churchland. [1982] Functionalism, Qualia, and Intentionality. In J. I. Biro & R. W. Shahan (eds.), *Mind, Brain, and Function: Essays in the Philosophy of Mind*. Norman: University of Oklahoma Press. Pp. 121–145.

Churchland, P. S. [1986] *Neurophilosophy: Toward a Unified Science of the Mind/Brain*. Cambridge, Mass.: MIT Press.

Clark, A. J. [1987] Connectionism and Cognitive Science. In J. Hallam & C. S. Mellish (eds.), *Advances in Artificial Intelligence*. London: Wiley. Pp. 3–15.

Clark, H. H. [1979] Responding to Indirect Speech Acts. *Cognitive Psychology*, 11, 430–477.

Clark, H. H., R. Schreuder & S. Buttrick. [1983] Common Ground and the Understanding of Demonstrative Reference. *J. Verbal Learning and Verbal Behavior*, 22, 245–258.

Clowes, M. B. [1969] Pictorial Relationships – A Syntactic Approach. In B. Meltzer & D. Michie (eds.), *Machine Intelligence 4*. Edinburgh: Edinburgh University Press. Pp. 361–383.

Clowes, M. B. [1971] On Seeing Things. *Artificial Intelligence*, 2, 79–116.

Clowes, M. B. [1973] Man the Creative Machine. In J. Benthall (ed.), *The Limits of Human Nature*. London: Allen Lane. Pp. 192–207.

Cohen, L. J. [1981] Can Human Irrationality Be Experimentally Demonstrated? *Behavioral and Brain Sciences*, 4, 317–345.

Cohen, P. R., C. R. Perrault, & J. F. Allen. [1982] Beyond Question Answering. In W. G. Lehnert & M. H. Ringle (eds.), *Strategies for Natural Language Processing*. Hillsdale, N.J.: Erlbaum. Pp. 245–274.

Colby, K. M. [1981] Modeling a Paranoid Mind. *Behavioral and Brain Sciences*, 4, 515–533.

Colby, K. M., & J. P. Gilbert. [1964] Programming a Computer Model of Neurosis. *J. Mathematical Psychology*, 1, 405–417.

Collins, A. M., & M. R. Quillian. [1972] Experiments on Semantic Memory and Language Comprehension. In L. W. Gregg (ed.), *Cognition in Learning and Memory*. New York: Wiley. Pp. 117–138.

Cowper, E. A. [1976] Constraints on Sentence Complexity: A Model for Syntactic Processing. Ph.D. thesis, Brown University.

Craik, K. J. W. [1943] *The Nature of Explanation*. Cambridge: Cambridge University Press.

Crick, F. H. C., & C. Asanuma. [1986] Certain Aspects of the Anatomy and Physiology of the Cerebral Cortex. In D. E. Rumelhart & J. L. McClelland (eds.), *Parallel Distributed Processing: Explorations in the Microstructure of Cognition*, Vol. 2: *Psychological and Biological Models*. Cambridge, Mass.: MIT Press. Pp. 333–371.

Cutler, A. (ed.). [1982] *Slips of the Tongue and Language Production*. Amsterdam: Mouton.

Davey, A. C. [1978] *Discourse Production: A Computer Model of Some Aspects of a Speaker.* Edinburgh: Edinburgh University Press.

Davies, D. J. M., & S. D. Isard. [1972] Utterances as Programs. In B. Meltzer & D. Michie (eds.), *Machine Intelligence 7.* Edinburgh: Edinburgh University Press. Pp. 325–340.

Davis, M. [1980] The Mathematics of Non-monotonic Reasoning. *Artificial Intelligence,* 13, 73–80.

Davis, R., & J. J. King. [1977] An Overview of Production Systems. In E. Elcock & D. Michie (eds.), *Machine Intelligence 8.* Chichester: Ellis Horwood. Pp. 300–333.

Dennett, D. C. [1969] *Content and Consciousness.* London: Routledge & Kegan Paul.

Dennett, D. C. [1971] Intentional Systems. *J. Philosophy,* 68, 87–106. Reprinted in D. C. Dennett, *Brainstorms: Philosophical Essays on Mind and Psychology.* Cambridge, Mass.: MIT Press, 1978. Pp. 3–22.

Dennett, D. C. [1978] *Brainstorms: Philosophical Essays on Mind and Psychology.* Cambridge, Mass.: MIT Press.

Dennett, D. C. [1983] Styles of Mental Representation. *Proc. Arist. Soc.,* n.s., 83, 213–226.

Doyle, J. [1979] A Truth Maintenance System. *Artificial Intelligence,* 12, 231–272.

Doyle, J. [1983] What Is Rational Psychology? *AI Magazine,* 4, 50–54.

Draper, S. W. [1981] The Use of Gradient and Dual Space in Line-Drawing Interpretation. *Artificial Intelligence* (special issue on vision), 17, 461–508.

Dresher, E., & N. Hornstein. [1976] On Some Supposed Contributions of Artificial Intelligence to the Scientific Study of Language. *Cognition,* 4, 321–378.

Dreyfus, H. L. [1979] *What Computers Can't Do: The Limits of Artificial Intelligence.* Revised edn. New York: Harper & Row.

Dreyfus, S. E., & H. L. Dreyfus. [In press] Towards a Reconciliation of Phenomenology and AI. In D. Partridge & Y. A. Wilks (eds.), *Foundational Issues in Artificial Intelligence.* Cambridge: Cambridge University Press.

Dyer, M. G. [1983] *In-Depth Understanding: A Computer Model of Integrated Processing for Narrative Comprehension.* Cambridge, Mass.: MIT Press.

Erman, L. D., & V. R. Lesser. [1980] The HEARSAY-II Speech Understanding System: A Tutorial. In W. A. Lee (ed.), *Trends in Speech Recognition.* Englewood Cliffs, N.J.: Prentice-Hall. Pp. 361–381.

Erman, L. D., P. E. London & S. F. Fickas. [1981] The Design and an Example Use of HEARSAY-III. *Proc. Seventh Int. Joint Conf. Artificial Intelligence,* Vancouver, 409–415.

Falk, G. [1972] Interpretation of Imperfect Line Data as a Three-dimensional Scene. *Artificial Intelligence,* 3, 101–144.

Feigenbaum, E. A., & J. Feldman (eds.). [1963] *Computers and Thought.* New York: McGraw-Hill.

Fernald, M. R. [1912] The Diagnosis of Mental Imagery. *Psychological Monographs,* 14, no. 58, 1–169.

Fikes, R. E. [1970] REF-ARF: A System for Solving Problems Stated as Procedures. *Artificial Intelligence,* 1, 27–120.

Finke, R. A., & M. J. Schmidt. [1977] Orientation-specific Color After-Effects Following Imagination. *J. Experimental Psych.: Human Perception and Performance,* 3, 599–606.

Fodor, J. A. [1976] *The Language of Thought.* Hassocks, Sussex: Harvester Press.

Fodor, J. A. [1978] Tom Swift and His Procedural Grandmother. *Cognition,* 6, 229–247. Reprinted in J. A. Fodor, *Representations: Philosophical Essays on the Foundations of Cognitive Science.* Brighton: Harvester Press, 1981. Pp. 204–224.

Fodor, J. A. [1979] Reply to Johnson-Laird. *Cognition,* 7, 201–205.

Fodor, J. A. [1980] Methodological Solipsism Considered as a Research Strategy in

Cognitive Psychology. *Behavioral and Brain Sciences*, 3, 63–110. Reprinted in J. A. Fodor, *Representations: Philosophical Essays on the Foundations of Cognitive Science*. Brighton: Harvester Press, 1981. Pp. 225–256.

Fodor, J. A. [1983] *The Modularity of Mind: An Essay on Faculty Psychology*. Cambridge, Mass.: MIT Press.

Fodor, J. A. [In press] *Psychosemantics: The Problem of Meaning in the Philosophy of Mind*. Cambridge, Mass.: MIT Press.

Fodor, J. A., & T. G. Bever. [1965] The Psychological Reality of Linguistic Segments. *J. Verbal Learning and Verbal Behavior*, 4, 414–420.

Fodor, J. A., T. G. Bever & M. F. Garrett. [1974] *The Psychology of Language: An Introduction to Psycholinguistics and Generative Grammar*. New York: McGraw-Hill.

Fodor, J. A., & M. F. Garrett. [1966] Some Reflections on Competence and Performance (with peer-commentary). In J. Lyons & R. J. Wales (eds.), *Psycholinguistic Papers*. Edinburgh: Edinburgh University Press. Pp. 135–182.

Funt, B. V. [1980] Problem-Solving with Diagrammatic Representations. *Artificial Intelligence*, 13, 201–230.

Funt, B. V. [1983] A Parallel-Process Model of Mental Rotation. *Cognitive Science*, 7, 67–93.

Gazdar, G. J. M. [1981a] Speech Act Assignment. In A. K. Joshi, B. L. Webber & I. A. Sag (eds.), *Elements of Discourse Understanding*. Cambridge: Cambridge University Press. Pp. 64–83.

Gazdar, G. J. M. [1981b] On Syntactic Categories. In H. C. Longuet-Higgins, J. Lyons & D. E. Broadbent (eds.), *The Psychological Mechanisms of Language*. London: The Royal Society & The British Academy. Pp. 53–69.

Gazdar, G. J. M., E. Klein, G. Pullum & I. Sag. [1985] *Generalized Phrase Structure Grammar*. Oxford: Blackwell Publisher.

Geach, P. T. [1957] *Mental Acts*. London: Routledge & Kegan Paul.

Gergen, K. J. [1973] Social Psychology as History. *J. Personality and Social Psychology*, 26, 309–320.

Gibbs, R. W. [1981] Your Wish Is My Command: Convention and Context in Interpreting Indirect Requests. *J. Verbal Learning and Verbal Behavior*, 20, 431–444.

Goodwin, C. [1979] The Interactive Construction of a Sentence in Natural Conversation. In G. Psathas (ed.), *Everyday Language: Studies in Ethnomethodology*. New York: Irvington. Pp. 97–122.

Grape, G. R. [1969] *Computer Vision Through Sequential Abstractions*. Stanford, Calif.: Stanford University AI Department.

Gray, J. A. [1982] The Neuropsychology of Anxiety: An Enquiry into the Functions of the Septo-Hippocampal System. *Behavioral and Brain Sciences*, 5, 469–484.

Gregory, R. L. [1967] Will Seeing Machines Have Illusions? In N. L. Collins & D. Michie (eds.), *Machine Intelligence 1*. Edinburgh: Edinburgh University Press. Pp. 169–180.

Gregory, R. L. [1977] *Eye and Brain*. Third edn. London: Weidenfeld & Nicolson.

Gregory, R. L., & L. G. Wallace. [1963] *Recovery from Early Blindness: A Case-Study*. Experimental Psychology Soc. Monographs, No. 2. Cambridge: Cambridge University Press.

Grey Walter, W. [1953] *The Living Brain*. London: Duckworth.

Grice, P. [1975] Logic and Conversation. In P. Cole & J. L. Morgan (eds.), *Syntax and Semantics*, Vol. 3: *Speech Acts*. New York: Academic Press. Pp. 41–58.

Grosz, B. [1981] Focusing and Description in Natural Language Dialogues. In A. K. Joshi, B. L. Webber & I. A. Sag (eds.), *Elements of Discourse Understanding*. Cambridge: Cambridge University Press. Pp. 84–105.

Guzman, A. [1969] Decomposition of a Visual Field into Three-Dimensional Bodies. In A.

Grasselli (ed.), *Automatic Interpretation and Classification of Images*. New York: Academic Press. Pp. 243–276.

Haas, A. R. [1986] A Syntactic Theory of Belief and Action. *Artificial Intelligence*, 28, 245–292.

Hamlyn, D. W. [1978] *Experience and the Growth of Understanding*. London: Routledge & Kegan Paul.

Hand, D. J. [1985] *Artificial Intelligence and Psychiatry*. Cambridge: Cambridge University Press.

Haugeland, J. [1978] The Nature and Plausibility of Cognitivism. *Behavioral and Brain Sciences*, 1, 215–226. Reprinted in J. Haugeland (ed.), *Mind Design: Philosophy, Psychology, Artificial Intelligence*. Cambridge, Mass.: MIT Press, 1981. Pp. 243–281.

Haugeland, J. [1981] Analog and Analog. In J. I. Biro & R. W. Shahan (eds.), *Mind, Brain, and Function: Essays in the Philosophy of Mind*. Norman: University of Oklahoma Press. Pp. 213–226.

Haugeland, J. [1985] *Artificial Intelligence: The Very Idea*. Cambridge, Mass.: MIT Press.

Hayes, P. J. [1974] Some Problems and Non-Problems in Representation Theory. *Proc. AISB Summer Conference*, University of Sussex, 63–79. Reprinted in R. J. Brachman & H. J. Levesque (eds.), *Readings in Knowledge Representation*. Los Altos, Calif.: Morgan Kaufmann, 1985. Pp. 3–22.

Hayes, P. J. [1979] The Naive Physics Manifesto. In D. Michie (ed.), *Expert Systems in the Micro-Electronic Age*. Edinburgh: Edinburgh University Press. Pp. 242–270.

Hayes, P. J. [1985] The Second Naive Physics Manifesto. In J. R. Hobbs & R. C. Moore (eds.), *Formal Theories of the Commonsense World*. Norwood, N.J.: Ablex. Pp. 1–36. Reprinted in R. J. Brachman & H. J. Levesque (eds.), *Readings in Knowledge Representation*. Los Altos, Calif.: Morgan Kaufmann. Pp. 467–486.

Hayes-Roth, B., & F. Hayes-Roth. [1979] A Cognitive Model of Planning. *Cognitive Science*, 3, 275–310.

Hebb, D. O. [1949] *The Organization of Behavior: A Neuropsychological Theory*. New York: Wiley.

Hewstone, M. (ed.). [1983] *Attribution Theory: Social and Functional Extensions*. Oxford: Blackwell Publisher.

Hill, D. R. [1980] Spoken Language Generation and Understanding by Machine: A Problems and Applications Oriented Overview. In J. C. Simon (ed.), *Spoken Language Generation and Recognition*. Dordrecht: Reidel. Pp. 3–38.

Hillis, W. D. [1985] *The Connection Machine*. Cambridge, Mass.: MIT Press.

Hinton, G. E. [1979] Some Demonstrations of the Effects of Structural Descriptions in Mental Imagery. *Cognitive Science*, 3, 231–251.

Hinton, G. E. [1981a] Shape Representations in Parallel Systems. *Proc. Seventh Int. Joint Conf. Artificial Intelligence*, Vancouver, 1088–1096.

Hinton, G. E. [1981b] Implementing Semantic Networks in Parallel Hardware. In G. E. Hinton & J. A. Anderson (eds.), *Parallel Models of Associative Memory*. Hillsdale, N.J.: Erlbaum. Pp. 161–188.

Hinton, G. E. [1984] Parallel Computations for Controlling an Arm. *J. Motor Behavior*, 16, 171–194.

Hinton, G. E., & J. A. Anderson (eds.). [1981] *Parallel Models of Associative Memory*. Hillsdale, N.J.: Erlbaum.

Hinton, G. E., J. L. McClelland & D. E. Rumelhart. [1986] Distributed Representations. In D. E. Rumelhart & J. L. McClelland (eds.), *Parallel Distributed Processing: Explorations in the Microstructure of Cognition*, Vol. 1: *Foundations*. Cambridge, Mass.: MIT Press. Pp. 77–109.

Hinton, G. E., & T. J. Sejnowski. [1983] Optimal Perceptual Inference. *Proc. IEEE Computer Society Conference on Computer Vision and Pattern Recognition*, 448–453.

Hinton, G. E., & T. J. Sejnowski. [1986] Learning and Relearning in Boltzmann Machines. In D. E. Rumelhart & J. L. McClelland (eds.), *Parallel Distributed Processing: Explorations in the Microstructure of Cognition,* Vol. 1: *Foundations.* Cambridge, Mass.: MIT Press. Pp. 282–317.

Hodges, A. [1983] *Alan Turing: The Enigma.* London: Burnett Books.

Hofstadter, D. R. [1979] *Gödel, Escher, Bach: An Eternal Golden Braid.* New York: Basic Books.

Hofstadter, D. R. [1985] Waking Up from the Boolean Dream, or, Subcognition as Computation. In D. R. Hofstadter, *Metamagical Themas: Questing for the Essence of Mind and Pattern.* New York: Viking. Pp. 631–665.

Holland, J. H. [1984] Genetic Algorithms and Adaptation. In O. G. Selfridge, E. L. Rissland & M. A. Arbib (eds.), *Adaptive Control in Ill-Defined Systems.* New York: Plenum. Pp. 317–334.

Howe, J. A. M., T. O'Shea & F. Plane. [1980] Teaching Mathematics through LOGO Programming: An Evaluation Study. In R. Lewis & E. D. Tagg (eds.), *Computer Assisted Learning: Scope, Progress, and Limits.* Amsterdam: North-Holland. Pp. 85–102.

Hubel, D. H., & T. N. Wiesel. [1959] Receptive Fields of Single Neurones in the Cat's Striate Cortex. *J. Physiology,* 148, 579–591.

Hubel, D. H., & T. N. Wiesel. [1979] Brain Mechanisms of Vision. *Scientific American,* 241 (3), 150–162.

Huffman, D. A. [1971] Impossible Objects as Nonsense Sentences. In B. Meltzer & D. Michie (eds.), *Machine Intelligence 6.* Edinburgh: Edinburgh University Press. Pp. 295–325.

Hunt, E. B., J. Marin & P. T. Stone. [1966] *Experiments in Induction.* New York: Academic Press.

Inhelder, B., & J. Piaget. [1964] *The Early Growth of Logic in the Child.* London: Routledge & Kegan Paul.

Isard, S. D. [1986] Levels of Representation in Computer Speech Synthesis and Recognition. In M. Yazdani (ed.), *Artificial Intelligence: Principles and Applications.* London: Chapman & Hall. Pp. 111–121.

Johnson-Laird, P. N. [1977] Psycholinguistics Without Linguistics. In N. S. Sutherland (ed.), *Tutorial Essays in Psychology,* Vol. 1. Hillsdale, N.J.: Erlbaum. Pp. 75–136.

Johnson-Laird, P. N. [1978] What's Wrong with Grandma's Guide to Procedural Semantics: A Reply to Jerry Fodor. *Cognition,* 6, 262–271.

Johnson-Laird, P. N. [1981] Cognition, Computers, and Mental Models. *Cognition,* 10, 139–143.

Johnson-Laird, P. N. [1983] *Mental Models: Towards a Cognitive Science of Language, Inference, and Consciousness.* Cambridge: Cambridge University Press.

Joshi, A. K., B. L. Webber & I. A. Sag (eds.). [1981] *Elements of Discourse Understanding.* Cambridge: Cambridge University Press.

Julesz, B. [1960] Binocular Depth Perception of Computer Generated Patterns. *Bell Systems Technology Journal,* 39, 1125–1162.

Julesz, B. [1975] Experiments in the Visual Perception of Texture. *Scientific American,* 232 (April), 34–43.

Kanizsa, G. [1974] Contours Without Gradients or Cognitive Contours? *Italian J. Pyschol.,* 1, 93–112.

Kaplan, R. M. [1972] Augmented Transition Networks as Psychological Models of Sentence Comprehension. *Artificial Intelligence,* 3, 77–100.

Kaplan, R. M. [1975] On Process Models for Sentence Analysis. In D. A. Norman & D. W. Rumelhart (eds.), *Explorations in Cognition.* San Francisco: Freeman. Pp. 117–135.

Kaplan, R. M. [1981] Appropriate Responses to Inappropriate Questions. In A. K. Joshi,

B. L. Webber & I. A. Sag (eds.), *Elements of Discourse Understanding*. Cambridge: Cambridge University Press. Pp. 127–144.

Karmiloff-Smith, A. [1979] Micro- and Macro-developmental Changes in Language Acquisition and Other Representational Systems. *Cognitive Science*, 3, 81–118.

Karmiloff-Smith, A. [1986] From Meta-Processes to Conscious Access: Evidence from Children's Metalinguistic and Repair Data. *Cognition*, 23, 95–147.

Karmiloff-Smith, A. [1987] Why Developmental Studies Are Needed to Understand Consciousness. Lecture to British Psychological Society, University of Sussex, April.

Karmiloff-Smith, A., & B. Inhelder. [1975] If You Want to Get Ahead, Get a Theory. *Cognition*, 3, 195–212.

Katz, J. J., & J. A. Fodor. [1963] The Structure of a Semantic Theory. *Language*, 39, 170–210.

Kempen, G. [1977] On Conceptualizing and Formulating in Sentence Production. In S. Rosenberg (ed.), *Sentence Production*. Hillsdale, N.J.: Erlbaum. Pp. 259–274.

Kempson, R. M. [1977] *Semantic Theory*. Cambridge: Cambridge University Press.

Kosslyn, S. M. [1973] Scanning Visual Images: Some Structural Implications. *Perception and Psychophysics*, 14, 90–94.

Kosslyn, S. M. [1975] Information Representation in Visual Images. *Cognitive Psychology*, 7, 341–370.

Kosslyn, S. M. [1980] *Image and Mind*. Cambridge, Mass.: Harvard University Press.

Kosslyn, S. M. [1981] The Medium and the Message in Mental Imagery: A Theory. *Psychological Review*, 88, 46–66.

Kosslyn, S. M. [1983] *Ghosts in the Mind's Machine: Creating and Using Images in the Brain*. New York: Norton.

Kosslyn, S. M., & J. R. Pomerantz. [1977] Imagery, Propositions, and the Form of Internal Representations. *Cognitive Psychology*, 9, 52–76.

Kuhn, T. S. [1962] *The Structure of Scientific Revolutions*. Chicago: University of Chicago Press.

Kurland, D. M., R. D. Pea, C. Clement & R. Mawty. [1986] A Study of the Development of Programming Ability and Thinking Skills in High School Students. *J. Educational Computing Research*, 2, 429–458.

Lakatos, I. [1970] Falsification and the Methodology of Scientific Research Programmes. In I. Lakatos & A. Musgrave (eds.), *Criticism and the Growth of Knowledge*. Cambridge: Cambridge University Press. Pp. 91–196.

Langley, P. [1982] Language Acquisition Through Error Recovery. *Cognition and Brain Theory*, 5, 211–255.

Langley, P., H. A. Simon, G. L. Bradshaw & J. M. Zytkow. [1987] *Scientific Discovery: Computational Explorations of the Creative Processes*. Cambridge, Mass.: MIT Press.

Larkin, J. H. [1979] Information Processing Models and Science Instruction. In J. Lochhead & J. Clement (eds.), *Cognitive Process Instruction: Research on Teaching Thinking Skills*. Philadelphia: Franklin Institute Press. Pp. 109–118.

Larkin, J. H., J. McDermott, D. P. Simon & H. A. Simon. [1980] Models of Competence in Solving Physics Problems. *Cognitive Science*, 4, 317–345.

Lashley, K. S. [1951] The Problem of Serial Order in Behavior. In L. A. Jeffress (ed.), *Cerebral Mechanisms in Behavior: The Hixon Symposium*. New York: Wiley. Pp. 112–135.

Latané, B., & J. M. Darley. [1970] *The Unresponsive Bystander: Why Doesn't He Help?* New York: Appleton-Century-Crofts.

Lehnert, W. G. [1978] *The Process of Question Answering*. Hillsdale, N.J.: Erlbaum.

Lehnert, W. G., & M. H. Ringle (eds.). [1982] *Strategies for Natural Language Processing*. Hillsdale, N.J.: Erlbaum.

Lenat, D. B. [1982] The Nature of Heuristics. *Artificial Intelligence*, 19, 189–249.

Lenat, D. B. [1983a] Theory Formation by Heuristic Search. The Nature of Heuristic II: Background and Examples. *Artificial Intelligence*, 20, 61–98.

Lenat, D. B. [1983b] The Role of Heuristics in Learning by Discovery: Three Case Studies. In R. Michalski, J. G. Carbonell & T. M. Mitchell (eds.), *Machine Learning: An Artificial Intelligence Approach*, Vol. 1. Palo Alto, Calif.: Tioga. Pp. 243–305.

Lenat, D. B., & J. S. Brown. [1984] Why AM and Eurisko Appear to Work. *Artificial Intelligence*, 23, 269–294.

Lettvin, J. Y., H. R. Maturana, W. Pitts & W. S. McCulloch. [1959] What the Frog's Eye Tells the Frog's Brain. *Proc. Inst. Radio Engineers*, 47, 1940–1959.

Lichtenstein, E. H., & W. F. Brewer. [1980] Memory for Goal-directed Events. *Cognitive Psychology*, 12, 412–445.

Lindsay, P. H., & D. A. Norman. [1977] *Human Information Processing: An Introduction to Psychology*. New York: Academic Press.

Longuet-Higgins, H. C. [1972] The Algorithmic Description of Natural Language. *Phil. Trans. Royal Society London*, B, 182, 255–276. Reprinted in Longuet-Higgins [1987], pp. 193–216.

Longuet-Higgins, H. C. [1979] The Perception of Music. *Proc. Royal Society London*, B, 205, 307–322. Reprinted in Longuet-Higgins [1987], pp. 169–189.

Longuet-Higgins, H. C. [1987] *Mental Processes: Studies in Cognitive Science*. Cambridge, Mass.: MIT Press.

Longuet-Higgins, H. C., & K. Prazdny. [1980] The Interpretation of a Moving Image. *Phil. Trans. Royal Society London*, B, 208, 385–397. Reprinted in Longuet-Higgins [1987], pp. 295–309.

Longuet-Higgins, H. C., & M. J. Steedman. [1971] On Interpreting Bach. In B. Meltzer & D. Michie (eds.), *Machine Intelligence 6*. Edinburgh: Edinburgh University Press. Pp. 221–242.

McCarthy, J. [1968] Programs with Common Sense. In M. L. Minsky (ed.), *Semantic Information Processing*. Cambridge, Mass.: MIT Press. Pp. 403–418.

McCarthy, J. [1980] Circumscription: A Form of Non-monotonic Reasoning. *Artificial Intelligence*, 13, 27–40.

McCarthy, J. [1986] Applications of Circumscription to Formalizing Common-Sense Knowledge. *Artificial Intelligence*, 28, 89–116.

McCarthy, J., & P. J. Hayes. [1969] Some Philosophical Problems from the Standpoint of Artificial Intelligence. In B. Meltzer & D. Michie (eds.), *Machine Intelligence 4*. Edinburgh: Edinburgh University Press. Pp. 463–502.

McClelland, J. L., & D. E. Rumelhart. [1981] An Interactive Model of Context Effects in Letter Perception–I: An Account of Basic Findings. *Psychological Review*, 88, 375–407.

McClelland, J. L., D. E. Rumelhart & G. E. Hinton. [1986] The Appeal of Parallel Distributed Processing. In D. E. Rumelhart & J. L. McClelland (eds.), *Parallel Distributed Processing: Explorations in the Microstructure of Cognition*, Vol. 1: *Foundations*. Cambridge, Mass.: MIT Press. Pp. 3–44.

McCulloch, W. S. [1965] *Embodiments of Mind*. Cambridge, Mass.: MIT Press.

McCulloch, W. S., & W. H. Pitts. [1943] A Logical Calculus of the Ideas Immanent in Nervous Activity. *Bull. Mathematical Biophysics*, 5, 115–133. Reprinted in W. S. McCulloch, *Embodiments of Mind*. Cambridge, Mass.: MIT Press, 1965. Pp. 19–39.

McDermott, D., & J. Doyle. [1980] Non-Monotonic Logic I. *Artificial Intelligence*, 13, 41–72.

Mackworth, A. K. [1973] Interpreting Pictures of Polyhedral Scenes. *Artificial Intelligence*, 4, 121–138.

Mackworth, A. K. [1976] Model-driven Interpretation in Intelligent Vision Systems. *Perception*, 5, 349–370.

Mackworth, A. K. [1983] Constraints, Descriptions, and Domain Mappings in Computational Vision. In O. J. Braddick & A. C. Sleigh (eds.), *Physical and Biological Processing of Images*. New York: Springer-Verlag. Pp. 33–40.

Mandler, J. M. [1984a] *Stories, Scripts, and Scenes: Aspects of Schema Theory*. Hillsdale, N.J.: Erlbaum.

Mandler, J. M. [1984b] Representation and Recall in Infancy. In M. Moscovitch (ed.), *Infant Memory*. New York: Plenum. Pp. 75–102.

Mandler, J. M., & N. S. Johnson. [1976] Remembrance of Things Parsed: Story Structure and Recall. *Cognitive Psychology*, 9, 11–151.

Marcus, M. P. [1980] *A Theory of Syntactic Recognition for Natural Language*. Cambridge, Mass.: MIT Press.

Marr, D. [1969] A Theory of Cerebellar Cortex. *J. Physiology*, 202, 437–470.

Marr, D. [1977] Artificial Intelligence: A Personal View. *Artificial Intelligence*, 9, 37–48. Reprinted in J. Haugeland (ed.), *Mind Design: Philosophy, Psychology, Artificial Intelligence*. Cambridge, Mass.: MIT Press, 1981. Pp. 129–142.

Marr, D. [1982] *Vision: A Computational Investigation into the Human Representation and Processing of Visual Information*. San Francisco: Freeman.

Marr, D., & H. K. Nishihara. [1978] Visual Information Processing: Artificial Intelligence and the Sensorium of Sight. *Technology Review*, 81 (October), 1–23.

Marslen-Wilson, W. D. [1980] Speech Understanding as a Psychological Process. In J. C. Simon (ed.), *Spoken Language Generation and Recognition*. Dordrecht: Reidel. Pp. 39–67.

Marslen-Wilson, W. D., & L. K. Tyler. [1981] Central Processes in Speech Understanding. In H. C. Longuet-Higgins, J. Lyons & D. E. Broadbent (eds.), *The Psychological Mechanisms of Language*. London: The Royal Society & The British Academy. Pp. 103–117.

Mayhew, J. E. W. [1983] Stereopsis. In O. J. Braddick & A. C. Sleigh (eds.), *Physical and Biological Processing of Images*. New York: Springer-Verlag. Pp. 204–216.

Mayhew, J. E. W., & J. P. Frisby. [1981] Psychophysical and Computational Studies Towards a Theory of Human Stereopsis. *Artificial Intelligence* (special issue on vision), 17, 349–386.

Mayhew, J. E. W., & J. P. Frisby. [1984] Computer Vision. In T. O'Shea & M. Eisenstadt (eds.), *Artificial Intelligence: Tools, Techniques, and Applications*. London & New York: Harper & Row. Pp. 301–357.

Miller, G. A. [1956] The Magical Number Seven, Plus or Minus Two. *Psychological Review*, 63, 81–97.

Miller, G. A., & N. Chomsky. [1963] Finitary Models of Language Users. In R. D. Luce, R. Bush & E. Galanter (eds.), *Handbook of Mathematical Psychology*, Vol. 2. New York: Wiley. Pp. 419–492.

Miller, G. A., E. Galanter & K. H. Pribram. [1960] *Plans and the Structure of Behavior*. New York: Holt, Rinehart & Winston.

Miller, G. A., & P. N. Johnson-Laird. [1976] *Language and Perception*. Cambridge: Cambridge University Press.

Minsky, M. L. [1961] Steps Toward Artificial Intelligence. *Proc. Inst. Radio Engineers*, 49, 8–30. Reprinted in E. A. Feigenbaum & J. Feldman (eds.), *Computers and Thought*. New York: McGraw-Hill, 1963. Pp. 406–450.

Minsky, M. L. [1975] A Framework for Representing Knowledge. In P. H. Winston (ed.), *The Psychology of Computer Vision*. New York: McGraw-Hill. Pp. 211–277. Reprinted in J. Haugeland (ed.), *Mind Design: Philosophy, Psychology, Artificial Intelligence*. Cambridge, Mass.: MIT Press, 1981. Pp. 95–128.

Minsky, M. L. [1980] K-Lines: A Theory of Memory. *Cognitive Science*, 4, 117–133.

Minsky, M. L. [1986] *The Society Theory of Mind*. New York: Simon & Schuster.

Minsky, M. L., & S. Papert. [1969] *Perceptrons: An Introduction to Computational Geometry.* Cambridge, Mass.: MIT Press.

Minsky, M. L., & O. G. Selfridge. [1961] Learning in Random Nets. In C. Cherry (ed.), *Information Theory: Fourth Symposium (Royal Institution).* London: Butterworth. Pp. 335–347.

Mitchell, T. M., & R. M. Keller. [1983] Goal Directed Learning. *Proc. International Machine Learning Workshop,* University of Illinois, 117–118.

Mitchell, T. M., P. E. Utgoff & R. Banerji. [1983] Learning by Experimentation: Acquiring and Refining Problem-Solving Heuristics. In R. Michalski, J. G. Carbonell & T. M. Mitchell (eds.), *Machine Learning: An Artificial Intelligence Approach,* Vol. 1. Palo Alto, Calif.: Tioga. Pp. 163–190.

Montague, R. [1974] *Formal Philosophy: Selected Papers.* New Haven: Yale University Press.

Morgan, M. J. [1984] Computational Theories of Vision. *Quarterly Journal of Experimental Psychology,* 36, 157–165.

Morgan, M. J., G. Mather, B. Moulden & R. J. Watt. [1984] Intensity-Response Nonlinearities and the Theory of Edge Localization. *Vision Research,* 24, 713–719.

Movshon, J. A., I. D. Thompson & D. J. Tolhurst. [1978] Spatial Summation in the Receptive Fields of Simple Cells in the Cat's Striate Cortex. *J. Physiology (London),* 283, 53–77.

Neisser, U. [1967] *Cognitive Psychology.* New York: Appleton-Century-Crofts.

Newell, A. [1973] You Can't Play Twenty Questions with Nature and Win. In W. G. Chase (ed.), *Visual Information Processing.* New York: Academic Press. Pp. 283–308.

Newell, A. [1980] Physical Symbol Systems. *Cognitive Science,* 4, 135–183.

Newell, A. [1982] The Knowledge Level. *Artificial Intelligence,* 18, 87–127.

Newell, A., J. C. Shaw & H. A. Simon. [1957] Empirical Explorations with the Logic Theory Machine. *Proc. Western Joint Computer Conference,* 15, 218–239. Reprinted in E. A. Feigenbaum & J. Feldman (eds.), *Computers and Thought.* New York: McGraw-Hill, 1963. Pp. 109–133.

Newell, A., & H. A. Simon. [1961] GPS – A Program That Simulates Human Thought. In H. Billing (ed.), *Lernende Automaten.* Munich: Oldenbourg. Pp. 109–124. Reprinted in E. A. Feigenbaum & J. Feldman (eds.), *Computers and Thought.* New York: McGraw-Hill, 1963. Pp. 279–296.

Newell, A., & H. A. Simon. [1972] *Human Problem Solving.* Englewood Cliffs, N.J.: Prentice-Hall.

Nisbett, R. E., & L. Ross. [1980] *Human Inference: Strategies and Shortcomings and Social Judgment.* Englewood Cliffs, N.J.: Prentice-Hall.

Norman, D. A. [1976] *Memory and Attention: An Introduction to Human Information Processing.* Second edn. New York: Wiley. (First edn. 1969.)

Norman, D. A. [1986] Reflections on Cognition and Parallel Distributed Processing. In D. E. Rumelhart & J. L. McClelland (eds.), *Parallel Distributed Processing: Explorations in the Microstructure of Cognition,* Vol. 2: *Psychological and Biological Models.* Cambridge, Mass.: MIT Press. Pp. 531–546.

Norman, D. A., & D. E. Rumelhart. [1970] A System for Perception and Memory. In D. A. Norman (ed.), *Models of Human Memory.* New York: Academic Press. Pp. 21–66.

Norman, D. A., & D. E. Rumelhart. [1975] *Explorations in Cognition.* San Francisco: Freeman.

Oatley, K. G., G. D. Sullivan & D. A. Hogg. [In press] Drawing Visual Conclusions from Analogy: Preprocessing, Cues, and Schemata in the Perception of Three-dimensional Objects. *J. Intelligent Systems,* 1. (Freund Publishing House.)

Ortony, A. (ed.). [1979] *Metaphor and Thought.* Cambridge: Cambridge University Press.

O'Shea, T., & J. Self. [1984] *Teaching and Learning with Computers*. Brighton: Harvester Press.

O'Shea, T., & R. M. Young. [1978] A Production Rules Account of Errors in Children's Subtraction. *Proc. AISB Conference*, Hamburg, 1978, 229–237.

Paivio, A. [1971] *Imagery and Verbal Processes*. New York: Holt, Rinehart & Winston.

Papert, S. [1980] *Mindstorms: Children, Computers, and Powerful Ideas*. Brighton: Harvester Press.

Pea, R. D., & D. M. Kurland. [1984] On the Cognitive Effects of Learning Computer Programming. *New Ideas in Psychology*, 2, 137–168.

Pea, R. D., D. M. Kurland & J. Hawkins. [In press] LOGO and the Development of Thinking Skills. In J. Lochhead & D. N. Perkins (eds.), volume based on Second International Conference on Thinking, Harvard Graduate School of Education, 1984.

Pellionisz, A., & R. Llinas. [1979] Brain Modeling by Tensor Network Theory and Computer Simulation. The Cerebellum: Distributed Processor for Predictive Coordination. *Neuroscience*, 4, 323–348.

Pellionisz, A., & R. Llinas. [1985] Tensor Network Theory of the Metaorganization of Functional Geometries in the Central Nervous System. In A. Berthoz & G. Melvill Jones (eds.), *Adaptive Mechanisms in Gaze Control*. Amsterdam: Elsevier. Pp. 223–232.

Pentland, A. P. [1986] Perceptual Organization and the Representation of Natural Form. *Artificial Intelligence*, 28, 293–332.

Perrett, D. I., M. Harries, A. J. Mistlin & A. J. Chitty. [1986] Three Stages in the Classification of Body Movements by Visual Neurons. Paper given at the Rank Prize Funds International Symposium *Images and Understanding*, Royal Society, London. (Publication forthcoming.)

Perrett, D. I., P. A. J. Smith, D. D. Potter, A. J. Mistlin, A. S. Head, A. D. Milner & M. A. Jeeves. [1985] Visual Cells in the Temporal Cortex Sensitive to Face View and Gaze Direction. *Phil. Trans. Royal Society London*, B, 223, 293–317.

Piaget, J. [1952] *The Origins of Intelligence in the Child*. London: Routledge & Kegan Paul.

Pichert, J. W., & R. C. Anderson. [1977] Taking Different Perspectives on a Story. *J. Educational Psychology*, 69, 309–315.

Pinker, S. [1980] Explanations in Theories of Language and of Imagery. *Behavioral and Brain Sciences*, 3, 147–148.

Popper, K. R. [1963] *Conjectures and Refutations: The Growth of Scientific Knowledge*. London: Routledge & Kegan Paul.

Power, R. J. D. [1979] The Organization of Purposeful Dialogues. *Linguistics*, 17, 107–152.

Power, R. J. D., & H. C. Longuet-Higgins. [1978] Learning to Count: A Computational Model of Language Acquisition. *Phil. Trans. Royal Society London*, B, 200, 391–417. Reprinted in H. C. Longuet-Higgins [1987], *Mental Processes: Studies in Cognitive Science*. Cambridge, Mass.: MIT Press. Pp. 249–280.

Putnam, H. [1975] The Meaning of "Meaning". In H. Putnam, *Mind, Language and Reality* (Philosophical Papers, Vol. 2). Cambridge: Cambridge University Press. Pp. 215–271.

Pylyshyn, Z. W. [1973] What the Mind's Eye Tells the Mind's Brain: A Critique of Mental Imagery. *Psychological Bulletin*, 80, 1–24.

Pylyshyn, Z. W. [1984] *Computation and Cognition: Toward a Foundation for Cognitive Science*. Cambridge, Mass.: MIT Press.

Quine, W. V. O. [1960] *Word and Object*. Cambridge, Mass.: MIT Press.

Quinlan, J. R. [1979] Discovering Rules from Large Collections of Examples: A Case

Study. In D. Michie (ed.), *Expert Systems in the Micro-Electronic Age*. Edinburgh: Edinburgh University Press. Pp. 168–201.

Quinlan, J. R. [1982] Semi-autonomous Acquisition of Pattern-based Knowledge. In D. Michie (ed.), *Machine Intelligence 10*. Chichester: Ellis Horwood. Pp. 159–172.

Quinlan, J. R. [1983] Learning Efficient Classification Procedures and Their Application to Chess End-Games. In R. Michalski, J. G. Carbonell & T. M. Mitchell (eds.), *Machine Learning: An Artificial Intelligence Approach*. Palo Alto, Calif.: Tioga. Pp. 463–482.

Reichman, R. [1978] Conversational Coherency. *Cognitive Science*, 2, 283–327.

Reitman, W. R. [1965] *Cognition and Thought: An Information-Processing Approach*. New York: Wiley.

Ringle, M. H., & B. C. Bruce. [1982] Conversation Failure. In W. G. Lehnert & M. H. Ringle (eds.), *Strategies for Natural Language Processing*. Hillsdale, N.J.: Erlbaum. Pp. 203–222.

Rips, L. J. [1986] Mental Muddles. In M. Brand & R. M. Harnish (eds.), *The Representation of Knowledge and Belief*. Tucson: University of Arizona Press. Pp. 258–286.

Ritchie, G. D., & F. K. Hanna. [1984] AM: A Case Study in AI Methodology. *Artificial Intelligence*, 23, 249–268.

Roberts, L. G. [1965] Machine Perception of Three-dimensional Solids. In J. T. Tippett, D. A. Berkowitz, L. C. Clapp, C. J. Koester & A. Vanderburgh (eds.), *Optical and Electro-Optical Information Processing*. Cambridge, Mass.: MIT Press. Pp. 159–198.

Robson, J. G. [1983] Frequency Domain Visual Processing. In O. J. Braddick & A. C. Sleigh (eds.), *Physical and Biological Processing of Images*. Berlin: Springer-Verlag. Pp. 73–87.

Rock, J. [1973] *Orientation and Form*. New York: Academic Press.

Rolls, E. T. [1987] Information Representation, Processing, and Storage in the Brain: Analysis at the Single Neuron Level. In J.-P. Changeux & M. Konishi (eds.), *The Neural and Molecular Bases of Learning*. New York: Wiley. Pp. 503–539.

Rosch, E. [1978] Principles of Categorization. In E. Rosch & B. B. Lloyd (eds.), *Cognition and Categorization*. Hillsdale, N.J.: Erlbaum. Pp. 28–49.

Rosenblatt, F. [1958] The Perceptron: A Probabilistic Model for Information Storage and Organization in the Brain. *Psychological Review*, 65, 386–407.

Rosenblatt, F. [1962] *Principles of Neurodynamics*. New York: Spartan.

Rosenfeld, A., R. A. Hummel & S. W. Zucker. [1976] Scene Labelling by Relaxation Operations. *IEEE Trans. Systems, Man, and Cybernetics*, 6, 420–433.

Rumelhart, D. E. [1975] Notes on a Schema for Stories. In D. G. Bobrow & A. Collins (eds.), *Representation and Understanding*. New York: Academic Press. Pp. 211–236.

Rumelhart, D. E. [1984] Schemata and the Cognitive System. In R. S. Wyer & T. K. Srull (eds.), *Handbook of Social Cognition*, Vol. 1. Hillsdale, N.J.: Erlbaum. Pp. 161–188.

Rumelhart, D. E., & J. L. McClelland (eds.). [1986a] *Parallel Distributed Processing: Explorations in the Microstructure of Cognition*, Vol. 1: *Foundations*; Vol. 2: *Psychological and Biological Models*. Cambridge, Mass.: MIT Press.

Rumelhart, D. E., & J. L. McClelland. [1986b] On Learning the Past Tenses of English Verbs. In D. E. Rumelhart & J. L. McClelland (eds.), *Parallel Distributed Processing: Explorations in the Microstructure of Cognition*, Vol. 2: *Psychological and Biological Models*. Cambridge, Mass.: MIT Press. Pp. 216–271.

Rumelhart, D. E., & D. A. Norman. [1975] The Active Structural Network. In D. A. Norman & D. E. Rumelhart (eds.), *Explorations in Cognition*. San Francisco: Freeman. Pp. 35–84.

Rumelhart, D. E., & D. A. Norman. [1982] Simulating a Skilled Typist: A Study of Skilled Cognitive–Motor Performance. *Cognitive Science*, 6, 1–36.

Rumelhart, D. E., P. Smolensky, J. L. McClelland & G. E. Hinton. [1986] Schemata and

Sequential Thought Processes in PDP Models. In D. E. Rumelhart & J. L. McClelland (eds.), *Parallel Distributed Processing: Explorations in the Microstructure of Cognition*, Vol. 2: *Psychological and Biological Models*. Cambridge, Mass.: MIT Press. Pp. 7–57.

Rumelhart, D. E., & D. Zipser. [1985] Feature Discovery by Competitive Learning. *Cognitive Science*, 9, 75–112.

Russell, B. A. W. [1905] On Denoting. *Mind*, 14, 479–493.

Ryle, G. [1949] *The Concept of Mind*. London: Hutchinson.

Sampson, G. [1983] Deterministic Parsing. In M. King (ed.), *Parsing Natural Language*. London: Academic Press. Pp. 91–116.

Schank, R. C. [1972] Conceptual Dependency: A Theory of Natural Language Understanding. *Cognitive Psychology*, 3, 552–631.

Schank, R. C. (ed.). [1975] *Conceptual Information Processing*. New York: American Elsevier.

Schank, R. C. [1982] Reminding and Memory Organization: An Introduction to MOPS. In W. G. Lehnert & M. H. Ringle (eds.), *Strategies for Natural Language Processing*. Hillsdale, N.J.: Erlbaum. Pp. 455–494.

Schank, R. C. [1983] *Dynamic Memory: A Theory of Learning in Computers and People*. Cambridge: Cambridge University Press.

Schank, R. C. [1986] *Explanation Patterns: Understanding Mechanically and Creatively*. Hillsdale, N.J.: Erlbaum.

Schank, R. C., & R. P. Abelson. [1977] *Scripts, Plans, Goals, and Understanding*. Hillsdale, N.J.: Erlbaum.

Schumer, R. A., & J. A. Movshon. [1984] Length Summation in Simple Cells of Cat Striate Cortex. *Vision Research*, 24, 565–571.

Searle, J. R. [1969] *Speech Acts: An Essay in the Philosophy of Language*. Cambridge: Cambridge University Press.

Searle, J. R. [1980] Minds, Brains, and Programs. *Behavioral and Brain Sciences*, 3, 417–457. Reprinted (without peer-commentary) in J. Haugeland (ed.), *Mind Design: Philosophy, Psychology, Artificial Intelligence*. Cambridge, Mass.: MIT Press, 1981. Pp. 282–306.

Searle, J. R. [1983] *Intentionality: An Essay in the Philosophy of Mind*. Cambridge: Cambridge University Press.

Searle, J. R., & D. Vanderveken. [1985] *Foundations of Illocutionary Logic*. Cambridge: Cambridge University Press.

Sejnowski, T. J. [1977] Statistical Constraints on Synaptic Plasticity. *J. Theoretical Biology*, 69, 385–389.

Selfridge, O. G. [1959] Pandemonium: A Paradigm for Learning. In D. V. Blake & A. M. Uttley (eds.), *Proceedings of the Symposium on Mechanisation of Thought Processes*. London: H.M. Stationery Office. Pp. 511–529.

Selfridge, O. G., & U. Neisser. [1960] Pattern Recognition by Machine. *Scientific American*, 203 (3), 60–68.

Selfridge, O. G., E. L. Rissland & M. A. Arbib (eds.). [1984] *Adaptive Control in Ill-defined Systems*. New York: Plenum.

Shepard, R. N., & J. Metzler. [1971] Mental Rotation of Three-dimensional Objects. *Science*, 171, 701–703.

Sleeman, D. H., & J. S. Brown (eds.). [1982] *Intelligent Tutoring Systems*. London: Academic Press.

Sloman, A. [1978] *The Computer Revolution in Philosophy: Philosophy, Science, and Models of Mind*. Brighton: Harvester Press.

Sloman, A. [1979] What About Their Internal Languages? *Behavioral and Brain Sciences*, 1, 602–603.

Sloman, A. [1983] Image Interpretation: The Way Ahead? In O. J. Braddick & A. C.

Sleigh (eds.), *Physical and Biological Processing of Images*. New York: Springer-Verlag. Pp. 380–402.

Sloman, A. [1985] Why We Need Many Knowledge Representation Formalisms. In M. Bramer (ed.), *Research and Development in Expert Systems*. Cambridge: Cambridge University Press. Pp. 163–183.

Sloman, A. [1986a] Reference Without Causal Links. In B. du Boulay and L. J. Steels (eds.), *Seventh European Conference on Artificial Intelligence*. Amsterdam: North Holland. Pp. 369–381.

Sloman, A. [1986b] What Sorts of Machines Can Understand the Symbols They Use? *Proc. Aristotelian Soc.*, Supp., 60, 61–80.

Sloman, A. [In press] Motives, Mechanisms, and Emotions. *J. of Emotion and Cognition*, 1.

Sloman, A. [In preparation] *Artificial Intelligence: The Philosophical Foundations*. To be published – Chichester: Ellis Horwood.

Sloman, A., & M. Croucher. [1981] Why Robots Will Have Emotions. *Proc. Seventh Int. Joint Conf. Artificial Intelligence*, Vancouver, 197–202.

Smith, B. C. [1982] *Reflection and Semantics in a Procedural Language*. Cambridge, Mass.: MIT. (Ph.D. dissertation and Technical Report LCS/TR-272).

Smith, B. C. [In press] *Is Computation Formal?* Cambridge, Mass.: MIT Press.

Smolensky, P. [1987] Connectionist AI, Symbolic AI, and the Brain. *AI Review*, 1, 95–110.

Stabler, E. P. [1983] How Are Grammars Represented? *Behavioral and Brain Sciences*, 6, 391–402.

Stevens, A. L., & D. E. Rumelhart. [1975] Errors in Reading: Analysis Using an Augmented Transition Network Model of Grammar. In D. A. Norman & D. E. Rumelhart (eds.), *Explorations in Cognition*. San Francisco: Freeman. Pp. 136–156.

Stich, S. C. [1983] *From Folk Psychology to Cognitive Science: The Case Against Belief*. Cambridge, Mass.: MIT Press.

Strawson, P. F. [1950] On Referring. *Mind*, 59, 320–344.

Sullivan, G. D. [1983] Perceptual Filters. In O. J. Braddick & A. C. Sleigh (eds.), *Physical and Biological Processing of Images*. New York: Springer-Verlag. Pp. 115–126.

Sussman, G. J. [1975] *A Computer Model of Skill Acquisition*. New York: American Elsevier.

Sutherland, N. S. [1957] Visual Discrimination of Orientation and Shape by the *Octopus*. *Nature (London)*, 179, 11–13.

Sutherland, N. S. [1968] Outlines of a Theory of Visual Pattern Recognition in Animals and Man. *Phil. Trans. Royal Society London*, B, 171, 297–317.

Thorndyke, P. W. [1977] Cognitive Structures in Comprehension and Memory of Narrative Discourse. *Cognitive Psychology*, 9, 77–110.

Thorne, J. P., P. Bratley & H. M. Dewar. [1968] The Syntactic Analysis of English by Machine. In D. Michie (ed.), *Machine Intelligence 3*. Edinburgh: Edinburgh University Press. Pp. 281–309.

Thornton, S. P. [1982] Challenging "Early Competence": A Process-Oriented Analysis of Children's Classifying. *Cognitive Science*, 6, 77–100.

Thornton, S. P. [Forthcoming] Mechanisms of Self-Modification in Young Children's Problem-Solving. Submitted to *Cognitive Science*.

Touretsky, D. S., & G. E. Hinton. [1985] Symbols Among the Neurons: Details of a Connectionist Inference Architecture. *Proc. Ninth Int. Conf. Artificial Intelligence*, Los Angeles, 238–243.

Turing, A. M. [1936] On Computable Numbers, with an Application to the Entscheidungsproblem. *Proc. London Mathematical Society*, series 2, 42, 230–265.

Turing, A. M. [1950] Computing Machinery and Intelligence. *Mind*, n.s., 59, 433–460. Reprinted in E. A. Feigenbaum & J. Feldman (eds.), *Computers and Thought*. New York: McGraw-Hill, 1963. Pp. 11–35.

Tversky, A., & D. Kahnemann. [1974] Judgment under Uncertainty: Heuristics and Biases. *Science*, 125, 1124–1131.

Uhr, L., & C. Vossler. [1963] A Pattern Recognition Program that Generates, Evaluates, and Adjusts Its Own Operators. In E. A. Feigenbaum & J. Feldman (eds.), *Computers and Thought*. New York: McGraw-Hill. Pp. 251–268.

Van Dijk, T. A. [1972] *Some Aspects of Text-Grammars*. The Hague: Mouton.

von Neumann, J. [1958] *The Computer and the Brain*. New Haven: Yale University Press.

von Neumann, J. [1960] The General and Logical Theory of Automata. In J. R. Newman (ed.), *The World of Mathematics*, Vol. 4. New York: Random Hieghts. Pp. 2070–2098.

Waltz, D. L. [1975] Understanding Line Drawings of Scenes with Shadows. In P. H. Winston (ed.), *The Psychology of Computer Vision*. New York: McGraw-Hill. Pp. 19–92.

Wanner, E. [1980] The ATN and the Sausage Machine: Which One Is Baloney? *Cognition*, 8, 209–225.

Wanner, E., R. Kaplan & S. Shiner. [1976] Garden Paths in Relative Clauses. Unpublished ms., Harvard University.

Wanner, E., & M. P. Maratsos. [1978] An ATN Approach to Comprehension. In M. Halle, J. W. Bresnan & G. A. Miller (eds.), *Linguistic Theory and Psychological Reality*. Cambridge, Mass.: MIT Press. Pp. 119–159.

Wason, P. C. [1977] The Theory of Formal Operations: A Critique. In B. A. Geber (ed.), *Piaget and Knowing: Studies in Genetic Epistemology*. London: Routledge & Kegan Paul. Pp. 119–135.

Waterman, D. A. [1970] Generalization Learning Techniques for Automating the Learning of Heuristics. *Artificial Intelligence*, 1, 121–170.

Watt, R. J., & M. J. Morgan. [1983a] Mechanisms Responsible for the Assessment of Visual Location: Theory and Evidence. *Vision Research*, 23, 97–109.

Watt, R. J., & M. J. Morgan. [1983b] The Recognition and Representation of Edge Blur: Evidence for Spatial Primitives in Human Vision. *Vision Research*, 23, 1465–1477.

Watt, R. J., & M. J. Morgan. [1985] A Theory of the Primitive Spatial Code in Human Vision. *Vision Research*, 25, 1661–1674.

Weir, S. [1987] *Cultivating Minds: A LOGO Casebook*. New York: Harper & Row.

Wiener, N. [1948] *Cybernetics, or Control and Communication in the Animal and the Machine*. New York: Wiley.

Wilensky, R. [1983] *Planning and Understanding: A Computational Approach to Human Reasoning*. Reading, Mass.: Addison-Wesley.

Wilks, Y. A. [1972] *Grammar, Meaning, and the Machine Analysis of Natural Language*. London: Routledge & Kegan Paul.

Wilks, Y. A. [1975] A Preferential, Pattern-seeking, Semantics for Natural Inference. *Artificial Intelligence*, 6, 53–74.

Wilks, Y. A. [1978] Good and Bad Arguments for Semantic Primitives. *Communication and Cognition*, 10, 181–221.

Wilks, Y. A. [1982] Some Thoughts on Procedural Semantics. In W. G. Lehnert & M. H. Ringle (eds.), *Strategies for Natural Language Processing*. Hillsdale, N.J.: Erlbaum. Pp. 495–516.

Wilson, H. R., & D. J. Gelb. [1984] Modified Line-Element Theory for Spatial-Frequency and Width Discrimination. *J. Optical Society of America*, A, 1, 124–131.

Winograd, T. [1972] *Understanding Natural Language*. New York: Academic Press.

Winograd, T. [1983] *Language as a Cognitive Process: Syntax*. Reading, Mass.: Addison-Wesley.

Winston, P. H. [1975] Learning Structural Descriptions from Examples. In P. H. Winston (ed.), *The Psychology of Computer Vision*. New York: McGraw-Hill. Pp. 157–210.

Woods, W. A. [1970] Transition Network Grammars for Natural Language Analysis. *Comm. Assn. Computing Machinery,* 13, 591–606.

Woods, W. A. [1975] What's in a Link: Foundations for Semantic Networks. In D. G. Bobrow & A. Collins (eds.), *Representation and Understanding: Studies in Cognitive Science*. New York: Academic Press. Pp. 35–82.

Woods, W. A. [1981] Procedural Semantics as a Theory of Meaning. In A. Joshi, B. N. Webber & I. A. Sag (eds.), *Elements of Discourse Understanding*. Cambridge: Cambridge University Press. Pp. 300–334.

Wyer, R. S., & T. K. Srull (eds.). [1984] *Handbook of Social Cognition,* Vol. 1. Hillsdale, N.J.: Erlbaum.

Yarbus, A. L. [1967] *Eye Movements and Vision*. New York: Plenum.

Young, R. M. [1976] *Seriation by Children: An Artificial Intelligence Analysis of a Piagetian Task*. Basel: Birkhauser.

Young, R. M., G. D. Plotkin & R. F. Linz. [1977] Analysis of an Extended Concept-Learning Task. *Proc. Fifth Int. Joint Conf. Artificial Intelligence,* Cambridge, Mass., 285.

Index of names

Index of subjects